The Glands Regulating Personality

Louis Berman, M.D.

Contents

THE GLANDS REGULATING PERSONALITY

BY

Louis Berman, M.D.

INTRODUCTION
ATTITUDES TOWARD HUMAN NATURE
THE CASE AGAINST HUMAN NATURE

Man, know thyself, said the old Greek philosopher. Man perforce has taken that advice to heart. His life-long interest is his own species. In the cradle he begins to collect observations on the nature of the queer beings about him. As he grows, the research continues, amplifies, broadens. Wisdom he measures by the devastating accuracy of the data he accumulates. When he declares he knows human nature, consciously cynical maturity speaks. Doctor of human nature--every man feels himself entitled to that degree from the university of disillusioning experience. In defense of his claim, only the limitations of his articulate faculty will curb the vehemence of his indictment of his fellows.

For all history provides the material, literature the critique, biology the inexorable logic of the case against human nature. The historical record is a spectacle of man destroying man, a collection of chapters on man's increasing cruelty to man. Limitations of time and space have been shortened and eliminated. Tools of production have been multiplied and complicated. The sources of energy and power have been systematically attacked and trapped. But the nature of man has remained so unchanged that clap trap about progress is easy target for the barrage of every cheap pamphleteer.

The naturalist probes into codes of conduct, systems of morality, structures of societies, variations in the scales of value that individuals, races and nations have subjected themselves to as custom, law and religion. Again and again the portrait is presented of man preying upon man, of cunning a parasite upon stupidity and of predatory strength enslaving the weakling intellect. Until finally are evoked reactions and consequences that overtake in catastrophe and cataclysm preyer and preyed upon alike.

Human nature is but part of the magnificent tree of beast nature. Man is linked by every tie of blood and bone and cell memories with his brethren of the sea, the jungle, the forest and the fields. The beast is a seeker of freedom, but a seeker for his own ego alone, and the satisfaction of his own instincts only. Thus he struggles to a sort of freedom which makes him the Ishmael of the Universe, everyone's hand against him, as his own hand is against everyone. The human animal has achieved no advance beyond the necessities of his ancestors, nor freed himself from his bondage to their instincts and automatic reflexes. And so the sociologist, the analyst of human associations, turns out to be simply the historian and accountant of slaveries.

Yet the history of mankind is, too, a long research into the nature of the machinery of freedom. All recorded history, indeed, is but the documentation of that research. Viewed thus, customs, laws, institutions, sciences, arts, codes of morality and honor, systems of life, become inventions, come upon, tried out, standardized, established until scrapped in everlasting search for more and more perfect means of freeing body and soul from their congenital thralldom to a host of innumerable masters. Indeed, the history of all life, vegetable and animal, of bacillus, elephant, orchid, gorilla, as well as of man is the history of a searching for freedom.

Freedom! What to a living creature is freedom? How completely has it dominated the life history of every creature that ever crawled upon the earth? Trace our cellular pedigree, descend our family tree to its rootlets, our amebic ancestors, and the craving for more freedom is manifest in the soul of even the lowest, buried in darkness and slime. When the first clever bit of colloidal ooze, protoplasm as the ameba, protruded a bit of itself as a pseudopod, it achieved a new freedom. For, accidentally or deliberately, it created for itself a new power--the ability to go directly for food in its environment, instead of waiting, patiently, passively, as the plant does, for food to just happen along. Therewith developed in place of the previous quietist pacifist, quaker attitude toward its surroundings, a new religion, a new tone: aggressive, predatory, careerist.

That adventure was a great step forward for the ameba--a miracle that freed it forever from the danger of death by starvation. But latent in that move were all the terrible possibilities of the tiger, the alligator, the wolf and all the varieties of predaceous beast and plant, parasitism and slavery. The device that enabled the ameba to change its position in space of its own will, and so increased its freedom immeasureably, meant the generation of infinite evil, pain, suffering and degradation for billions in the womb of time.

THE BREEDING OF INFERIORITY

Human history, being a continuation of vertebrate history, is full of similar instances. The invention of the stock company, for example, furnished a certain relative freedom to hundreds, a certain amount of leisure to think and play, and independence to travel and record, and immunity from a daily routine and drudgery. In turn, it bore fruit in miseries and horrors multiplied for millions, like those of the child lacemakers of Mid-Victorian England, who were dragged from their beds at two or three o'clock in the morning to work until ten or eleven at night in the services of a stock company.

A corporation is said to have no soul. The struggle for freedom of every living thing has no conscience. Throughout the living world, from ameba to man, parasitism and slavery together with their by-products, physical and spiritual degeneracy, appear as the after effects of the more vital individual's efforts to remain alive and free. The origins of slavery may be seen in the parasitisms of the infectious diseases which kill man. The change from parasitism to slavery was an inevitable step of creative intelligence. In the transition evolution made one of those breaks which it indulges in periodically as its mode of progress.

The natural effect of slavery has been a selection of two sorts of individuals along the lines of the survival of the adapted. It has tended to perpetuate in the breed the qualities of the strong which would make them stronger, and certain qualities in the weak which would increase their weakness. For parasitism and likewise slavery infallibly entail the degradation of certain structures and an overgrowth of others by the law of use and disuse. The type of organ which would function normally, were not its possessor parasitic in that function, invariably degenerates or disappears. Parasitic insects lose their wings. An entire anatomical system may even be lost. So the tapeworm, which feeds upon the digested food present in the intestines of its host, has no alimentary canal of its own because it needs none. On the other hand, the organs of attack and combat grow by a constant use into the most remarkable of efficient weapons.

In human society the process continues. Out of the tapeworm nature, the tiger nature, the wolf nature, the simian nature, human nature evolves. Repeated episodes of subjugation and suppression mixed with countless incidents of predaceous cupidity and rapacity have made Man what he is today. Indeed, by a sort of instinct, society has constructed its institutions upon empirical observations and assumptions agreeing with this principle. The deductions concerning human nature and human traits that an interplanetary visitor would draw from a study of our common law would be at least slightly humiliating to our incorrigible pride. Law courts, codes of civil contract and criminal procedure, the systems of subordination in armies and navies, castes and classes, men and women, employers and employees, teachers and pupils, parents and children, are based upon the fundamental, the conservative axiom that man, especially the common plain man (Lincoln's phrase), is a being incurably lazy, stupid, dishonest, muddled, cowardly, greedy, restless, obsessed with a low cunning and a selfish callousness and insensibility to the sufferings of his fellow creatures, animal and human.

Why is it that Man, the noblest creature of creation, made in the image of God, capable of the flights of attainment that distinguish a Christ, a Caesar, a Plato, a Shakespeare, a Shelley, a Newton, is so described, not alone by hopeless pessimists like Koheleth, Swift, and Mark Twain, but by the common law, the common opinion, the common assumptions of mankind? Because the development of slavery and parasitism in human society, the subjection of the weak to the strong, the dull and base to the clever and headstrong, set up a vicious cycle: the liberation of more energy for the making of more and more slaves and the propagation of slaves and slave qualities in a geometrically increasing proportion.

This might be called the ***Malthusian law of slavery***. For the qualities that I have named as man's own characterization of himself are the qualities of the slave and the slave-soul. Nietzche took great pains to repeat ad nauseam that these qualities were the qualities of the slave. But by burdening himself with the hypothesis, evolved from his inner consciousness, that the slaves imposed from below a morality of weakness upon their masters, he missed the really obvious process by which slaves beget more slaves, slavery begets more slavery, and the slave-soul becomes universal. That process is the simple action of physical and spiritual reproduction of the slaves. The subnormal begets the subnormal, the inferior begets the inferior.

Slavery appeared as an invention of the would-be-free. It was a brilliant flash of genius of a seeker after freedom. However, it became a boomerang. By multiplication and hereditary transmission, the inferiority and the number of the slaves created a new overwhelming problem for the superior few, the upper crust of the free. At last the problem grew into the problem of problems, the problem of government, that threatened all freedom, as an epidemic disease threatens even the most healthy. Government, at first organized for conquest and subjugation, had to change its character until it became more and more to consist of experiments in a new social machinery that would free somebody of the incubus. So through the centuries, one technique of liberty after another was tested in the laboratory of experience.

But always the attempts are so muddled, because the problem is not grasped. Muddledom is the essence of the slave-soul. And the essence infiltrates and poisons the whole atmosphere in which the would-be-free think and act. Kings' heads are chopped off, a whole class is guillotined, reform movements come and go, the masters fight every inch of their retreat, and pile stratagem upon stratagem, device upon device, to retain their spoils.

The democratic formula of freedom for all comes to the fore. So at last universal suffrage is introduced as the panacea. Freedom seems within grasp. Now it looks as if a method and an objective have been hit upon, that will lead both the free and the enslaved out of their mutual bondage, and release the handcuffs which have bound them together. All the trial and error tests to which history had subjected institutions appeared to culminate in the formula that would automatically yield Liberty. The French wanted a little more and added Equality and Fraternity. The Americans put it quite definitely as the formula that would assist the Pursuit of Life, Liberty, and Happiness. That formula is: the ***democracy of the normals***.

To be sure, a civilization might be organized for the breeding and the glorification of the supernormals. Such a civilization may yet have to be tried. But as the supernormals, as we know them today, are merely biologic sports, in a sense, simple accidents, no one can tell whether they will turn out true shots or just flashes in the pan. So it looks the better course to stick to the plan of nature, which seems to be the raising of the level of the normals, and the gradual increase of their faculties and powers.

WHAT THE STATESMAN IS UP AGAINST

Under the terms of the democratic formula the problems of the statesman seem to become enormously simplified. That is, if one assumes that he has worked out a perfectly clear idea of what a democracy means and what the normal means. Assuming these unassumables, his problem simplifies into the definite object of producing and developing the greatest possible number of normals--or if you will, the greatest happiness of the greatest number of normal lives.

Furthermore you then begin to have the entirely novel possibility in the world: some sort of collective effort for a collective purpose, beyond the personal greeds and fears, factions and hatreds. So the state, instead of fulfilling its old function of serving as the tool of certain powerful individuals, latterly known as the Big Men, might be transformed into an instrument toward freedom. With the ideal of a democracy of the normals ever before him, the statesman could go on to construct and modify his social machinery. That would entail the satisfaction not alone of the animal needs, but also the highest aspirations and therefore the provision of the finest conditions of life for the normal: those most favorable, stimulative, and assistant to creative activity. For what else is the content of the idea of freedom?

Without committing the intellectual sin which William James named Vicious Abstractionism, the goal of the clearest progressive and liberal thought and forces of the twentieth century might be summed up as this freedom in a democracy of normals. A good formula which coincides with the technique of nature in the evolution of species. A fair fight, a free-for-all who are unhandicapped, is the motto of natural selection. Where civilization shakes hands with natural instinct, what but the happiest of results can be expected?

Unfortunately, the formula in human society possesses an Achilles' heel. Again it is slavery. Where slavery has become bred into the bone, the standard of the normal becomes reduced so tremendously that the average of normals, the majority, are hopelessly inferior. In effect, they are really subnormal. So the ideal of our ideal statesman is bound to be defeated because of the inadequacy of his material.

No matter how interested in his main business: the promotion of freedom for creative activities in a democracy of the normals, he is bound to be beaten by the majority consisting of subnormals. There is nothing left for him but to cater to the minority of careerists, the one-eighth of the electorate representing superior intelligence. The intelligence tests employed in the War showed that and also that forty-five per cent of the examined, or about one half the total population, had a mental capacity, or natural ability that would never develop beyond the stage normal to a twelve-year-old child. They are doomed to remain forever subnormal.

THE CAREERISTS AS THE ABNORMALS

The careerists are those who practice the careerist religion. The careerist religion is the religion par excellence of modernity. Someone once said, with the perfect candor of the North American, that America is the land of opportunity. He meant that America is the land of the Careerist or, as it has also been put, it is the land of the man on the make. The careerist, or the man on the make, is of a thousand genera and species, varieties and subvarieties, with transition links between. One finds him at every level of society.

Excepting a negligible minority, the feminine career of today (as of the last ten thousand years of the race's history) consists in the acquisition of a husband. After that she is so identified with him that her own life, as something distinct, individual and unique, becomes blurred and then completely erased. The feminine careerist, the careeristina, if you will, is a definite type. Consider the unimportance of a collective purpose to the woman whose career is the mate, and then the mate's career. All the kinks and twists of the feminine mind, resulting from the necessities of that fundamental primary problem, would form a multitudinous and interesting list. The most successful careeristinas are the absolutely unconscious ones because they are not passively besieged nor actively bombarded by any doubts as to what they want. They play their game exceedingly well as do not the quasi-rebels and faint-hearted revoltees that form no small percentage of the Newest Women. For a number of women the feminist movement has been an attempt to break away from the traditions of the wife-careerist, and to strike a line of auto-careerism. Can the careeristina instinct, the fruit of the practice of so many generations, be uprooted by the good intentions of a mere statesman?

But the masculine careerist is a marvelous creature. He is a biologic sport, an abnormal variation. New York is the place to watch and study him in his thousands and tens of thousands. You can observe him climbing, climbing, climbing, precisely as an ant climbs a tree. Nothing can really discourage or sway him from his chosen path. If he is not getting on financially, he is getting on socially, or he is using the one method of advance to help him with the other. How the line of least resistance and greatest advantage is determined for and taken by him is a fascinating process.

The careerist instinct, the inherited flair for a career, must not be confounded with the instincts of self-preservation, self-expansion or self-expression, because they are utterly different. Indeed, the careerist instinct is often their direct antagonist, clashing with and dominating them. The making of the career involves the distortion, the mutilation, degradation, degeneration or even the complete suppression of the true personality. But it is all instinctive. To consider the life of the careerist as an expression of instinct will explain too the success of so many who have no inner awareness of what they want. These go straight for the career, looking neither to the right nor to the left, without doubt or hesitation, just as they go for the respiration business as soon as they are born.

Then there is the Super-Careerist. Ordinarily, the careerist is rather obvious, easily recognizable, with diaphanous motives and conduct. But there is another and rarer bird, the careerist of talent, even the careerist of genius, whom it is not so easy to see through. Clever and brainy, he may be a good all around trifler, or his specific gift for some line of achievement may make him more effective. There is nothing he may not call himself: conservative, liberal, progressive, or radical. Often he is an agnostic about social and political affairs and problems, which passes for the indecision of the open mind, and is quite handy to render him all things to all men. But perpetually, the underlying careerist instinct drives him to use all men and women, all ideas and movements and forces he comes in contact with for his own personal advancement, just as the slave making instinct guides the red ant in all its activities to procure its captives. Ideas do not make a hero out of him, but he makes heroes of ideas, because they serve him in his ascent.

Because he is the most subtle, the most complex and the most deceptive type of careerist, he is the most dangerous to the adventure and speculation in intellect which mankind is. To say that he is a wolf in sheepskin is to be unjust to him, since he is most successful when he is most unaware of his own charlatanry. He is most sincere when he is most insincere, and most truthful when he lies best. A little self-consciousness of hypocrisy is a corrupting thing, much of it completely incompatible with the most successful careerism. Tartuffe is always applauded by the world when he plays Hamlet, if he really believes in himself as Hamlet. And, as all he has to do, if he is at all talented, is to look into his glass and see himself in the part, he carries it off very well.

WHY THE STATESMAN FAILS

Slaves and careerists, subnormals and abnormals, are the important elements of the constituency of every modern statesman. The financial and social careerists as business men, professionals, artists, publicists, presidents of countries, politicians, philosophers dominate his outlook, his plans, his horizon. The slaves, the inferiors, the subnormals exist merely to be exploited by them. No one questions the causes of the multiplicity of them. No one asks why there are so many little lives. For a fundamentally minded statesman the control of the production of the careerist, why he is produced, and how he may be prevented, becomes the primary problem of his art.

Well, you say, what are you going to do about it? That is human nature. The Evils of Human Nature! There is the perpetual answer to be repeated by our clever editors unto Eternity. You cannot get away from human nature. It is human nature to be a careerist. It is human nature to put the immediate triumphs of the self and its pleasures above the more indirect, the more remote and distant benefits of a great, wonderful, free community. We are all careerists. In so far as democracy has succeeded as a form, it has persisted because there was in it for the common man the promise of his getting more out of life that way than any other way. For himself. And the devil take the others. The myopia of such crude selfishness continues to determine his politics to this very day. And so he proceeds to vote for favors bestowed and patronage past or potential. That is, when he does not throw his ballot away altogether into the fire of family habit, sectional inertia, or race prejudice.

Again you say, that is human nature. It is human nature for us to be narrow, to be confined within the circle of personal thought and desire, without imagination for the beyond. So the calf is limited in its wanderings to the radius of the rope by which it is tethered. The servile soul will always be submissive and docile, greedy and stupid. What else could you expect from the descendant of the solitary beast who once lived for thousands of years in caves? Without servility of the soul, without chains for the spirit of the wild animal against the world, men could never have been driven to live together for twenty-four hours in communities.

The conception of human quality out of which all social machinery has been devised and built is a conception of slave quality and careerist quality. As we are all caught in the net, as the unconscious memories of our slave and careerist ancestors flow in our blood and echo in our cells, all we can do is accept it and work with it. Human nature is an incurable disease. Like Jehovah's definition of Himself, it is, it has been, and ever will be. Everywhere the same, always the same, forever the same, there is no way out.

POOR HUMAN NATURE

All of these strictures upon poor human nature are exceedingly delightful to our careerists. Every unpleasant social fact, every outrage to our best instincts, every exhibition of incapacity, incompetency, inefficiency, indifference, every example of super-criminal negligence is pardoned as an effect of that universal sin, human nature. Take the case of the statesman and the diplomats who failed to prevent the Great War, though they saw it coming for years, and who should therefore all, Entente as well as German, American as well as Japanese, be indicted for their criminal negligence, precisely as a physician would be for failure to report and stop the spread of an epidemic disease. All these crimes of omission and commission are excused on the plea that it was all due to human nature, and that what can be blamed on human nature in general can be blamed on no one in particular.

Poor human nature! Flagellated on every hand, what are we to do with it? Why is the careerist so numerous and ubiquitous? Why does the slave-soul infiltrate like a cancer the soul of society with its black fluid? Is freedom, the divine idea, nothing but the toy of an orator to the majority, a distant star in the night to a helpless minority? Yet the instinct to freedom, the appetite for freedom, flickers through the centuries as a fitful flame, though snuffed out by every gust of class passion, every wind of mob resentment, and every storm of national jealousy. Though the inferior subnormals multiply into great sheep majorities, and the careerists, like Napoleon, morbid variants, involve millions in their disease, the idea of freedom persists obstinately. Have we any reason for regarding it as other than an illusion?

If freedom is an illusion, we must admit the doom of democracy. And no Wagnerian crashes of orchestration mitigate the tragedy of the scene as our eyes are opened to the twilight of our new gods. For what other social methods are there left to us? In the struggle against nature's barriers upon human aspiration for perfect satisfactions, it looks as though every other method has failed us.

In the past, refined aristocracies and benevolent despotisms have failed as miserably as our democracies are now failing and as we are sure crude anarchism and communism would. Their inferiority has thrown them on the scrap heap. As for our present ways of government as a permanent method, the storage of power in the hands of the Clever Few. War burns in the lesson of how little the careerist regards either the subnormal or supernormal. He condemns them all sooner or later to wholesale slavery and carnage.

Is man then never to be the architect of his own destiny? Are we to surrender our faith in the future of our kind to the spectacle of a miserable species sentenced by its own nature to self-destruction? We thought to rise upon the wings of knowledge and beauty, lured by the mysteries of color and the magic of design and the might of the intellect and its words, that have transfigured life into the greatest adventure ever attempted in time and space. But we find ourselves merely another experiment, intricate and rather long drawn out, to be sure, with marvelous pyrotechnics, magnificent effects here and there, but bound to eliminate itself in the end, to make stuff for the museums of the real conqueror of the stars yet to come. We are condemned to be classed with the dodo and the mammoth by the coming discoverer of an escape from the slave and careerist. And so let us resign ourselves to fate. Let us eat of the humble bread of the stoic's consolation in the face of the mocking laughter of the gods, let us admit that Mind in Man has unconsciously but irretrievably willed its own self-annihilation. What remains for us except to beat our breasts and proclaim: So be it, O Lord, so be it?

MAN AS A TRANSIENT

Yet, true as it is that the human animal has achieved no advance beyond the necessities of his ancestors, nor freed himself from his bondage to their instincts and automatic reflexes, is there no way out anywhere? Is there perhaps some ground for hope and consolation in the thought that we, of the twentieth century, no longer see ourselves, Man, as something final and fixed? Darwin changed Fate from a static sphinx into a chameleon flux. Just as certainly as man has arisen from something whose bones alone remain as reminders of his existence, we are persuaded man himself is to be the ancestor of another creature, differing as much from him as he from the Chimpanzi, and who, if he will not supplant and wipe him out, will probably segregate him and allow him to play out his existence in cage cities.

The vision of this After-man or From-man is really about as helpful to us as the water of the oasis mirage is to the lost dying of thirst in the desert. The outcries of the wretched and miserable, the gray-and-dreary lived din an unmanageable tinnitus in our ears. Like God, it may be but a large, vague idea toward which we grope to snuggle up against. It seems implicit in the doctrines of evolution. But how do we know that in man the spiral of life has not reached its apex, and that now, even now, the vortices of its descent are not beginning? How do we know that the From-man is to be a Superman and not a Subman? How can we dare to hope that the slave-beast-brute is to give birth to an heir, fine and free and superior?

We do not know and we have every indication and induction for the most oppositely contrary conclusions. Life has blundered supremely, in, while making brains its darling, forgetting or helplessly surrendering to the egoisms of alimentation. So it has spawned a conflict between its organs, and a consequent impasse in which the lower centres drive the higher pitilessly into devising means and instruments for the suicide of the whole.

As War shows plainly to the most stupidly gross imagination, the germs of our own self-destruction as a species saturate our blood. The probability looms with almost the certainty of a syllogistic deduction, that such will be the outcome to our hundreds of thousands of years of pain upon earth. In the face of that, speculations upon a comet or gaseous emanations hitting the planet, or the sun growing cold, become babyish fancies. How clearly the possibility is pointed in the discussions about the use in the next War of bacterial bombs containing the bacilli of cholera, plague, dysentery and many others! What influenza did in destroying millions, they can repeat a thousand times and ten thousand times. What else the laboratories will bring forth, of which no man dreams, in the way of destructive agents acting at long distance, upon huge masses and over any extent of territory, is presaged in that single example. But besides thus willing, by an inner necessity, its own annihilation, Life, in the very structure and machinery of its being, seems caught into the entanglements of an inescapable net, an eternity-long bondage it can never rip, to flee and remake itself into the immortal image that is its God.

And so there go by the board the last alleviations of those unbeatable optimists who would soothe their aching souls with at least the drop of comfort: that if man is a mortal species, with not the slightest prospect of a continuing immortality, not to mention a glorious future and destiny, there are others. Man, after all, may be simply a bad habit Life will succeed in shaking off. No philosophy or religion can afford to be anthropocentric merely. It must include all life and all living things to which we are blood-related. There are other species or latent species to take up the torch that burned poor homo sapiens and ascend the heights. The ant and bee may yet mutate along certain lines that would make them the masters of the universe.

But no matter what species or variety gets the upper hand in the struggle for survival and power, the implications of the qualities necessary to victory in conflicts of individual separate pieces of protoplasm will be there. Besides, life is always begotten of life. That is why synthetic protoplasm is nothing but a phrase. It is impossible to conceive of something alive, possessed of the property of remembering, that is not possessed of a store of past experiences. You can no more think of getting rid of these unconscious memories of protoplasm than you can think of getting rid of the wetness of water. They are imbedded in the most intimate chemistry of the primeval ameba as well as in our most complex tissues.

The memories of the cold lone fish and the hot predatory carnivor who were our begetters, may haunt us to the end of time. The bee and the ant, too, have woven inextricably into the woof of their cells the instincts that sooner or later would send their brain ganglia, even when evolved to the pitch of perfection, to elaborating the self-and-species murdering inventions and discoveries that are apparently destined to slay us. The powers of unconscious memory and unlearnable technique of reaction to experience, once grooved, thus prove the great gift and the eternal curse of protoplasm. Making it possible for it to be and become what it is and has, they have also made it forever impossible for it to be or become its own contradiction.

Add to this unsloughable remembrance of the past, for better, for worse, the secretive consciousness of its present needs every living thing, as against every other living thing, is obsessed with. As a peregrinating, finite, spatially limited being, it is separated from all other living beings by inorganic, dead masses, and yet driven to contact with them by a fundamental impulse to assimilate them into itself, and make them part of itself. That assimilatory urge is present in every activity from coarse ingestion as food to the moral metabolism of the hermit-saint who would influence others to do as he.

FATE AND ANTI-FATE

In effect the history of Life resembles the life history of the smallest things we know of, the electrons, and the largest, the great suns and stars of space. The electron begins, perhaps, as a swirl in the primeval ether, joins other electrons, forms colonies, cities, empires, elements of an increasing complexity, through stages of a relative stability, like lead or gold. Until it reaches the stage of integration which wills its own disintegration, that we have been taught to look upon with proper awe and reverence as radium. And we are told that nebulae wander until they collide and give birth to stars, stars wander and collide and give birth to nebulae. Life begins as a quivering colloid, goes on painfully to build a brain, which automatically refines itself to the point of discovering and using the most efficient methods of destroying others, and by a boomerang effect, itself. Fate!

The conception of Fate was a Greek idea. The classic formula for tragedy, the struggle of Man with the sequence of cause and effect within him and without, that is so utterly beyond his grasp and ken, or power to modify, originated with them. But they must also be given the credit for having conceived an idea and started a process which, at first slowly and gropingly, now slipping and falling, torn and bleeding among the thorns of the dark forest of human motives, presently goes on, with a firmer, more practiced, more confident step, to emerge into the light as the deliberate Conqueror of Fate. That idea-process, this Anti-Fate is Science.

Science began with the adventures of free-thinking speculators, who revolted against religious cosmogonies and superstitions. Sceptics concerning the knowledge that was the accepted monopoly of the priesthood must have existed in the oldest civilization we know anything of, more than twenty-five thousand years ago, the Aurignacians. But it was to the Greeks that we owe that amalgamation of curiosity delivered of fear, that merger of systematic research and critical thinking untrammelled by social inhibitions which is the essence of modern science. Out of them has come the great Tree of Knowledge of our time, which is, too, the only Ygdrasil of Life, undying because it lives upon successive generations of human brain cells.

Science, as the pursuit of the real, began with very small things by men with very small intentions. Inventories, collections of isolated data, something permanent for the mind out of the flux of transient sensations, little tracks and foot paths in the jungle of phenomena, were their goal. With no sense of themselves as the mightiest of master-builders, cultivating humility toward their material at any rate, the little men ploughed their little fields, striking the oil of a great generalization or classification or explanation with no fanfare of trumpets.

First as freaks and cranks, then as scholars and pedants, then protected and perhaps stimulated under the competitive royal patronage as societies and academies, they prepared for the harvest. Comparing them to pioneer farmers sowing an undeveloped territory is really totally inadequate and inaccurate. For the most part, they were like coral makers, laboriously constructing, with no vision, certainly no sustained vision, of the whole. To the practical men of affairs, the shopkeepers and traders, the land-owners and ship-owners, the soldiers and sailors, the statesmen and politicians, the people who specialized in maneuvering human beings and materials, they were, for this futile devotion to abstract knowledge, marked ridiculous and absurd weaklings, mollycoddles, babies, not to be trusted with the demands and dangers of public life.

But it so happened remarkably late in history that with the discovery of the possibilities of coal there was a great boom in the demand for industrial machinery. At the same time there were thrown up the most marvelous advances in physics and chemistry. Recurring War became not the clashes of mercenary armies, but the catapulting of whole nations at each other. New destructive devices out of the laboratories were raised into the commandants of the course of history. Then science acquired prestige.

Science as King, science as power, looms as the great new figure, the overshadowing novel factor, in practical statesmanship. Unlike the factor X in the traditional equation, it is the known factor par excellence, the factor by which the value of all the other factors of human life will be ascertained and solved. As knowledge of the conditions determining all life, it stands as the courageous David of the race against the Goliath territory of the uncontrollable and the inevitable, even the unknowable. Human history resolves itself into the drama: Science contra Fate. Quite a change from the vaudeville show of the restless personal ambitions of vindictive fools and greedy scoundrels, the mischief and adventures of half-witted geniuses and licensed rogues that have been figures of the prologue.

The future of science has become the future of the race. So much of an inkling of the truth is beginning to be appreciated. That is ordinarily taken to mean that the process by which the Wessex man became the New York and London man, the accumulation of accidental discoveries and inspired inventions of scattered individuals, will go on, providing a succession of marvels and miracles for the careerist and his retinue. Not only is he to be entertained and served by them, but any commercial value will also be exploited by him. The natural wonders of the laboratories have taken the place of the supernatural absurdities of the medieval mind as a fillip for the imagination of the man in the street. Even spiritualism apes the technique of the physicist. The credulity of reporters alone concerning developments in surgery, for example, is incredible. There is enough rot published daily for a brief to be made out against the idolatry of science.

THE RELIGION OF SCIENCE

Science also as a religion, as a faith to bind men together, as a substitute for the moribund old mythologies and theologies which kept them sundered, is commencing to be talked of in a more serious tone. The wonder-maker may have forced upon him, may welcome, the honors of the priest, though he pose as the humble slave of Nature and her secrets. Presently the foundations and institutes, which co-exist with the cathedrals and churches, just as once the new Christian chapels and congregations stood side by side with pagan temples and heathen shrines, may oust their rivals, and assume the monopoly of ritual. Should its spirit remain fine and clear, should it maintain the glorious promise of its dawn, should its high priests realize the perpetually widening intimations of its universal triumph, and escape the ossification that has overtaken all young and hopeful things and institutions, the real foundation for a future of the species would be laid, and so its ultimate suicide prevented.

The time has gone by, however, for any complacent assurance that the redemption of mankind is to be attained by a new religion of words. There is no doubt that the damnation or salvation of an individual has often been determined by a religious crisis, in which the magic of words have worked their witchery. There is plenty of evidence that a psychic conversion will effect an actual revolution in the whole way of living of the victim or patient, as you like it. William James, in his "Varieties of Religious Experience," established that pretty definitely. When it comes to groups, races, nations, the outlook is wholly different. There is a conflict of so many and diverse habits and interests, beliefs and prejudices, that hope for some common merely intellectual solvent for all of them is rather forlorn. If at all, the resolution of the conflict will come by a pooling of actual powers and interests, in which the religion of science will play the great part of the Liberator of mankind from the whole system of torments that have made the way of all flesh a path of rocks along which a manacled prisoner crawls to his doom.

SCIENCE AND HUMAN NATURE

Science has a future. The religion of science has a future. Can science assure us that human nature, in spite of its beast-brute-slave origins holds the possibility of a genuine transformation of its texture? Can Fate's stranglehold upon us be broken? There will be certainly a tremendous, an overwhelming increase in the general stock of informations we call physics and chemistry and biology. An abundance of new comforts, novel sensations, fresh experiences, and breath-bereaving devices that will thrill or heal, will follow of course in their wake. The religion of science will infiltrate and penetrate and permeate by its capillary action the barbaric super-stitions, the ridiculous rites, the unsanitary insanities of our social systems.

But what about the poor human soul itself, with its inherent vices and virtues, its fears and indulgences, audacities and nobilities, jealousies, shames, blunders, in-curable likes, cravings and diseases? Can science change the texture of the slave and careerist, if they represent the subnormal and the abnormal? What about the Becky Sharps, the Mark Tapleys, and Tom Pinches, not to speak of the Nicholas Nicklebys and the Hamlets, the Micawbers and the Falstaffs? What future have they as they recur in the generations? Indeed, does not the very fact of their recurrence, of them and of the hundreds of other types and temperaments, point implacably to the con-clusion to which the historian, the philosopher and the biologist have driven us: that in the grip of an endless chain of pasts the human soul has no future?

That may appear an irrelevant, an immaterial, and an incompetent question to our men of business and affairs. Human nature, as fallen angel or ape parvenu, has always looked upon itself as fixed for eternity. "Human nature never changes, and is everywhere and always will be the same." "As a man is built." "Bred in the bone." These are the axioms of our social and economic Euclids. Indeed, Man, assuming that his nature is as uncontrollable as the course of the stars, has limited his research into the substance of freedom to a groping for an understanding of the adequate ex-ternal conditions of liberty. Thus he set himself another of the insoluble problems he seems to delight in by neglecting the most important factor in the equation. Yet the invisible soul of man, ignored, as a variable, varying quantity, has upset all societies and constitutions, and all schemes of bondage as well as of freedom.

For freedom, it becomes obvious as soon as it is clearly stated, is sheer impossibility until the internal conditions of his nature are ascertained, and the way paved for their control. A simple illustration of the working of this principle is supplied by our democracies, grossly pretenders. How can a democracy be possible without a knowledge of the control of the individually and socially subnormal, who, since they offer themselves to exploitation by the careerists, prove themselves the weak links in the chain of co-operation with an equal opportunity for all, that is the democratic ideal? In what does the equality or inequality of men consist? Just what are the qualities necessary for successful competition, or if you will, co-living, of man with his fellow-men, and how and why do they operate? No freedom, independent of the servile repetitions of history and heredity, is conceivable until these inquiries have been elaborately carried out toward a certain working finality.

THE PROMISES OF EUGENICS

There are, to be sure, the claims and assertions and negative achievements of the youngest of the sciences, eugenics. They are invincible optimists, the eugenists: it is perhaps a case of a virtue born of necessity. Thus Francis Galton, in the preface to the "Bible of Eugenics," his essays on Hereditary Genius, declares: "There is nothing either in the history of domestic animals or in that of evolution to make us doubt that a race of sane men may be formed who shall be as much superior, mentally and morally, to the Modern European, as the Modern European is to the lowest of the Negro races." High hopes beat in this declaration. But Galton could not have foreseen that the signing of a scrap of paper by one of the Modern Europeans would let loose all the other Modern Europeans in a pandemonium of horrors the lowest of the Negro races could not but envy as a masterpiece of its kind. It seemed to be suspiciously easy for him to accept an excuse to slide down the dizzy height he had climbed from the African level.

The eugenists would put their trust in the encouraged breeding of the best and the compulsory sterility of the rest. But what is the best, and who are the best, and where will you find them when they are not inextricably emulsified with the worst? It's a long, long way to the day of a segregating out and in of Mendelian unit-characters. Besides, this is a strange world of choices. Nobody is to be considered worthy of parenthood until he has fallen in love properly. Nobody who would permit an outsider's decision as to when he was properly in love would be worth thirty cents as a parent. There is the ultimate dilemma of the eugenist--the dilemma which destroys forever the dream of a control of parenthood from the point of view of merely psychic values.

NEW PSYCHOLOGY

There are the claims and outcries and promises of the psychologists--the specialists in the probing of the human soul and human nature. In our time, the demand for a dynamic psychology of process and becoming, psychology with an energy in it, has split them into two schools--the emphasizers of instinct and the subconscious, the McDougallians, and the pleaders for sex and the unconscious, the Freudians. A synthesis between these two groups is latent, since their differences are those of horizon merely. For the McDougallians look upon the world with two eyes and see it whole and broad--the Freudians see through their telescope a circular field and exclaim that they behold the universe. It is true that they own a telescope.

But what has either to offer our quest for light on the future of the species? Nothing very much. Thus, to turn to the disciples of McDougall. In a recent volume entitled, "Human Nature and its Remaking," Professor William Ernest Hocking of Harvard contends that Man, all axioms about his nature to the contrary, is but a creature of habit, and so the most plastic of living things, since habit is self-controlled and self-determined. By the self-determination of the habits of the race will the new freedom be reborn. It sounds old, very old. And pathetic because it recognizes original and permanent ingredients of our composition in the words pugnacity, greed, sex, fear, as elements to be accepted in any system of the principles of civilization. It is the bubble of education all over again. What in our cells is pugnacity? What in our bones is greed? What in our blood is sex? What in our nerves is fear? Until these inquiries are respected, conscious character building or even stock breeding must remain the laughing stock of the smoking rooms and the regimental barracks.

Come the Freudians. To them we owe the aeroplanes to a new universe. They have opened up for us the geology of the soul. Layer upon layer, cross-section upon cross-section have been piled before us. And what a melodramatic cinema of thrills and shivers, villains and heroes, heroines and adventuresses have they not unfolded. Each motive, as the stiff psychologist of the nineteenth century, with his plaster-of-Paris categories and pigeon holes and classifications, labelled the teeming creatures of the mind, becomes anon a strutting actor upon a multitudinous stage, and an audience in a crowded playhouse. Scenes are enacted the febrile fancy of a Poe or a de Maupassant never could have conjured. The complex, the neurosis, the compulsion, the obsession, the slip of speech, the trick of manner, the devotion of a life-time, the culture of a nation all furnish bits for the Freudian mosaic. Attractions and inhibitions, repulsions and suppressions are held up as the ultimate pulling and pushing forces of human nature.

But is the problem solved? Is not human nature primarily animal nature? And do we so thoroughly understand this animal nature? Does not all this material of Freudianism consist of variations upon social burdens imposed on the original human nature? To be sure, at every moment of life, choices have to be made, and choice involves the clashing of instincts and motives, with victory for one or some, and defeat for the others. But the Freudian material per se--the sex material--is it not merely the by-product of a certain state of society? A sane society would eliminate nearly all of Freudian disease, but still have original human nature upon its hands. Why is it that of two individuals exposed to the same situation, one will develop a complex, the other will remain immune? The only soil we know of, the real foundation stones of our being and living, are the cells we are made of. Tell me the cellular basis of a complex, and I will grant that you have arrived at some real knowledge.

WAY FOR THE PHYSIOLOGIST

There has grown up, contemporaneously with the teachings of Freud, a body of discoveries and knowledge in physiology, concerning these factors, which is like a long sword of light illuminating a pitch-black spot in the night. The dark places in human nature seem to have become the sole monopoly of the Freudians and their psychology. But only seemingly. For all this time the physiologist has been working. Beginning with a candle and now holding in his hands the most powerful arc-lights, he has explored two regions, the sympathetic nervous system and the glands of internal secretion, and has come upon data which in due course will render a good many of the Freudian dicta obsolete. Not that the Freudian fundamentals will be scrapped completely. But they will have to fit into the great synthesis which must form the basis of any control of the future of human nature. That future belongs to the physiologist. Already his achievements provide the foundations. I propose in the following chapters to sketch the history and outline the elements of this new knowledge, and then to glimpse some of the larger human reactions to it. A good deal of this new knowledge is not altogether new. A number of the isolated facts have been known and talked about for more than two generations. But the newer additions, and the light they have thrown upon old problems present the opportunity for a synthesis, which must sooner or later be made.

THE CHEMISTRY OF THE SOUL

Besides, it is time that the secrets of the laboratories stepped out into the market place, unashamed. Imaginative man has played for ages immemorial with wondrous fairy tales and fancies of what he would achieve. The sciences of physics and chemistry have made everyday commonplace realities out of his radiant dreams. One need not repeat the cliches of our editors. But the analogy is there nevertheless. No control over heat and light and electricity, today our slaves, was possible until physics and chemistry took them in hand. No control of the human soul is possible until it too will be taken in hand by them. We may now look forward to a real future for mankind because we have before us the beginnings of a chemistry of human nature. The internal secretions, with their influence upon brain and nervous system as well as every other part of the body corporation, as essentially blood-circulating chemical substances, have been discovered the real governors and arbiters of instincts and dispositions, emotions and reactions, characters and temperaments, good and bad. A huge complex of evidence, as various, complicated and obscure as human nature itself, supports that fundamental law.

The chemistry of the soul! Magnificent phrase! It's a long, long way to that goal. The exact formula is as yet far beyond our reach. But we have started upon the long journey and we shall get there. Then will Man truly become the experimental animal of the future, experimenting not only with the external conditions of his life, but with the constituents of his very nature and soul. The chemical conditions of his being, including the internal secretions, are the steps of the ladder by which he will climb to those dizzy heights where he will stretch out his hands and find himself a God. Modern knowledge of these chemical substances, circulating in the blood, and affecting every cell of the body, dates back scarce half a century. But already the paths blazed by the pioneers have led to the exploration of great countries. The thyroid gland, the pituitary gland, the adrenal glands, the thymus, the pineal, the sex glands, have yielded secrets. And certain great postulates have been established. The life of every individual, normal or abnormal, his physical appearance, and his psychic traits, are dominated largely by his internal secretions. All normal as well as abnormal individuals are classifiable according to the internal secretions which rule in their make-up. Individuals, families, nations and races show definite internal secretion traits, which stamp them with the quality of difference. The internal secretion formula of an individual may, in the future, constitute his measurement which will place him accurately in the social system.

"More and more we are forced to realize that the general form and external appearance of the human body depends, to a large extent, upon the functioning, during the early developmental period, of the endocrine glands. Our stature, the kinds of faces we have, the length of our arms and legs, the shape of the pelvis, the color and consistency of the integument, the quantity and regional location of our subcutaneous fat, the amount and distribution of hair on our bodies, the tonicity of our muscles, the sound of the voice, and the size of the larynx, the emotions to which our exterior gives expression. All are to a certain extent conditioned by the productivity of our glands of internal secretion." (Llewellys F. Barker, Johns Hopkins University, 1st President of Association for Study of Internal Secretions.)

The implications for the statesman, the educator, the vocational expert, the student of the neurotic and of genius, of delinquents, deficients and criminals, the explorers of the exceptional and the commonplace, the understanding of the poetic and kinetic, base and dull types, as well as of those two master interests of mankind, Sex and War, are manifest. The mystery of the individual, in all his distinct uniqueness, begins to be penetrated. And so every phase of social life, in which the individual is at bottom the final determinant, must be reviewed in the light of the new knowledge. History may be examined from an entirely new angle. The biographies of our Heroes of the Past, in the Carlylean sense, will bear reinspection. Even Utopias will have to be revised.

The internal secretions constitute and determine much of the inherited powers of the individual and their development They control physical and mental growth and all the metabolic processes of fundamental importance. They dominate all the vital functions during the three cycles of life. They co-operate in an intimate relationship which may be compared to an interlocking directorate. A derangement of their function, causing an insufficiency of them, an excess, or an abnormality, upsets the entire equilibrium of the body, with transforming effects upon the mind and the organs. In short, they control human nature, and whoever controls them, controls human nature.

The control of the glands of internal secretion waits upon our knowledge of them, the nature and precise composition of the substances manufactured by them, and just what they do to the cells. Envisaging the future, that knowledge today is meagre. Looking back fifty years, it becomes an amazing achievement and revelation. It is worth our while to survey the accomplished, and to trace its general human significance. For a certain tangible degree of knowledge and control has been attained and should be part of the average citizen's equipment in dealing with the everyday problems of his life.

THE ATTITUDE OF THE LABORATORY

A certain number of so-called experimental physiologists, that is, the physiologists of the animal laboratory, who will have nothing but syllogistic deductions and quantitative determinations based upon animal experiments as the data of their science, will be apt to look askance upon the preceding paragraphs, and those which will follow. To them, any man who relates the internal secretions to anything, outside of the routineer's paths, puts his reputation at stake, if he has any reputation at all to start in with. They would have us deliver a Scotch verdict upon all the questions which arise as soon as one attempts to take in the more general significance of the glands of internal secretion. This, even though the more general implications concerning the effects of their products, the relations of them to growth and development, nutrition and energy, environmental reactions and resistance to disease, as well as the grand complex of intelligence, are admittedly well ascertained in some directions.

The method of absolute measurement in science has yielded miracles. For some thousands of years, an isolated individual, here and there or an isolated institution have devoted themselves to the task, struggling not only with their own weaknesses, but with religious and political dogmas which spoiled and vitiated even the beginnings of their efforts. When, in the seventeenth century, men associated themselves in research, for free communication and discussion of their findings, a great invention came alive. Close on its heels was born the exact experimental method. Amazing triumphs were born of that marriage which swept away before it ignorance and superstition and prejudice. Its children and grandchildren have flourished and grown strong and mighty. They have transmuted the material conditions of life. Certainly all the laurels belong to the method of absolute, measured observations.

Yet all this time the old method of inductive observation has not gone dead. Most magnificent triumph of nineteenth century science, the evolution theory of Charles Darwin, remains the most conspicuous instance of clarification of thought in human history. That work was the outcome of an attempt to relate and interpret a collection of observations on species and their variations, that had long lain to hand, a mixture without a solvent. Darwin saw certain generalizations as solvents, and behold! a clear solution out of the mud. But it was by piling evidence upon evidence, co-ordinating isolated facts not directly associated, that the towering structure was erected. There is no prettier sample extant of the powers of the inductive method.

Not that there are no triumphs of the quantitative method in store for the biologist. Already, the materials of the Mendelians have become basic parts of his structure. And today, in pursuit of the solutions of hundreds of the problems of living matter, chemists and physiologists are employing the most precise standards, units, and measures of the physical sciences. Blood chemistry of our time is a marvel, undreamed of a generation ago. Also, these achievements are a perfect example of the accomplished fact contradicting a priori prediction and criticism. For it was one of the accepted dogmas of the nineteenth century that the phenomena of the living could never be subjected to accurate quantitative analysis.

However desirable the purely quantitative experimental methods may be, they naturally need always to be preceded by the qualitative studies of direct observations. Inevitably there will be numberless errors, apparent and real inconsistencies and contradictions, and ideas that will have to be discarded. Just the same there is no other method of progress. Every bit of evidence points towards the internal secretions as the holders of the secrets of our inmost being. They are the well springs of life, the dynamos of the organism. In trailing their scent we appear to be upon the track not only of the chemistry of our bodies, but of the chemistry of our very souls. An increasing host of factors and studies marshal themselves solidly for that declaration. Endeavor to conceive the consequences and possibilities for the future. A synthesis of the known in the field provides even now a means of understanding and control of the perplexities of human nature and life that are like a vista seen from a mountain top after the lifting of a fog.

The most precious bit of knowledge we possess today about Man is that he is the creature of his glands of internal secretion. That is, Man as a distinctive organism is the product, the by-product, of a number of cell factories which control the parts of his make-up. Much as the different divisions of an automobile concern produce the different parts of a car. These chemical factories consist of cells, manufacture special substances, which act upon the other cells of the body and so start and determine the countless processes we call Life. Life, body and soul emerge from the activities of the magic ooze of their silent chemistry precisely as a tree of tin crystals arises from the chemical reactions started in a solution of tin salts by an electric current.

Man is regulated by his Glands of Internal Secretion. At the beginning of the third decade of the twentieth century, after he had struggled, for we know at least fifty thousand years, to define and know himself, that summary may be accepted as the truth about himself. It is a far-reaching induction, but a valid induction, supported by a multitude of detailed facts.

Amazingly enough, the incontestable evidence, that first pointed to, and then proved up to the hilt, this answer to the question: What is Man? has been gathered in less than the last fifty years. Darwin and Huxley, and Spencer, who first opened men's eyes to their origins, were ignorant of the very existence of some of them, and had not the faintest notion or suspicion of the real importance or function of any of them.

THE PREJUDICES OF PHILOSOPHERS

Now, there are certain prejudices and problems which appear to be rudely brushed away by the dogmatic arrogance of the principle stated. What, you say, is Man but an affair of his peculiar gland chemistry? But what of mind, soul, consciousness? Still another of these pathetically one-sided and superficial theories of man as a machine pure and simple which would make him the most complicated of mechanisms, a marvel of intricate parts, but would deprive him of his essence as self-conscious unique in the universe. Man, thinking man, at any rate, dreads to lose the cherished impregnable conviction that he is something apart, inherently, and therefore infinitely different from every other phenomenon in the range of his cosmos.

A thorough dissection of the relation and attitude toward psychic material of the consistent physiologist, who refuses to deal in contradictory terms, would lead us a little too far. So would the reconciliation between the claims of mind and the concept of the organism as a system of chemical reactions. The most fundamental aspects of that herculean task, warned by the sign, No Trespassing, we shall leave to the metaphysicians. The influence of the glands of internal secretion upon the mind we must consider, but at present postpone. Yet the hot-headed contenders on both sides may be reminded of certain facts.

We live in the most iconoclastic of ages. There are sane people alive today going quietly about their business who deny the very existence of consciousness. These heretics of course pooh-pooh absolutely the lions of metaphysics. On the other hand, it may be pointed out to our mechanists who believe in mechanism to the bitter end, that even if man can be described entirely as a mere transformer of energy, there is no reason why he cannot also be described as a transformer of energy plus someone who makes use of the transformer and of the energy transformed. The stone wall before the honest mechanist is the abolition of purpose, and design, an old insoluble problem upon his premises. Preach, until you are blue in the face, behaviorist tropisms, in which man is pushed and pulled about in his environment as are iron filings in a magnetic field. Think up objective physiologies in which your life and mine become a series of concatenated influences and compound reflexes. Play with words like the concentration reflex when you mean idea, and the symbolic reflex when you mean language. But your most rigid nomenclature will never abolish the mystic personal purpose in the equation, no matter how low the step in the animal series to which you descend. The declaration that a man is dominated by certain glands within his body should not be taken to give aid and comfort to those who would banish mind from the universe.

CHAPTER I
HOW THE GLANDS OF INTERNAL SECRETION
WERE DISCOVERED

Just what are the glands of internal secretion? And how have we become possessed of whatever information about them we have? A brief review of how the idea of a gland of internal secretion came into the human mind and of the contributions that have converged into a single body of knowledge is worth while.

A gland is a collection of cells (those viscous globules which are the units of all tissues and organs). It manufactures substances intended for a particular effect upon the body economy. The effect may be either local or upon the body as a whole.

Originally, a gland meant something in the body which was seen to make something else, generally a juice or a liquid mixture of some sort. A classical example is the salivary glands elaborating saliva. The microscope has shown us that every gland is a chemical factory in which the cells are the workers. The product of the gland work is its secretion. Thus the sweat glands of the skin secrete the perspiration as their secretion, the lachrymal glands of the eyes the tears as theirs. The collectivism of management and control is the only essential difference between them and the modern soap factory or T.N.T. plant.

Man as a carnivor, and as a consequent anatomist, has been acquainted with these more superficially placed glands for some thousands of years. During all this time and during the epoch of the achievements of gross anatomy, it was believed that the secretions of all glands were poured out upon some surface of the body. Either an exterior surface like the skin, or some interior surface, the various mucous membranes. This was supported by the discovery of canal-like passage ways leading from the gland to the particular surface where its secretion was to act. These corridors, the secretory or excretory ducts, are present, for example, in the liver, conducting the bile to the small intestine. Devices of transportation fit happily into a comparison of a gland to a chemical factory, corresponding thus closely to the tramways and railroads of our industrial centers.

Little more than a hundred years ago, it was observed that certain organs, like the thyroid body in the neck, and the adrenal capsules in the abdomen, hitherto neglected because their function was hopelessly obscure, had a glandular structure. As in so much scientific advance, the discovery or improvement of a new instrument or method, a fresh tool of research, was responsible. The perfection of the microscope was the reason this time.

If one wishes to trace the idea of internal secretion by cells to an individual, it is convenient, if not pedantic, to give the credit to Theophile de Bordeu, a famous physician of Paris in the eighteenth century. Bordeu came to Paris as a brilliant provincial in his early twenties and by the charm of his manner and daring therapy fought his way to the most exclusive aristocratic practice of the court. Naturally a courtier, taking to the intrigues of the royal court like a duck to water, making enemies on every hand as well as friends, and with a fastidious and impatient clientele, he yet found time to dabble in the wonders of the newly perfected microscope and to speculate upon the meaning of the novelties revealed by it in the tissues. ***He coined the thought of a gland secretion into the blood***.

It was in the year 1749 that he came to Paris from the Pyrenees, a young medical graduate, destined to become the most fashionable practitioner of his time. At the age of twenty-three he was holding the professorship of anatomy at his alma mater, Montpelier, where his father was a successful physician. At twenty-five he was elected corresponding member of the Royal Academy of Sciences. A handsome presence and a Tartarin de Tarascon disposition assured his success from the start. The medical world was then composed of the emulsion of charlatanry and science Moliere ridiculed. Success stimulated envy and jealousy. One of the richest of the older medical men set himself the job of procuring his scalp. On a trumped-up charge of stealing jewels from a dead patient--a favorite accusation against the doctors of the eighteenth century--he had Bordeu's license taken away from him. The good graces of certain women to whom Bordeu had always appealed, and who indeed supplied the funds to get him started in Paris, rammed through two acts of Parliament to reinstate him. Nothing daunted, he returned to his quest for a court clientele, and was rewarded finally by having the moribund Louis XV as a patient.

This was the man with whom the modern history of the internal secretions begins. Not content with adventures among the courtiers and desperadoes of the most corrupt court in the most corrupt city of the world, he went in for research. The high power microscope that came into vogue when he was studying, revealed vague wonders which he described in a monograph, "Researches into the mucous tissues or cellular organs." But what makes him interesting is a slender volume on the "Medical Analysis of the Blood," published in the year of the American Declaration of Independence. The sexual side of men and women aroused Bordeu's most ardent enthusiasms. Starting with observations on the characters of eunuchs and capons, as well as spayed female animals, he formulated a conception of sexual secretions absorbed into the blood, settling the male or female tint of the organism and setting the seal upon the destiny of the individual. Thus he must be donated the credit of anticipating the most modern doctrine on the subject.

The generation after him witnessed the triumph of the cell as the recognized unit of structure of the tissues, the brick of the organs. It was soon found that the cells of the more familiar glands, like the sweat or tear glands, resembled the cells of the more mysterious structures named the thyroid in the neck, or adrenal in the abdomen, of which the function was unknown. What had hitherto prevented classification of the latter as glands was the fact that they possessed no visible pathways for the removal of their secretion. So now they were set apart as the ***ductless*** glands, the glands without ducts, as contrasted with the glands normally equipped with ducts. Since, too, they were observed to have an exceedingly rich supply of blood, the blood presented itself as the only conceivable mode of egress for the secretions packed within the cells. So they were also called the blood or vascular glands.

The names which became most popular were those which represented a contrast of the glands with the ducts, conveying their secretion to the exterior, as the glands of EXTERNAL SECRETION and the glands without the ducts, the secretions of which were kept within the body, absorbed by the blood and lymph to be used by the other cells, as the glands of INTERNAL SECRETION. How different these two classes of glands are may be realized by imagining the existence of great factories manufacturing food products, which would diffuse through their walls into the atmosphere, to be absorbed by our bodies.

There are certain terms for the glands of internal secretion which are used interchangeably. They are spoken of often as the ***endocrine*** glands and as the ***hormone*** producing glands. Endocrine is most convenient for it stands for both the gland and its secretion. Hormone is employed a good deal in the literature of the subject. But it applies specifically to the internal secretion, and not to the gland.

THE EXPERIMENTAL PIONEER

All this clarification of the concept of the glands of internal secretion occurred in the first quarter of the nineteenth century. However, no inkling of their real importance to the body, of which quantitatively they form so insignificant a part, was apparently revealed to anyone. Not even the most daring speculation or brilliant guess work in physiology engaged them as material. Thus Henle, the great anatomist, calmly affirmed that these glands "have no influence on animal life: they may be extirpated or they degenerate without sensation or motion suffering in the least." Johann Mueller, the most celebrated physiologist of his day and contemporary of Henle, wrote in 1844 and coolly stated, "The ductless glands are alike in one particular--they either produce a different change in the blood which circulates through them or the lymph which they elaborate plays a special role in the formation of blood or of chyle." In other words, they were dismissed as curious nonentities, of no real significance to the running of the body. Laennec, the French founder of the Art of Diagnosis in Medicine, once said that nothing about a science is more interesting than the progress of that science itself. He might have added that nothing either was more interesting than the contradictions in that progress. For while these grand moguls of their sciences were enunciating their dogmas, pioneers here and there were already setting the mines that were to explode them.

The experimental method, to the value of which biologists were just beginning to awaken, was destined to be the vehicle of Time's revenges. An application of it to the mysteries of sex was the immediate occasion. Sex and sex differences have always more or less obsessed the imagination of mankind. The volumes of theories about them would constitute a respectable museum. Certain gross facts, however, were known. The effects of loss of the sex glands upon the configuration of the body and the predominating constitution in animals and eunuchs have always attracted attention. The proverbs and stories of all nations are full of references to them. But up to the nineteenth century no controlled experimental work was ever carried out regarding them. It was in 1849, that A.A. Berthold of Goettingen, a quiet, sedate lecturer, carried out the pioneer experiment of removing the testes of four roosters and transplanting them under the skin. It was Berthold's idea to test whether a gland with a definite external secretion, and a duct through which that secretion was expelled, but which yet had powers over the body as a whole that were to be attributed only to an internal secretion, could not be shown, by a clean-cut experiment, to possess such an internal secretion. He succeeded perfectly. For he found that, though, in thus separating the gland from its duct and so cutting off its external secretion, the action of the cells manufacturing that secretion was destroyed, the general effects upon the body were not those of castration. The animals retained their male characteristics as regards voice, reproductive instinct, fighting spirit and growth of comb and wattles. Whereas if the glands were entirely removed, these male traits, peculiar to the rooster, were completely lost. The inference was the existence of an internal secretion.

To Berthold belongs the honor of being the first experimental demonstrator who proved the reality of a gland with a true internal secretion and the power it exercised through the blood upon the entire organism. Besides, he showed that a typical gland of external secretion could also have an internal secretion, a possibility never before considered. That two kinds of cells could live within the same gland: one set usually recognized as producing the external secretion, the other evolving the internal secretion, was an astounding original conception.

ENTER CLAUDE BERNARD

Science is supposed to be immune to the personal prejudices and emotional habits of the vulgar. It is the tradition that a new contribution to knowledge emerging from no matter how obscure the source, should be hailed as a gift from the gods. But the sad truth of the matter is that a new finding in science requires as much backing as a new project in high finance or social climbing. Berthold, like Mendel, the founder of genetics, was a great pioneer. But there was no personage, no person of consequence, with no patronage by anyone of consequence, no wife or kin, to push him, and no audience to stimulate him. His poor four little pages of a report, published ten years before Darwin's "Origin of Species," attracted not the slightest notice. Buried in the print of a journal with a subscription list of possibly two or three hundred, of whom perhaps two dozen may have been interested enough to read it, but without any recorded reaction on the part of any of them, it was a flash in the pan. Though it was good, original, conclusive stuff, it was cut dead, absolutely, by the scientific world. As a result, forty years elapsed before the implications of his studies were rediscovered by the Columbus of the modern approach to the internal secretions, the American Frenchman, Brown-Sequard.

It took a first class man of genius in his field, in Paris, with a respected position in the whirl of its medical planetary system and a university appointment, to boom and advertise the doctrine of the internal secretions, so that people began to sit up and listen and take sides--on the wrong grounds. This Frenchman was Claude Bernard. At a series of lectures on experimental physiology delivered at the College of France, in 1855, he coined the terms internal secretion and external secretion and emphasized the opposition between them, on the basis of an incorrect example, the function of the liver in the supply of sugar to the blood.

Just as Columbus reached America, carried on a series of logical syllogisms, built upon unreal pictures of a straight path to the East, Claude Bernard opened up the continent of the internal secretions to the experimental enthusiasts of his time by a discovery which today is not grouped among the phenomena of internal secretion at all. In attempting to throw light upon the disease diabetes, in which there is a loss of the normal ability of the cells to burn up sugar, he examined the sugar content of the blood in different regions of the body. He found that the blood of the veins, in general, contained less sugar than the blood of the arteries, which meant that sugar was taken from the blood in passing through the tissues. But the venous blood of the right side of the heart contained as much sugar as the arterial blood. Evidently, somewhere, sugar was added to the blood in the veins before it got to the heart. The blood of the vein which goes from the liver to the right side of the heart was then found to contain a higher percentage of sugar than is present in the arteries. The vein which transmits the blood from the intestines to the liver had the usual lower percentage of sugar corresponding to the analysis established for the other veins. The liver, therefore, must add sugar to the blood on its way to the heart. Extraction of the liver then revealed the presence in it of a form of starch, an animal starch, which Bernard called glycogen, the sugar-maker. The origin of the sugar added to the blood on its way from the liver to the heart was thus settled. Bernard went on to hail glycogen and the sugar derivable as the internal secretions of the liver, and to erect, and then drive home, a theory of internal secretions and their importance in the body economy.

The case he had hit upon was exquisitely fortunate, as the liver had hitherto been regarded purely a gland of external secretion, the bile. Nowadays, glycogen and the blood sugar are not considered internal secretions, because they are classified as elementary reserve food, while the concept of the internal secretions has become narrowed down to substances acting as starters or inhibitors of different processes. Moreover, the process of liberation of sugar from glycogen itself in the liver, upon demand, is today set down to the action of an internal secretion, adrenalin. Claude Bernard's conception, like a novelist's characters, has turned upon its creator, taken on a life of its own, and evolved into something he never intended. He looked upon an internal secretion as simply maintaining the normal composition of the blood, which bathed alike and treated alike the democracy of cells. Today, the blood is believed merely the transporting medium for the internal secretion, destined for a particular group of cells.

ADDISON'S AS THE FIRST ENGLISH CONTRIBUTION

The years 1855-56 are red-letter years in the history of the glands of internal secretion. They witnessed, not only the publication of Claude Bernard's "Lectures on Experimental Physiology," but also the appearance of a monograph by Thomas Addison, an English physician, entitled "On the constitutional and local effects of disease of the suprarenal bodies." In this, he described a fatal disease during which the individual affected became languid and weak, and developed a dingy or smoky discoloration of the whole surface of the body, a browning or bronzing of the skin, caused generally by destructive tuberculous disease of the suprarenal or adrenal bodies. Addison promptly put down these constitutional effects of loss of the adrenal bodies to loss of something produced by them of constitutional importance. He was particularly struck by the change in the pigmentation of the skin, so much so that his own designation for the affection was "bronzed skin." Since then, however, the condition has been universally styled Addison's Disease.

There is something spectacularly mysterious and picturesque about most of the malign, insidious effects of the disease which appealed at once to a number of investigators. The most adventurous, the most daring, the most imbued with enthusiasm for the experimental method, was the American Frenchman, Brown-Sequard, who is acknowledged the father of modern knowledge of the glands of internal secretion, though to Claude Bernard belong the honors of the grandfather.

BROWN-SEQUARD THE GREAT

Brown-Sequard, as the outstanding figure in the history of the glands of internal secretion, deserves some notice as a personality. In the words of the note-makers for novels and plays, he was a card. He was born in 1817 at Port-Louis, on the island of Mauritius, off Africa, then French property. His father was a Mr. Brown, an American sea captain; his mother a Mme. Sequard, a Frenchwoman. Early in childhood, the father sailed away on one of his voyages and never came back. The mother thereafter supported herself and her son sewing embroideries. At fifteen, Brown-Sequard, with the physical appearance of an Indian Creole, was clerking in a colonial store by day, and composing poetry, romances and plays by night. The call of Paris was in his blood, which was indeed a supersaturated solution of wanderlust.

Soon he was landed there to make his fortune in literature, only too speedily to be disillusioned. Exhibition of manuscripts to a leading literary light merely evoked curt advice to learn a trade or go into business. He would have none of either and studied medicine instead, earning his way by teaching as he learned. In the laboratories, he made the acquaintance of people who more than once were to be his salvation in the ups and downs of his career. In 1848 he was one of the secretaries of the Society of Biology, newly founded by Claude Bernard.

Some trouble, perhaps some effect upon his health of cholera which then swept Paris, caused him to return to his native Mauritius, to encounter an epidemic of cholera. There he slaved manfully, for which a gold medal was afterward struck for him. That over with, he embarked in 1852 for New York, without a word of American, learning English on board. This was the first of a series of voyages. As he often boasted, he crossed the ocean sixty times, not a bad record for the days when the *Mauretania* was still in the womb of time. He made a hopeless failure out of practice in New York, became so poor as to practice obstetrics at five dollars a case, and married a niece of Daniel Webster. Then he went back to Paris. Back to America next as Professor of Physiology at the University of Richmond, Virginia, a job occupied for a few months only because of his opinions on slavery, ostensibly anyhow.

To Paris then the rolling stone meandered again. So that soon after he was offered and accepted the charge of a great newly opened hospital for epileptics in London. That proved merely an interlude and in 1863 we find him back in his fatherland (if we may hold France his motherland) as Professor of Neuropathology at Harvard. In New York fame preceded him now with a thousand trumpets, so that on the day of his arrival, he was kept busy seeing patients until night, when he had to desist because of exhaustion. But still he did not prosper. An unfortunate second marriage almost broke his heart, and an attempt to found in New York a new medical periodical, the ***Archives of Scientific and Practical Medicine and Surgery***, got him into hot water. Not until the death of Claude Bernard in 1878 left vacant the chair of physiology in the College of France, did he find peace and rest. He hastened to Paris, was appointed, and lived, in spite of the most erratic of existences, to the ripe old age of 78, working up to the last minute.

Addison's monograph stimulated Brown-Sequard, in the year after its printing, to reproduce the fatal disease experimentally by excising the suprarenal capsules in animals. Addison was very modest in his monograph. He stated that the first case of the malady had been reported by his great predecessor at Guy's Hospital, London, Richard Bright, the describer of Bright's Disease. Then he talks about the "curious facts" he had "stumbled upon" and refers to an "ill-defined impression" that these suprarenal bodies, in common with the spleen and other organs, "in some way or other minister to the elaboration of the blood." In the preface to his work he had spoken more confidently of the fact that Nature, as an experimenter and a vivisector, can beat the physiologist to a frazzle. Indeed, he begins like this: "If Pathology be to disease what Physiology is to health, it appears reasonable to conclude that, in any given structure or organ, the laws of the former will be as fixed and significant as those of the latter: and that the peculiar characters of any structure or organ may be as certainly recognized in the phenomena of disease as in the phenomena of health. Although pathology, therefore, as a branch of medical science, is necessarily founded on physiology, questions may nevertheless arise regarding the true character of a structure or organ, to which occasionally the pathologist may be able to return a more satisfactory and decisive reply than the physiologist--these two branches of medical knowledge being thus found mutually to advance and illustrate each other. Indeed, as regards the functions of individual organs, the mutual aids of these two branches of knowledge are probably much more nearly balanced than many may be disposed to admit: for in estimating them we are very apt to forget how large an amount of our present physiological knowledge respecting the functions of these organs has been the immediate result of casual observations made on the effects of disease." William James expressed the same thought some decades later, when he emphasized that the abnormal was but the normal exaggerated and magnified, played upon by the limelight, and therefore the best teacher and indicator of the exact definition and limitations of the normal.

Addison, speaking before the South London Medical Society in 1849, declared that in all of three afflicted individuals there was found a diseased condition of the suprarenal capsules, and that in spite of the consciousness "of the bias and prejudice inseparable from the hope or vanity of an original discovery ... he could not help entertaining a very strong impression that these hitherto mysterious organs--the suprarenal capsules--may be either directly or indirectly concerned in sanguification (the making of the blood): and that a diseased condition of them, functional or structural, may interfere with the proper elaboration of the body generally, or of the red particles more especially...." A modern, acquainted with after developments, would say that Addison was very hot upon the trail indeed. But withal, though he must have been well aware of John Hunter's advice to Jenner on vaccination, "Don't think, make some observations," his training in the indirect reasoning and deductions of the clinician prevented him from going right on to a direct experimental test of his theories.

This Brown-Sequard proceeded to do. Removing the adrenal glands in several species of animals, he found, meant a terrible weakness in twenty-four to forty-eight hours, and death shortly after. If only one were removed, there was no change apparent in the normal animal, but death occurred rapidly upon removal of the other, even after a long interval. Furthermore, transfusion of blood from a normal into one deprived of its suprarenals prevented death for a long time, indicating that the suprarenals normally secreted something into the blood necessary to life.

The years 1855-1856 beheld two other important glands of internal secretion, the thyroid, the gland in the neck astride the windpipe, and the thymus, in the chest above the heart, make their debut.

The thymus was introduced by the great classic monograph of Friedleben on the "Physiology of the Thymus," in which he mentioned the usual forgotten pioneers: Felix Plater, a Swiss physician, who in 1614 had found an enlarged thymus in an infant dying suddenly, and Restelli, an Italian, who interested himself in the effects of removal of the thymus more than ten years before. Friedleben believed that in the young without a thymus, there occurred a softening of the bones, and general physical and mental deterioration. He started the ball rolling for a number of researches.

Moritz Schiff, of Frankfort-on-the-Main, showed that excision of the thyroid gland in dogs is invariably fatal. A number of physicians in the first half of the century had reported certain remarkable symptoms associated with enlargement of the thyroid gland, as goitre. In 1825 the collected posthumous writings of Caleb Perry, an eminent physician of Bath, England, recorded eight cases, in which, together with enlargement of the gland, there developed enlargement and palpitation of the heart, a distinct protrusion of the eyes from their sockets and an appearance of agitation and distress. Schiff's paper was the first to throw any light on the subject. But for some reason, probably the same as in Berthold's forlorn experiments with the sex glands, the work of a person of no importance was ignored, or perhaps the more charitable view is that it was forgotten. Yet the tide of observation kept sweeping in relevant data.

In 1850, Curling, an English pathologist, studying the cretinous idiots of Salzburg, written about centuries before by Paracelsus, discovered that with their defective brain and mentality there was associated an absence of the thyroid body, and accompanying symmetrical swellings of fat tissue at the sides of the neck. Then Sir William Gull in 1873 painted the singular details of a cretinous condition developing in adult women, a condition to which another Englishman, William Ord, of London, five years later donated the title of myxedema, because of a characteristic thickening and infiltration of the skin that is one of its features.

Surgery then enters upon the scene. The great Swiss surgeon. Theodore Kocher, performed the first excision of the thyroid gland in human beings for goitre, in the same year. In 1882, J.L. Reverdin, another surgeon of Geneva, noticed that in man complete removal of the thyroid was followed by symptoms identical with those collected under the name of myxedema, and used the phrase "operative myxedema" to emphasize his conviction of the connection between them. Then Schiff, in 1884, neglected twenty-five years, came back, with an array of demonstrations, proving that the various symptoms, tremors, spasms and convulsions, following removal of the thyroid, could be prevented by a previous graft of a piece of the gland under the skin, or by the injection of thyroid juice into a vein or under the skin, or by the ingestion of thyroid juice or the raw thyroid by mouth.

A crystallization of ideas about the true function of the thyroid was now inevitable. In 1884, Sir Victor Horsley produced an experimental myxedema by removal of the thyroid in monkeys, resembling closely in its symptom-picture the disease as it occurs in human beings. Moebius, a German neurologist, came out boldly for the conception that a number of ailments could be due to qualitative and quantitative changes in the secretion of the thyroid, and that just as myxedema and cretinism were due to an insufficiency of the secretion, Parry's disease was to be ascribed to an excessive outpouring of it. The next steps were easy. In 1888, Sir Felix Semon, as an outcome of a collective investigation, established for all time that cretinism, myxedema and post-operative myxedema were one and the same.

It was bound to occur to someone that if human myxedema and animal experimental myxedema were one and the same, Schiff's procedure of prevention and cure by feeding thyroid gland by mouth in the latter could be applied to the former. The idea occurred to two men, Murray and Howitz, in 1891. Murray's patient, a Mrs. H., was shown before the Northcumberland and Durham Medical Society, an English country medical organization, in February, 1891. She was forty-two years old and had borne nine children. The illness attacking her had begun insidiously, with a gradual enlargement and thickening of her face and hands. She had become very slow in speech and gait, sensitive to cold, and languid and depressed in spirit to the point of inability to go about alone. Murray, employing the glycerin extract of the thyroid gland of a freshly killed sheep, injected twenty-four drops hypodermically, twice a week. There was an immediate and marvelous improvement, which continued steadily, Murray finding that it could be maintained by feeding the gland by mouth. The features and skin returned to the normal, speech quickened and she became able to walk about and live her life without hesitation or assistance. She lived to the age of seventy-four, dying in 1919. In the twenty-eight years, during which it was always necessary to administer the thyroid, she consumed over nine pints of thyroid, comprising the glands of 870 sheep.

Giants and dwarfs and fat people have always interested people as freaks, departures from the usual and the normal, and have formed the stock of popular museum, circus and country fair. Every mythology has concerned itself with them. The Titans among the Greeks, Og, Gog and Magog among the Hebrews, are examples of the fascination of the superlarge. John Hunter, the founder of experimental surgery, spent a fortune in chasing after the skeleton of a famous Irish Giant in 1783. Dwarfs have also fascinated--witness the short-limbed satyrs of the Greeks and the dwarf gods (Ptah and Bes) of Egypt, as well as the vogue of the court dwarf-buffoons, of whom Velasquez has left us some portraits. Fat people, obesity as a manifestation of personality, have aroused wonder and amusement the world over. The Fat Boy has always furnished good sport to the Sam Wellers.

All these characters, tall or short, fat or lean, are related to the activity of a gland of internal secretion in the head, the pituitary, which became a centre of interest in the late eighties. Because of its situation, the opinion of the ancients was that it was the source of the mucus of the nose, an opinion reinforced by the greatest anatomist of the Dark Ages, Galen, and held up to the seventeenth century. In other words, it was considered simply a gland of external secretion. Experimental removal of the pituitary was essayed by Horsley in 1886, the same man who two years before had reproduced myxedema successfully in monkeys. Others succeeded his attempt. But the conclusions drawn were uncertain or contradictory, resulting from the difficulties of the operative technique of getting at a gland placed at the base of the brain. Not until 1908 was the problem solved by Paulesco of Bucharest, who devised a way of reaching it by trepanning the skull. He was thus able to prove beyond a doubt that the pituitary gland was essential to life, and that without it no animal could continue to live for any length of time. Soon after, Harvey Gushing and his associates at Johns Hopkins Hospital discovered that removal of part of the gland was followed by a pronounced obesity and sluggishness. A basis for the understanding of obesity and growth was then established.

In the eighties, there came to the clinic of Pierre Marie in Paris, a pupil of the great Charcot, various women complaining of headache. They also told him about an enlargement of their hands and feet, and an alarming change in the bones of the face. He differentiated the affection from its imitators, and created its present designation of "acromegaly" (enlargement of the extremities). Also he correlated their relationship to the giants who have been mentioned. Acromegalics have been also likened to the Neanderthal Man, who had probably, as the gorillas may have, an excess of the pituitary in their systems. For four years he studied the morbid phenomena in the tissues of these sufferers at last consigned to their end. First one, and then another, and then a third and a fourth exhibited a striking hypertrophy of the pituitary body and a consequent widening of the portion of the base of the skull which cradles the gland. He proceeded to say so in the graduating thesis of his pupil, Souza Leite. The inference was inevitable that the entire process was to be put down to an overactivity of the pituitary. Ever since, too, the growth of the skeleton has been accepted as controlled by that gland.

About this time another set of old observations came to life again, related to those of Docent Berthold on the auto-grafting of the testes of a cock, with complete retention of its sexual characters, which he said, must be due "to the productive action of the testes, i.e., to its effect upon the blood, and thence to the corresponding effect of such blood upon the entire organism." Of course, stock raisers and poultry fanciers have noted the interesting outcome of castration for about as long as their professions have existed. And for ages the diminution of sexual activity as a predecessor to the decadence of senility has been harped upon. Rejuvenation, especially in connection with sexual activity, as well as with tissue and spiritual elasticity, has been one of the haunting phantoms of the imagination for as long as we have records of articulate humanity. Together with El Dorado, the Elixir of Youth has shared the honors with the Philosopher's Stone. The idea of employing the chemical materials of the sex glands, the testes or the ovaries, to bring back youth, to restore juvenility, had not, as far as we know, occurred to anyone who at any rate put himself on record, by word or deed, until 1889. The hero of the new departure was the hero of so many daring adventures among speculative experiments, Brown-Sequard.

At this time the wanderer was an aged sage, seventy-two years old, fit, as custom goes, only for retirement and resignation to the fate of all flesh. The old passion of experimenting upon himself as well as upon the guinea-pigs, dogs, cats and monkeys, by which he was always surrounded, was as alive and kicking as ever. I suppose he had been thinking for years concerning some method for the resumption of youth, for we find him exclaiming, when the opportunity loomed of a great laboratory on Agassiz Island, Long Island, on one of his recurrent flights to New York: "Would that I were thirty!" And other passages in his personal communications refer again and again to his consciousness of growing old. The miracles that were being performed by injecting thyroid and feeding thyroid in animals probably acted as the spark to an inflammable mass of ideas long smouldering in the subcellars of his mind. The effects were reported to the Society of Biology in Paris, one memorable evening, June 1, 1889, in two notes on the results of the hypodermic injection in man of the testis juice of monkeys and dogs, and certain generalizations deduced therefrom. Such juices, he stated, had a definite energy-mobilizing or, as he put it, dynamogenic action upon the subject himself, stimulating amazingly his general health, muscular power and mental activity.

These experiments, their nature, the manner in which they were conducted, the character and age of the experimenter, and the results claimed, were exquisitely good stuff for ridicule. Cartoonists and reporters leaped upon the theme with the avidity of the true-blue interviewer. Paris, where to be ridiculed is to be killed in public with the most ignominious of deaths, reacted as only the French temperament can react. The wits of the salons crackled, the bourgeoisie chortled, the proletariat roared. The Elixir of Life had been discovered and it was excellent sport.

But Brown-Sequard remained unshaken. He had all the roues of Paris running to him, and consequent charges of quackery and charlatanism. How much of these unsavory epithets really applied to him will not be determined until we have a better acquaintance with his more intimate life. A biography and collection of his letters is needed. But it is certain that the general principles he arrived at, aided as much by the wings of intuition as by the clues of incomplete and incompletely controlled experiments, survive as the foundations of whatever we know about the internal secretions, and all our present viewpoints. He summed these up in 1891 as follows:

"All the tissues, in our view, are modifiers of the blood by means of an internal secretion taken from them by the venous blood. From this we are forced to the conclusion that, if subcutaneous injections of the liquids drawn from these parts are ineffectual, then we should inject some of the venous blood supplying these parts.... We admit that each tissue, and, more generally, each cell of the organism, secretes on its own account, certain products or special ferments, which, through this medium (the blood), influence all other cells of the body, a definite solidarity being thus established among all the cells through a mechanism other than the nervous system.... All the tissues (glands and other organs) have thus a special internal secretion, and so give to the blood something more than the waste products of metabolism. The internal secretions, whether by direct favorable influence, or whether through the obstacles they oppose to deleterious processes, seem to be of great utility in maintaining the organism in its normal state."

The only part of this statement not conceded today is that relating to the formation of internal secretions by tissues other than those of which the cells are definitely glandular, that is secretory: as can be determined under the microscope. Brown-Sequard added to the concept of internal secretions, fathered by Claude Bernard, the idea of a correlation, a mutual influencing of them and of the different organs of the body through them. The nervous system had hitherto been regarded as the sole means of communication between cells, by its telegraphic arrangements of nerve filaments reaching out everywhere, interweaving with each other and the cells. The Brown-Sequard conception inferred the existence of a postal system between cells, the blood supplying the highway for travel and transmission of the post, the post consisting of the chemical substances secreted by the glands. To be sure, the doctrine was only an inference, though well-founded, of which the direct experimental proof was not to be obtained until the researches of Bayliss and Starling. Yet to Brown-Sequard belongs the immortal credit, if not of the originator, at any rate of the resurrector of the idea of using gland extracts to influence the body. The unwarranted hopes aroused by his enthusiastic reports of rejuvenating miracles have long since been dissipated. Moreover, they smeared the whole subject with a disrepute which clings to certain narrow and unreasonable minds to this day. But as every physiologist since has acknowledged, he was and remains the great pathbreaker in the conquest of the internal secretions.

THE HORMONES

The problem of the internal secretions was now attacked from another angle. A great Russian physiologist, Pawlow, called attention to the fact that the introduction of a dilute mineral acid, such as the hydrochloric acid, normally a constituent of the stomach digestive fluid, into the upper part of the intestine, provoked a secretion of the pancreas, which is so important for intestinal digestion. He explained the phenomenon as a reflex, a matter of the nerves going from the intestine to the pancreas.

His pupil, Popielski, threw doubt upon so easy an explanation, by proving that the same reaction could be elicited even after all the nerve connections between the gut and the spinal cord were severed. If the relation was a reflex, it would have to be classed now as one of those local nerve circuits, which are pretty common among the viscera, a local call and reply as it were, without mediation of the great long distance trunk lines in the spinal cord and the medulla oblongata.

The work of Bayliss and Starling, two English physiologists, was commenced then to test the hypothesis. They soon found that the experiment could be so devised as to exclude any influence whatever on the part of the nervous tissues, and yet result positively. Thus, if a loop of intestine was so prepared as to be attached to the rest of the body only by means of its blood vessels, all the nerves being cut, putting some acid into it was still followed by a flow of pancreatic juice, no less marked than when none of the parts about the piece of gut had been disturbed. It was evident that the stimulus to the pancreas was carried by way of the blood stream. That the stimulating substance was not the acid itself, was shown by the failure of the reaction to occur when the acid was injected directly into the blood stream. Since there was this difference in the effects between acid in the intestine and acid in the blood, it was manifest that the active substance must be some material elaborated in the intestinal mucous membrane under the influence of the acid. So they scraped some of the lining of the bowel, rubbed it up with acid, and injected the filtered mixture into the blood. They were rewarded by a flow of pancreatic juice greater in amount than any obtained in their other experiments. From the filtered mixture they isolated in an impure form, a solid substance which, when introduced into the circulation, has a similar action. To this, of which the exact chemical make-up is as yet an unknown, they gave the name secretin.

Secretin and its properties they used to generalize as a perfectly direct and amply demonstrable example of an internal secretion. Metaphors are no less valuable in physiology than in poetry. They declared that the internal secretions appeared to them to be chemical messengers, telegraph boys sent from one organ to another through the public highways, the blood (really more like a moving platform). So they christened them all hormones, deriving the word from the Greek verb meaning to rouse or set in motion. As a science is a well-made language, a new word is an event. It sums up details, economizes brain-work and so is cherished by the intellect. The study of the internal secretions has advanced by leaps and bounds since it became convenient to speak of them as hormones. Withal, the brilliant work of Bayliss and Starling stands as the third great foundation stone, the first Claude Bernard's and the second Brown-Sequard's, in the architecture of the modern concepts of the internal secretions.

CHAPTER II
THE GLANDS: THYROID AND PITUITARY

The glands of internal secretion, the history of which, as tools of thought, I reviewed in the previous chapter, have each an interesting evolutionary story. Without some acquaintance with that story, the rough outline of their physical architecture, and the particular work they are called upon to perform in the body, no adequate understanding of their influence upon types of human nature and personality is possible.

THE THYROID GLAND

This gland consists of two maroon colored masses astride the neck, above the windpipe, close to the larynx. These are bridged by a narrow isthmus of the same tissue. They remind one of the flaps of a purse opened up. The gland has always attracted much attention because its enlargement constitutes the prominent deformity known as goitre.

To begin with, the thyroid was once a sex gland, pure and simple. In the lowest vertebrates and in the homologous tissues of the higher invertebrates, the fractions of the thyroid are intimately connected with the ducts of the sexual organs. They are indeed accessory sexual organs, uterine glands, satellites of the sex process. From Petromyzon upward that relationship is lost, the thyroid migrates more and more to the head region, to become the great link between sex and brain. How alive that function still is, is grossly shown by the swelling of the gland with sexual excitement, menstruation and pregnancy.

Relative to the body weight it is largest in the mammalia, and smallest in the fishes. It therefore grows larger as the vertebrate ascends in the scale. It has, in fact, developed in direct proportion to and side by side with the fundamental, differentiating vertebrate characteristics. Of these, the possession of a dry hairy skin instead of a moist or mucus bearing, chitinous skin, the ownership of an internal bony skeleton and a large skull, and a complicated development of brain, are the diagnostic signs. Thyroid internal secretion has a very definite controlling relation to all of them: to skin, its hairiness, moisture and amount of mucus, to the growth and size of the bones, especially the bones of the extremities and the skull, and to intelligence and the complexity of the convolutions of the brain. Injury to the thyroid, especially in growing animals, is followed by profound retrogression or arrest of development in skin, skeleton and brain.

In the fishes and the cyclostomes the thyroid is represented only by some small scrubby patches, little larger than the heads of pins, scattered along the aorta, the great blood vessels from the heart, and out a little way along each gill. It becomes larger and more compact among the amphibians and reptiles, but still remains quite small. Large and prominent among the birds and mammalia, it is largest and most prominent among the primates and man. It is hence permissible to think of the thyroid as a dictator of evolution, to crown it as the vertebrate gland par excellence, and to call the typical vertebrate brand marks secondary *thyroid* characteristics in precisely the sense of Darwin classing the horns of cattle as secondary *sexual* characteristics.

In such enthusiasm for the thyroid as a determinant of evolution, its pillar of cloud by day and column of fire by night, one should not forget the other glands of internal secretion. In them all, we may suppose, Life, tired of inventing merely prehensile, destructive and reproductive organs, hit upon the happy thought of contrivances which are in essence chemical factories to speed up the rate of variation and so of a higher evolution.

CREATOR OF THE LAND ANIMAL

According to this conception the thyroid played a fundamental part in the change of sea creatures into land animals. Experimentally, thyroid has been used to transform one into the other. Thus the occasional change of a Mexican axolotl, a purely aquatic newt, breathing through gills, into the amblystoma, a terrestrial salamander, with spotted skin, breathing by means of lungs, has long been known. Feeding the axolotl on thyroid gland produces the metamorphosis very quickly, even if the axolotl is kept in water. In the reptile house at the London Zoological Gardens full-grown examples of the common black axolotl and the pretty white variety are exhibited. Some are nearly three inches long. Alongside are shown several examples of the amblystoma stage, produced in one of the laboratories of Oxford University and at the gardens by thyroid feeding. A variation of the thyroid in the direction of increased secretion was probably responsible for the first land animals.

THYROXIN, SECRETION OF THE THYROID

Under the microscope, as in the test tube, the thyroid shows remarkable and unique features. Closed spherules lined by a single layer of cells enclosing a gelatinous material known as colloid, which stains deeply with acid dyes, comprise the units of its architecture. Essentially, it may be pictured as a series of jelly bubbles secreted by outlying cells.

A relatively high percentage of iodine is the unique distinctive fact in its chemistry. Discovered by Baumann in 1895, the presence of the element has focused the intelligence of chemists upon the gland, with the consequent demonstration of arsenic also in it. It was soon manifest that the secretion of the gland was dependent upon the iodine content for its activity. Active extracts of the thyroid like thyreoglobulin and iodothyrin were proven to contain iodine, and to become inactive when the iodine was removed. Efforts to isolate the iodine containing active principle in pure form were fruitless until the work of Kendall at the Mayo Foundation. He obtained it as a white, finely crystalline, odorless and tasteless substance, heat stable, and analyzable. The free form separates as a sheaf of fine needles. Kendall at first called it the a-iodine compound, then named it thyroxin.

There are other internal secretions of the thyroid, with a function of their own, that have no iodine. But they are secondary, and obscure. Thyroxin is accepted today as the purified internal secretion of the thyroid because all the effects of the whole gland may be elicited with it. Thyroxin produces results with doses amazingly minute compared with the quantity of whole gland necessary. Moreover, a dose of thyroxin appears to last an organism in need of it over a period of time; the other has to be administered continuously.

Studies with thyroxin carried on in recent years have rounded out the whole concept of the business of the thyroid in the body economy. One may sum it up by saying that the thyroid secretion is the *great controller of the speed of living*. The more thyroid one has, the faster one lives; the less one has, the more slowly one lives.

That is not to imply any direct proportion between the amount of thyroid secretion in an individual, and the length of life to which he is destined. The speed of living, in the chemical sense (which is the fundamental sense), and the rate at which the chemical reactions go on that constitute the process of life, are dependent upon the thyroid. When the reactions go faster, more oxygen and food material are burned up or oxidized, more energy is liberated, the metabolic wheel rotates more quickly, the individual senses, feels, thinks and acts more quickly.

Likening one energy machine to another, the thyroid may be compared to the accelerator of an automobile. That is a rough and superficial comparison because an accelerator lets in more of the fuel to be burned up, while the thyroid makes the fuel more combustible. It thus resembles more the primer, for a rich mixture of gasoline and air burns at a greater velocity than a poor one. But the action of thyroid could really be simulated only by some substance that could be introduced into the best possible of gasoline mixtures, to increase its combustibility by a hundred per cent or more. For that is what thyroid will do to our food. Nor has it only this destructive or combustion side. Withal there is at the same time a constructive action, for the process frees energy to be used for heat, motion or other need. The thyroid, therefore, in addition to its role as an accelerator, acts, too, as the efficient lubricator for energy transformations. So we see it as accelerator, lubricator and transformer of our energies.

THE GLAND OF ENERGY PRODUCTION

The isolation of thyroxin has made possible the determination of the influence of the thyroid hormone upon the evolution of energy in any higher animal organism. There is, for every individual, a constant, known as the metabolic rate, or the combustion rate, a reading of the rate at which his cells are consuming material for heat. The metabolic rate is thus a gauge of the energy pressure within the organism. It may be calculated by measuring the amount of carbon dioxide gas exhaled during a unit of time, and the number of calories of heat radiated by the skin simultaneously. A simplified device has lately rendered it practicable to make actual determinations by a few five-minute readings of the rate of oxygen absorption by the lungs. Plummer, also connected with the Mayo Foundation, has shown that what would amount to less than a grain of the thyroxin would more than double the amount of energy produced in a unit of time. To be exact, one milligram of thyroxin increases the metabolic rate two per cent. That illustrates some of the power of the internal secretion of the thyroid and its importance to normal life.

THE MOBILIZATION OF ENERGY

But not only is the height of pressure of energy in the cells controlled by the thyroid. The mobility of that energy is also controlled. Without it, rapid and large fluctuations of energy output, and elasticity and flexibility of energy mobilization for any sudden mental or muscular act, let alone an emergency, become impossible. A woman suffering with myxedema, the condition described by the English physician Gull as a cretinoid state supervening in the adult life of woman, has an insufficient amount of thyroxin in her blood and tissues. She is clumsy and awkward and will stumble when endeavoring to walk upstairs. Any effort is almost paralyzed because the range of fluctuation of energy, the ability to mobilize energy, in turn dependent upon an ability to increase the metabolic rate, is limited. In slang phrase, she cannot step on it. Her existence is set to go at a rate in the neighborhood of forty per cent below the normal. By the administration of thyroxin, her metabolic rate can be raised to any desired figure, the spark can be adjusted, so to speak, to any point we like, and it can be so maintained for years.

In the normal animal, to be sure, the internal secretion of the thyroid is not absolutely essential to life. So it contrasts with the hormone of the minute parathyroids placed so closely to it, a minimum dose of which is absolutely a prerequisite for continued life. The fundamental chemical reactions within the cells occur in the complete absense of thyroxin. But they go on in a relatively fixed, rigid and unvarying way, confined within the narrow limits of a constant figure. Under such conditions, the level of energy production is bound to be low, and to remain low, and the modus of its mobilization slow and unwieldy. With thyroid is introduced the trick of *catalysis*, or the speeding up of the vital chemical reactions, through the agency of an *intermediate* which accelerates the process. It is par excellence the great catalyst of energy in the body. (A catalyst is an intermediary like the trace of water, which will bring about an explosion between dry oxygen and hydrogen that without it have stayed inert with the strongest currents of electricity.) Thus it supplies a mechanism not only for quantity output of that subtle reality we label energy, but also an apparatus for varying the available amount of it, and for permitting the maximum range in ease and rapidity of its utilization. The thyroid is still another device of life for procuring more and more variation and differentiation, its goal, as far as we can peer through the opalescent screen upon which its manifestations quiver.

From another point of view, the thyroid may be looked upon as the organ evolved for maintaining the same amount of iodine in the blood as there is in sea water. Sea water was our original habitat, since, like Venus, we have all come up out of the sea.

The more intimate study of the composition of the blood has revealed the most astonishing parallelism between it and the compounds of sea water. The blood is sea water, to which has been added hemoglobin as a pigment for carrying oxygen to the cells not in direct contact with the atmosphere, nutrients to take the place of the prey our marine ancestors gobbled up frankly and directly, and white cells to act as the first line of defense. To keep the concentration of iodine in the blood a constant, the thyroid evolved, since there is no iodine in most foods and very little in those which do contain it.

That a minimum amount of iodine in the food is necessary to health is shown by the existence of goitre regions. Around some of the Great Lakes in the United States, for instance, the water does not contain enough iodine. As a result, numerous cases of goitre occur. Iodine in the form of sodium iodide in small doses will act as a prophylactic. The amount of iodine in the blood is about one or two parts to ten millions, and that of the liver is about three or four parts to ten millions. Since the liver is the most complex and active chemical factory in the body, its appropriation of a greater amount of iodine for itself is understandable.

When thyroxin is administered in a single dose, there is a distinct lag in the absorption of it by the tissues. A single dose does not generate its maximum effect until the tenth day. This effect continues for about ten days. Then there is a gradual decrease in the intensity of reaction for another ten days. So that the length of time a single administration of thyroxin functions within the body is about three weeks. Again we have occasion to notice a protective device of the cells. Since the presence of thyroxin in the tissues determines the rate at which they burn themselves up, it is obvious that if there were no mechanism for retarding its action, and at need varying it, they really would set fire to themselves. That is to say, if the tissues held a maximum of the thyroid internal secretion, and had to take up more and more as it was fed out to them by the thyroid through the blood, the pressure of energy production would attain the state of a boiler without a safety valve. Even if self-destruction were avoided by the ingestion of the largest quantities of energy-bearing foods, rest for the cells would be difficult, if not impossible.

The thyroxin in the tissues diminishes after a period of great exertion, the thyroxin probably being carried back to the thyroid gland and kept there as reserve until further demand. So it has been discovered that during the winter months, the thyroid glands of beef, sheep and hogs all contain much less iodine than during the summer months. During the winter months, manifestly, more energy is required to maintain body temperature, hence the gland surrenders more of its secretion to the tissues and so keeps less of it itself. There must be, too, a certain wearing out of the potency of the iodine with time. Even dead inorganic catalysts, made of simple elements, wear out after having been used time and time again.

Though the thyroid is the supreme energizer, life is incompatible with a certain excess of it. Death can be produced by successive daily injections of its internal secretion. But it has, besides the energizing effect, certain formative and nervous influences equally marvelous. As illustrations, there are the cases of thyroid deprivation in human beings, cretinism and myxedema, as well as those in which it is believed there occurs an excess of the thyroid secretion in the blood and tissues, the condition of *hyper*thyroidism.

CRETINISM AS THYROID DEFICIENCY

Not that there is any arresting contrast of startling difference between the phenomena presented by different species. The younger the animal, the grosser the morbid symptoms witnessed. The animal fails to grow. The bones and cartilage, except of the skull, fail to develop. The abdomen projects and becomes large and flabby. The sex organs atrophy. There is sterility. Pregnant rabbits abort, hens produce very small eggs or none at all. These are the results of removing the thyroid in animals.

Apathetic, indifferent, dirty, awkward, apparently idiotic, describe the human cretins. Their skin is rough and coarse, peeling in sheets. In some it is considerably knarled and creased as in the aged, and in others swollen, hard and resistant. The hair becomes shaggy and rough, losing all luster, and tends to grow irregularly and fall out. The temperature becomes subnormal and an anemia supervenes. There is a distinct reduction in the resistance to infections and intoxications.

Cretinism in the human is a condition in which the burning taper we call Life flickers and smoulders and smokes. Thirty years ago it was an example of the most hopeless idiocy. Whole populations were afflicted with it. But neither man of science, nor bigot-fanatic, assured by the Divine Confidence of its meaning as a visitation, believed it could be modified an iota. Today, that inept word "cure" may be applied to our power of attack upon it, provided it is permitted to attack early enough. Modification, in the direction of the most surprising betterment, is the miracle that has been wrought.

The history of a cretin runs somewhat as follows: A baby is born, which in all appearances seems normal. Perhaps the nose is a trifle squatter than even the average new-born's flat nose. There may also be abnormal sleepiness, greater even than that of the normal baby in the first month or two in that there is no spontaneous awakening from the coma for food. But in most cases this is put down to normal variability, or maybe to that limbo of all a baby's troubles: weakness. After some months, it is noticed that the infant is failing to grow at the normal rate, either physically or mentally. Examination at this time reveals a curious thickening of the dental ridges. Then the tongue takes the centre of the scene, by becoming unusually thick and prominent, to the point of projecting beyond the mouth at all times, and interfering with breathing, when the infant is in a recumbent position.

More and more of the characteristics of the affection turn up. The queer, repulsive, pitiful face of the cretins, which makes them all seem brothers or twins, shapes itself. A yellowish, white or waxy pallor; rough, dry, scaly, bloated skin; swollen, often wrinkled brow; watery eyes, often almost concealed by the thickened eyelids; the depressed pug nose with its wide, thick nostrils; large, erect ears; the wobbly, drooling tongue, sticking out at one, yet not in derision; the hair thin, and like tow in texture rather than human; eyebrows and eyelashes are scant, and often absent; the nails short, thin and brittle; the teeth, very late in coming, may be represented by a few sharp points, irregular, decaying quickly, sometimes not succeeded at all by those of the second dentition.

Whatever growth occurs is irregular and disproportionate. The trunk, though small compared with the head, appears massive against the background of the diminutive extremities. The back is somewhat humped, arching at the waist-line, while the abdomen protrudes like a balloon, with a hernia, often, at the navel. The extremities are short, bowed, cold, and livid, covered with rolls of the infiltrated skin, rolls which cannot be smoothed out. Hands and feet are broad, pudgy, and floppy, the fingers stiff, square and spade-like, the toes spread apart, like a duck's, by the solid skin. Above the collar bones there are frequently great pads of fat which sometimes encircle the narrow bull neck.

The mental state varies with the degree of deprivation of the internal secretion of the thyroid. In the worst cases it is repulsively vegetable. Even the intelligence common to the higher animals is wanting. The cretins of the "human plant" kind, as they have been nicknamed, will not recognize mother or father or any person about them, or even a person from an object, and manifest no interest in anything or anybody, not even toys. Hunger and thirst they manifest by grunts and inarticulate sounds, or by screaming. They neither smile, cough, nor laugh, but sit like sphinxes, breathing, but not reacting.

There are, of course, all grades and varieties. There are those who recognize parents and familiar faces, and exhibit some evidence of affection for them, acquire a limited vocabulary, and then cease, no progress possible even with the alphabet. They attain the size and age of two or three years and there stop altogether, as if a permanent brake were applied to the wheels of their growth. Some higher types may even come to speak connected sentences, and exhibit a certain mild spontaneity, though stupid and slow and abnormally deliberate, resembling the acquired form of thyroid deprivation or insufficiency, for which Ord invented the name myxedema.

I have filled in with some detail this thumbnail sketch of thyroid deprivation as it occurs in infancy to illustrate how wide a sweep the gland's lariat embraces. Skin, hair, bones, muscle and fat, brain and intelligence, growth and development, are modified precisely as the size and shape of certain crystals are modified by the presence or absence of ingredients in an apparently homogeneous solution. A fertilized ovum, in which the predecessor of the thyroid gland is present, that is to say, in which there is the seed and soil for its sprouting, looks the same as one without that formative material. Yet, when the time comes for the internal secretion of the thyroid to put in its oar in the metabolic game, its presence or absence makes all the difference in the world to the individual.

In the middle of the nineteenth century, when the concentration of phosphorus in the brain was established as significant, the cry for the emphasis of that fact was--without phosphorus no thought is possible. We can much more relevantly declare that without thyroid, no thought, no growth, no distinctive humanity or even animality is possible. For the epigram about phosphorus was bombast, since it can be declaimed with equal truth that without oxygen, without carbon, without nitrogen, without any of the food elements that go to make up the chemical composition of brain matter, no thought is possible. Indeed, if one were set upon the indictment of a single chemical element as the begetter of consciousness, the prisoner at the bar would have to be copper. There is more copper in the brain by a considerable degree than in any other organ of the body. Which perhaps will be exceedingly regretted by the patrons of the aristocracy of the soul who would have it as an emanation of a deposit in the brain of silver at least, if not gold. They are like the old lady who would never permit herself to be cured of her ailments except by gold plated pills. Copper, however, is not necessary to intelligence. Without thyroid there can be no complexity of thought, no learning, no education, no habit-formation, no responsive energy for situations, as well as no physical unfolding of faculty and function, and no reproduction of kind, with no sign of adolescence at the expected age, and no exhibition of sex tendencies thereafter.

EFFECTS OF FEEDING THYROID

How subtly the internal secretion affects every phase and aspect of child as well as adult, by doing something to the speed of activities in their cells, is told straightway by the effects of it when eaten or introduced into the skin or blood of various people. A cretin, idiotic, dwarfish, deformed, hopeless, an incessantly prodding burden of sorrow to the mother, who looks upon the masterpiece she had labored to bring forth, and beholds a terrible gargoyle, becomes transformed when fed thyroid.

In a few days the cretin will get warmer, and require much less wrapping and bed-clothing. With the improvement in circulation, the color becomes better and the extremities lose their coldness. In a week or so, irritability and resentment at disturbance appear. He will begin to recognize and know his parents, smile and play. There is a gradual return to the normal of the facial appearance, and a resumption of growth. All kinds of marvelous growth effects occur. Twenty teeth may be cut in six months. Coarse, rough dry, shaggy hair becomes fine, silken, long and curly. The skin becomes soft, moist and roseate. Inches in height may be added every month. Bright, active, even talkative, are the descriptive terms an observer would apply after a few months. A complete remaking of body and soul is apparently affected.

Yet, should the administration of the thyroid cease, an almost immediate reversion to the original vegetative condition is inevitable. After a few days, reactiveness slows down, the child will speak only when spoken to, will sit quietly in a chair all day and act semi-anesthetized. Gradually hair and skin return to the previous cold-blooded animal state, and the whole picture of the cretin is in full bloom. Supplying the internal secretion of the gland promptly repeats the transformation.

One wonders what is to be the ultimate fate of these reformed cretins. Since the tale of the opening of life to them, once considered hopeless idiots, is scarce a generation old, we have no data, as yet, as to the character of their children or grandchildren, their adventures and vicissitudes, in short, their life history. Those of whom we have any record are normal and healthy school children or workers, alive to the interests of childhood or their occupation and social circles. No one outside their family knows that they are cretins, and the most acute observer would be hard put to it to suspect. What a theme for the reflections upon appearances the eminent Victorians loved!

There are possibilities the imagination may envisage. One may suppose such a cretin, with all his other ductless glands intact, grown successfully to manhood under careful medical guidance. No one but himself is aware of his affliction, outside of his medical advisers. Luck aids him to rise in the world, or perhaps he has been born with a spoon of the precious metals in his mouth. Adolescence, love and marriage dance their sequence. Our hero of course keeps his dread secret to himself. Whether such an omission of confidence would entitle his wife to a divorce is something courts will be called upon to decide sooner or later. But, without anticipating, the honeymoon involves a trip to the South Seas. A storm and a wreck throws them alone on an island, tropical, easy to live on, and rescue in the course of a few months certain. The man, to his horror, discovers that he has saved of his medicaments only a pill box containing half a dozen of thyroid tablets, his requirement being one a day. He sees them go day by day. Finally they are all gone. He feels his faculties slipping hour by hour. Shall he tell her? Indecision grips him, and he delays until the day when his consciousness sinks to the point where his mind no longer grasps his problem. The wife must endure the spectacle of the enchantment of her husband, and his change from gallant lover to dull animal ogre. A new version of Beauty and the Beast!

Cretinism as one manifestation of a soul without thyroid or without enough thyroid is not all. The first great successes with thyroid were achieved in adults, particularly adult women, exhibiting a peculiar obesity, coldness, loss of hair and teeth and a remarkable lassitude and torpor that might be summed up as a chronic drowsiness, like a saturation of the blood with some narcotic drug. Or there may be a melancholia, or a lack of ability to seize the finer points of a mental process, or an argument treated in the abstract. Children are said to be lazy, slow or dull. They experience an irritating difficulty in understanding questions and expressing their wants and desires, and so are declared to be vicious, or stupid.

All these are grades of the degeneration which Ord, the Englishman, named myxedema. At its worst it is a sort of bloating and drying of the body and the mind. Then there is infantilism, which is helped by the giving of thyroid extract. It differs from the ordinary cretinism in that, while one is reminded of the latter by the physical stunting and the other stigmata, there is a certain amount of intelligence which enables the individual to hold his own while he is a child. He becomes a grown-up baby: at twenty prefers the company of children of ten, and passes under the evil influence of designing so-called normal persons. So dominated he will lie, steal, start fires, commit almost any crime, with no inherent flair for criminality, but because of a lack of independent judgment and inability to resist suggestion, and a desire to please friends. He is simply an overgrown child who still loves to play with toys, laughs and cries, becomes angry or afraid, unreasonably and ridiculously, and yells for mamma when thwarted or scared.

So much for what happens when there is not sufficient of the thyroid secretion in the blood and tissues. Now to consider the effects of an excess of it, the condition called hyperthyroidism, as the insufficiency of it is labelled subthyroidism. Too much thyroxin can be introduced into the system of a normal individual, or even a cretin by the simple administration of too large doses or over too long a time. Also a train of symptoms similar to those evoked by an oversecretion of the thyroid may be mobilized by the taking of too much iodine. Great sorrow, great joy, a sudden severe jolt to the nervous equilibrium, sexual excitement, an overwhelming anger or grief may leave in their wake a permanent hyperthyroidism. The symptoms are the reverse of cretinism and myxedema. There is an over-excitability of the nerves in place of sluggishness, and an over-reactivity of the whole organism to its environment. The heart's action is too fast, and under the slightest stimulus gets faster to the point of obtruding itself into the conscious mind as a palpitation. Instead of the lowered temperature and coldness of the cretin, there is a heightened temperature, one or two degrees above the normal, and a feeling of heat. The individual has a high warm color, does not sleep well, becomes or remains thin no matter how much he or she eats, is abnormally susceptible sexually, may suffer from a definite insomnia, is emotional, and perspires freely. Alert, neurotic or high-strung, magnetic, and imaginative are some of the descriptive adjectives applicable. The eyes are bright and prominent, large and beautiful, when they have not reached the stage entitled "pop-eyed." Or they may even become so protuberant and bulging as to develop the expression of one staring aghast at some ineffable horror. The latter is the feature of only the severest types, when there is an associated goitre, the combination designated as exopthalmic goitre.

There are, too, individuals in whom hyperthyroidism and hypothyroidism are mixed, or rather alternate. At one time they present the phenomena of the one, at another of the other. They are the people who complain of the cyclic quality of their moods and purposes. Their mood will be a heaven of exaltation and exhilaration, and then descend into a slough of despond from which they feel themselves inextricable. They are always talking about the ups and downs of their mental states. Headache and languor and fatigability, dry skin and lack of appetite for food or exertion on one day or for one week, give way on the next day, or for the next week, to an energetic gayety, and sweaty, flushed skin, a prominent appetite for food and every sort of activity. Driven to be forever on the go, for one period, in the next they feel like lying down most of the day, with no inclination for any life whatever. The stage of depression may go as far as a melancholia, the stage of stimulation as far as mania. They may simulate manic-depressive or cyclic insanity. Something restrains them, and holds them bound as in a vise in the one cycle. And then they are driven on beyond themselves by some invisible whip in the next.

THYROID AS DIFFERENTIATOR

Besides the action of the thyroid as energizer, lubricator, and growth catalyzer, it has a remarkable power as a differentiator of tissues. It determines the embryonic etchings of the different organs which in their totality comprise the unique individual. Every multicellular animal must first have existed as a single cell, the impregnated ovum. With the body and personality of the ovum, the creature is one and continuous, literally something the single cell has made of itself by sub-dividing and differentiating. In the process, the cell mass often goes through stages which stand out as individualities in themselves, that appear on the surface absolutely unrelated. So the caterpillar and the butterfly, to the naive child, seem as far apart as worm and bird. In the case of the frog, the tadpole as a first sketch seems completely an impossible and wild absurdity. Yet we know that there is an orderly progression of events, a propagation of cells, a forward going arrangement of chemical reactions, that results in expansion and intricate complication of the organism. Just what the forces at work in this most mysterious of all natural processes are, has been an intellectual mystery that the best minds of the race have attempted to get rid of with words like pangenesis (Darwin). Words of Black (Mediterranean or Greek and Latin) origin, as Allen Upward has named them, always cover a multitude of ignorances. The glands of internal secretion, here, as in so many other dark places, provide the open sesame to certain long closed doors of biology. They offer themselves to us as the first definitely tangible agents which are known to keep the process of growth going, and undoubtedly initiate the marvelous unfolding of tissues and functions, organs and faculties summed up as development or differentiation.

Thus by the direct feeding of thyroid at particular points in the differentiating history most curious effects have been elicited. If the gland is made part of the nutriment, the bathing environment, of the tadpole, a hastening of its metamorphosis is attained. The tadpole lives not out its day as a tadpole, but precociously turns into a frog. But such a frog! It is a miniature frog, a dwarf frog, a frog seen by looking through the wrong end of the telescope, a frog not magnified, but micrified. Frogs have been so created the size of flies. There has occurred a splitting of the two reactions which ordinarily go hand in hand: the reaction of growth which is just brute increase of total mass or weight and volume, and the reaction of differentiation which is the finer process. The picture is a frog, but a frog the size of a tadpole, a frog which has missed its childhood, adolescence and youth, skipping over these transition stages into the adult age, as a pigmy.

It is all as if a baby were suddenly to grow a beard and moustache, evolve and shed teeth, and acquire the manner of an earnest citizen, and yet retain the height and weight of a baby. That the spectacle of such a superbaby is not quite the most fantastic of all improbabilities is shown by the condition of progeria, first recorded by the Briton, Hastings Guilford. A queer spectacle in which a child incontinently grows old without having lived--in the course of a few weeks or months. You look upon him and see senility on a small scale, but with all its peculiarities: wrinkled skin, apathy, gray hair and all the rest of it. All we can say about it is that it is probably due to a paralysis of all the glands of internal secretion, a removal of their influence upon the cells. Contrariwise to the feeding of thyroid, removal of the thyroid of tadpoles will prevent their development into frogs. If iodine is then fed to them, say mixed with flour, normal metamorphosis will occur. If Body is the tool chest which we carry about with us, as Samuel Butler said, then to the thyroid belongs the name of tool-maker.

Another function of thyroid that must be taken into consideration is what has been spoken of as its antitoxic function--in plainer English, its power to prevent poisoning, or to increase resistance against poisons, including the bacteria and other living agents which cause the infectious diseases. Each molecule of food, ingested for assimilation into our substance, accumulates a history of wanderings and pilgrimages, attachments and transformations beside which the gross trampings of a Marco Polo become the rambling steps of a seven-league booted giant. In the course of its peregrinations, it becomes a potential poison, potential because it is never allowed to grow in concentration to the danger point. The thyroid plays its role of protector like all the internal secretory machines. In an animal deprived of a thyroid the feeding of meat shortens life--a single sample of how it works to guard against intoxication from within. The feeding of thyroid will also raise the ability of the cells to stand poisons introduced from without--intoxications of all sorts. Alcohol and morphine will affect in much smaller doses the subthyroid person than the normal or the hyperthyroid. As regards the infections, which directly or indirectly kill most of us, the injection of thyroid will increase the content in the blood of the protective antibodies which preserve us, temporarily at any rate, against malignant invaders. The opsonins, for example, those substances which butter the bacteria so that the appetite of the white cells for them is properly roused, are mobilized by thyroid feeding or injection. Other substances in the blood which destroy and dissolve bacteria are also increased. The thyroid probably performs these functions by sending its secretion to the cells directly responsible for the immunity reactions, and stimulating them to activity.

A sketch of the thyroid like the foregoing shows it as the wondrous controller of vitality and growth, and indefatigable protector against intoxicants and injuries. When it is sufficiently active, life is worth while; when it is defective, life is a difficult threatening blackness. That would make it out as the gland of glands. It is tremendously important, without a doubt, in normal everyday life. But no more so than the other members of the cast. The position of star it may claim, but in vain. The other glands of internal secretion to be sketched will each, when the marvels of its business in the cell-corporation are considered, present itself as candidate for the honors of the president. Justice should give fair credit to all the organs which fabricate the reagents of individuality, and the regulators of personality.

THE PITUITARY

In the human skull, the pituitary is a lump of tissue about the size of a pea lying at the base of the brain, a short distance behind the root of the nose. It is of a grayish-yellow color, unpretentious and insignificant enough in appearance, and so long neglected by the scientists who boast their immunity to the glamor of the spectacular. Guesses at its nature date back to Aristotle.

Like most of its colleagues among the glands of internal secretion, it is really two glands in one, two glands with but a single name. At least it consists of two different parts, distinct in their origin, history, function and secretions, but juxtaposed and fused into what is apparently a homogeneous entity. They are conveniently spoken of as the anterior gland and the posterior gland.

In the embryo, the anterior gland is derived by a proliferation of cells from the mouth area. The posterior gland represents an outgrowth of the oldest part of the nervous system. When it is traced back along the tree of the vertebrate species, it is found to be present in all of them. An ancient invention, its precursor has been identified in worms and molluscs and even among the starfish. "The pituitary is practically the same, from myxine to man." A trusted veteran, therefore, among the internal secretory organs, its importance can be surmised.

To understand the story of the pituitary, variously acquired bits of information concerning it have been assembled and fitted together like the fragments of a picture puzzle, as Cushing has so well put it. Here and there pieces stick out, obviously out of place. The relations of some of them to one another or to the whole design are not at all clear. Parts appear to have been irrevocably lost, or not yet to have turned up. Chance bystanders will select odd figures and articulate them into a new harmony. Yet out of the jumble of fragments, a fairly respectable insight has been gained in less than a half century.

The pituitary is cradled in a niche at the base of the skull which, because of its form, is known as the Sella Turcica or Turkish saddle. So situated, an operative approach to it is overwhelmingly difficult. On the other hand, X-ray studies are favored. "Nature's darling treasure" it might be called, since there has been provided a skull within the skull to shelter it.

Under the most highly magnifying lenses of the microscope, three kinds of cells have been distinguished. The anterior gland is a collection of solid columns of cells, surrounded by blood spaces into which their secretion is undoubtedly directly poured. A gelatinous material, presumed to be the internal secretion of the gland, has, in fact, been observed emerging from the cells into the blood spaces. The posterior lobe, or gland, consists of secreting cells producing a glassy substance which finds its way into the spinal fluid that bathes the nervous system. The spinal fluid itself is a secretion of another gland at the base of the brain, the choroid. Nerves and internal secretion are associated here with a closeness symbolic of their general relations.

From each portion of the gland (to stick to the accepted nomenclature of speaking of the two glands as one) an active substance has been isolated. Robertson, an American chemist, separated from the anterior lobe a substance soluble in the fat solvents, like ether and gasoline, which he christened tethelin. But P.E. Smith has shown that the active material is soluble neither in boiling water nor in boiling alcohol, the typical fat solvent. A number of facts favor the idea of the anterior lobe cells as stimulants of growth of bone and connecting and supporting tissues generally. From the posterior lobe, pituitrin, believed its internal secretion, has been obtained in solution.

Pituitrin is a substance of many marvelous functions. In general, it controls the *tone* of the tissues, of involuntary or smooth muscle fibres of the blood vessels and the contractile organs of the body like the intestines, the bladder and uterus. When injected, it will slowly raise the blood pressure and keep it raised for some time, and will increase the flow of urine from the kidneys and of milk from the breasts. It will also cause an intense continued contraction of the bladder and the uterus. It is also said to control the salt content of the blood upon which its electrical conductivity and other properties depend. Normally, there is a certain fixed ratio of the salts in the blood, which keeps them like the ratio in sea-water. Again, we have an example of the curious atavism of the internal secretions. The thyroid, remember, keeps the iodine concentration of the blood like that of the ocean, our original habitat. Pituitrin likewise does its part to maintain our internal environment as near as possible to what was once the surrounding medium. A substance somewhat similar has been found in the skin glands of toads.

The extraordinarily well protected position of the pituitary, its persistence throughout life, and its abundant blood supply, emphasize its vital importance. No other gland of internal secretion can adequately substitute for it. Complete expiration means death, in two or three days, with a peculiar lethargy, unsteadiness of gait and loss of appetite, emaciation, and a fall of temperature, so that the animal becomes cold-blooded, its temperature the same as that of the atmosphere it occupies. If only part of the anterior lobe is taken away, there occurs a remarkable degeneration of the individual. The degeneration is not a mucinous infiltration of the skin and the internal organs which occurs with thyroid deprivation, but a fatty degeneration, with a tendency to inversion of sex. A singular somnolence, a dry skin, loss of hair, a dull mentality, sometimes epilepsy, and a noticeable craving for and tolerance of sweets appear. These are but a few of the observations obtained in experimental sub-pituitarism, that is, underaction or insufficient secretion of the pituitary, produced by removing part of the anterior gland.

If such an experimental sub-pituitarism is started in infancy, for instance in puppies, there is a cessation, or marked hindering and slowing of growth. That is, dwarfs are artificially created. Apropos, pathologists have shown that in several true human dwarfs the gland is rudimentary or inadequate. All of which goes hand in hand with the evidence that the skeleton stands directly under the domination of the pituitary.

REGULATOR OF ORGANIC RHYTHMS

There are certain other singular by-effects of the gland in its relation to the periodic phenomena of the organism like hibernation, sleep, and the critical sex epochs of both sexes. In hibernation, or winter sleep, the animal in cold weather passes into a cataleptic state in which it continues to breathe, more deeply but more slowly than when awake, but shows no other signs of consciousness or life. A lowered blood pressure and a marked insensitivity to painful and emotional stimuli go with it. There is a preliminary storage of starch in the liver, and of fat throughout the fat depots of the body. These are so like what happens after part of the pituitary is removed, that a comparison of the two becomes inevitable. Common to both conditions is a drop in the rate of tissue combustion or metabolism, which can be relieved by injection of an extract of the pituitary, a rise of temperature occuring simultaneously. Moreover, examination of the glands of internal secretion of hibernating species, like the woodchuck, during the period of hibernation, shows changes in all of them, but most marked in the pituitary, the shrunken cells staining as if they too were asleep, or in a resting stage. The characteristic alive qualities of these cells return, without relation to food or climate, when the animal comes to in the spring, at the vernal equinox. Hibernation may, perhaps, be put down to a seasonal wave of inactivity of the pituitary gland.

Now winter sleep may be looked upon as an exaggeration of ordinary night sleep, the latter differing from the former only in its brevity. In the natural sleep of non-hibernating species there occurs, too, a fall in temperature. Moreover, they all, even man, have a certain capacity for winter sleep, as the experiences of travellers and explorers in the arctic regions indicate. In certain parts of Russia, where there is a scarcity of food during the winter months, the peasants pass weeks at a time in a somnolent state, arousing once a day for a scant meal. Just as the sex glands influence the body and mind profoundly with a certain cyclic periodicity of activity and inactivity (rut, heat, menstrual period and so on), which has been demonstrated to have a very close functional relationship with the pituitary, so sleep and hibernation will bear interpretation as products of a temporary dormancy of the same gland. We have, then, to set up in the place of Morpheus and Apollo, the new gods of the internal secretion of a chemical-making bit of the brain, as an explanation of the rhythms of sleep and wakefulness.

There are individuals who go about outside of hospital walls, quasi-normally, who are semi-hibernators or partial hibernators, and who are really in a state of subpituitarism. They are people who may have something wrong or inferior with their pituitary, but not to the extent of interference with their daily life. They go about with their type stamped upon them for the seeing eye. The classical type is obese, with fat distributed everywhere, but more so in the lower abdomen and the lower extremities. They are slow and dull, and sexually inactive, often impotent. They are sometimes tall, but most often dwarfish, and may be subject to epileptic seizures. They recall the picture of what happens to young dogs partially deprived of the pituitary. Dickens delivered a perfect likeness of an extreme degree of the condition in the Fat Boy of the "Pickwick Papers," whose employment with Mr. Wardle consisted in alternate sleeping and eating.

WHEN THE PITUITARY OVERACTS

All grades of overaction of the pituitary exist. Then its peculiar power to act as a stimulant to the growth of bone and the soft supporting and connecting tissues like tendons and ligaments comes into play. If the overaction or excess of secretion begins in childhood or adolescence, that is, before puberty, there results a great elongation of the bones, so that a giant is the consequence. Now giants have always appealed to the imagination of the little man, and have had all kinds of wonderful abilities ascribed to them by him. The giants and ogres of folk-lore and fairy tales are favored with the most extraordinary mental advantages. Direct and analytic acquaintance with the giants of our own day, as well as a probing of their conduct in the past, has shown that normal giants--persons of exceptional size free from physical or mental deformities--are rare. There are people with *hyper*-pituitarism who exhibit the highest mental powers. In them is an increased activity of the posterior lobe in association with enlargement and hyperfunction of the anterior, overgrowth is not so marked, and the individual is lean and mentally acute. But the ordinary giant is one in whom there is degeneration of the pituitary after too much action of the anterior and too little of the posterior glands. A tumor or disease process in the gland is most often responsible.

If the overaction of the anterior happens after puberty, when the long bones have set, and can not grow longer, a peculiar diffuse enlargement of the individual occurs, especially of his hands and feet and head. The nose, ears, lips and eyes get larger and coarser. As these people are rather big and tall to begin with, the effect produced is that of a heavy-jawed, burly, bulking person, with bushy overhanging eyebrows, and an aggressive manner. For there is, too, something distinctive about their mentality which has been as often portrayed as those of the pathologic giant. Rabelais' most famous character, Gargantua, belongs to the group. We recruit more drum-majors than prime ministers from among these people. They often suffer much from torturing boring headaches, and a consequent despondency and feeling of hopelessness which colors gray the entire spiritual spectrum. Up to a certain point these sufferers have a remarkable alertness and capacity. When conscious of the malady, they often meet it with a doggedly courageous optimism, which is another characteristic, although women occasionally commit suicide.

In both the semi-hibernators who remind one of cattle, and in the giant or acromegalic types who remind one of the anthropoid ape, there develops a distinct diminution of sexual life. An abnormal process in the anterior gland, whether of oversecretion or of undersecretion, may interfere with the proper functioning of the posterior gland, the secretion of which is tonic not only to the brain cells, but also to the sex cells. Thus, young animals deprived of the pituitary will not, if male, grow spermatozoa, nor ripe ova in the female. Moreover, the feeding of pituitary increases sexual activity. In the case of hens, this has been demonstrated to be about thirty per cent by a pretty experiment. At a time of the year when eggs diminish, six hundred and fifty-five hens laid two hundred and seventy-three eggs upon an ordinary diet. When pituitary was added to their food for four days, the number of eggs rose to three hundred and fifty-two, an increase of seventy-nine. In addition, the fertility of the chicks born of these eggs was augmented, especially if both parents had been fed on pituitary. There are other aspects of the relation of the pituitary to sex, which will be treated in another chapter.

THE BONY CRADLE OF THE PITUITARY

Always, in attempting to understand the pituitary, it is necessary to remember that it is tightly packed in the bony cradle, the Turkish Saddle or Sella Turcica. Should some stimulus, local, or in the blood, arouse the gland to growth, a good deal will depend upon whether it has room to grow in, or it will make room by eroding the bone. With space for the formation of a large anterior and posterior pituitary gland, there will be created the long, lean individual, with a tendency to high blood pressure and sexual trends, great mental activity, initiative, irritability and endurance. An outstanding trait of these favorites of fortune is that they remain thin no matter how much food they consume, and they have the best of appetites. They often are subject to severe headaches because of intermittent swelling of the gland against the bone of its container.

If the bony container is or becomes too small for its contents, it is interesting that along with the other signs of pituitary insufficiency, such as undersize, obesity, and asymmetry, there developes conspicuous moral and intellectual inferiority. The unfortunates suffer from compulsions and obsessions and lack inhibitions. They are the pathological liars with little or no initiative or conscience--amoral, not merely theoretically, but instinctively and unconsciously, with all the certitude and perfection of the unconscious accomplishment.

THYROID AND PITUITARY

The thyroid and the pituitary have often been compared. The anterior gland and the thyroid arise from almost the same spot in the embryonic oesophagus, the thyroid being an outgrowth in front, the anterior pituitary an outgrowth behind of the same soil. They both control growth marvelously, also the differentiation, the mass and intricacy of the tissues. But they differ in the site of their control. The thyroid bears more directly upon the inner and outer coverings of the body, the skin, the skin glands and the hair, the mucous membranes, and the irritability and the preparedness for response of the nerves. The pituitary acts more upon the framework of the body, the skeleton and the mechanical supports and movers. Bone and ligament, muscle and tendon seem to be within its immediate sway. The secretion or secretions of the pituitary diffuse directly into the fluid bathing the nervous system, supplying beneficent stimulants and aiding in the abstraction of harmful waste. So while the thyroid raises the energy level of the brain, and the whole nervous system, as a byproduct of its general awakening effect upon all the cells of the body, the pituitary probably stimulates the brain cells more directly, perhaps in the manner of caffeine or cocaine.

The difference between the thyroid and the pituitary might be put this way: that while the thyroid increases energy evolution and so makes available a greater supply of crude energy, by speeding up cellular processes, the pituitary assists in energy transformation, in energy expenditure and conversion, especially of the brain, and of the sexual system. In short, the thyroid facilitates energy production, the pituitary its consumption. The pituitary appears therefore as the gland of continued effort. Hence fatigability, an inability to maintain effort, is one of the prominent complaints when there is destruction or an insufficiency of it for one reason or another. As such, it contrasts with the glands of emergency effort, known as the adrenals.

CHAPTER III
THE ADRENAL GLANDS, THE GONADS, AND THYMUS

Like the pituitary, each adrenal gland is a double gland, that is, consists of two distinct portions, united together, one might say, by the accident of birth. It would be confusing, however, to speak of each as two glands, because there are, as a matter of fact, two separate adrenal glands, one in the right side of the abdomen, and the other in the left. Each gland is composite, or duplex. How the two parts came to be united is a long story, interesting but too long to be recounted here. In fishes they are apart and independent.

Each adrenal is a cocked hat shaped affair, astride the kidneys, easily recognized because of its yellowish fatty color. Indeed, for centuries the glands were not given a separate status as organs, but were passed up as part of the fat ensheathing the kidney. In childhood and youth, in common with the other glands, they are relatively larger and more prominent than in the adult. Also, at every age, the amount of blood passing through them is very large compared to their size. Their tremendous importance in the body economy accounts for their being so favored.

The two parts of which each gland is composed, are known as the cortex or outer portion (literally the bark) and the medulla or inner portion (literally the core). No clean-cut boundary sharply delimits the two, as strands and peninsulas of tissue of one portion penetrate the other. In the history of their development in the species and the individual, and in their chemistry and function, a sharp difference contrasts them.

In the embryo, the cortex is derived from the same patch that gives rise to the sex organs, the ovaries in the female, and the testes in the male, described as the germinal epithelium. How intimately the two sets of glands are connected is neatly pointed by this fact of a common ancestor. All vertebrates possess adrenal glands. In the lowest of the vertebrates, Petromyzon, the two parts are distinct, the cells of the cortex-to-be are situated in the walls of the kidney blood vessels, projecting as peninsulas in the blood stream, the blood sweeping over and past them. The medulla-to-be consists of cells accompanying the vegetative nerves. Among reptiles, the two become adjacent for the first time, and among birds one part occupies the meshes of the other. The size of the cortex varies directly with the sexuality and the pugnacity of the animal. The charging buffalo, for example, owns a strikingly wide adrenal cortex. The fleeing rabbit, on the other hand, is conspicuous for a narrow strip of cortex in its adrenal. Human beings possess a cortex larger than that of any other animal.

No definite chemical substance has as yet been isolated from the cortex. That remains a problem for the investigator of the future. But certain observations, especially concerning the relation between the development and behaviour of the so-called secondary sex characteristics, those qualities of skin, hair and fat distribution, physical configuration and mental attitudes, which distinguish the sexes, and the condition of the gland, indicate clearly that an internal secretion will be isolated, and that it will in its activity furnish certain predictable features.

Three different layers of cells, arranged in strings, that interpenetrate to form a network directly bathed by blood, that breaks in upon them from *open* blood vessels, compose the cortex. Most remarkable is this method of blood supply for it is exceedingly common among the invertebrates and rare among the vertebrates.

In certain disturbances of these glands, especially when there are tumors, which supply a massive dose of the secretion to the blood presumably, peculiar sex phenomena and general developmental anomalies and irregularities are produced. If the disease be present in the fetus, taking hold before birth, and so brought into the world with the child, there evolves the condition of pseudo-hermaphroditism. The individual, if a female, presents to a greater or less extent the external habits and character of the other sex. So that she is actually taken for a man, although the primary sex organs are ovaries, often not discovered to be such except when examined after an operation or death. How closely such an occurrence touches upon the problems of sex inversion and perversion comes at once to mind.

If the process involving the adrenal cortex attacks it after birth, the symmetrical correspondence and harmony of the primary sex organs and the secondary sex characters are not affected. But there follows a curious hastening of the ripening of body and mind summed up in the word puberty, a precocious puberty, with the most startling effects. A little girl of 2, 3, or 4 years of age perhaps will come to exhibit the growth and appearance of a girl of 14. She begins to menstruate, her breasts swell, she shoots up in height and weight, sprouts the hair distribution of the adult, and the mentality of the adolescent, restless, acquiring, doubting, emerge. A tot bewitched into puberty! A boy of six or seven may suddenly, in the course of a few weeks or months, become a little man, robust, rather short and stocky, but moustached, with the muscular strength and sexual powers of a man and thinking as a man. It is all as if into some fermentable medium or solution a little yeast were dropped that changed the quiet calm of its surface into a bubbling, effervescing revolution. It suggests at once that maturation, the transformation of the child into the man or woman, must be due to the pouring into the blood and the body fluids of some substance which acts like the yeast in the fermentable solution. The adrenal cortex is one source of the maturity-producing internal secretions.

If trouble in the adrenal cortex starts after puberty, phenomena of the same type, but of a different order, exhibit themselves. A woman, say in the thirties, becomes thus afflicted. Slowly or quickly her body will be covered by an abundant growth of hair, more or less of a beard and moustache appear upon the face, her voice will become deep and penetrating, her muscles will harden, and she will show a capacity for hard physical labor. Sexually she appears to be made over, masculinity now predominates in her make-up. Virilism is the name by which the French in particular have popularized the knowledge of the condition. Virilists have to shave or be shaved regularly and are not bothered in the least by the cares, responsibilities, jealousies and anxieties of personal beauty, for the change in their spirituality makes them immune to the preoccupations of the feminine. The cause of such a transformation in a previously entirely normal woman has been found to be a tumor of the adrenal cortex.

But not only is sexuality, and the conduct of the secondary sex characters, connected with the adventures of the adrenal cortex. The development of the master tissues of the body, the brain, the pride and darling of evolution, is in some subtle way correlated with it. The adrenal cortex contains more of the phosphorus-containing substances of the general nature of those found in the central nervous system than any other gland or non-nervous tissues in the body. During human intrauterine life the adrenal glands are large and conspicuous, in the first half of the second month being twice as large as the kidneys. Most of this relatively huge size, which happens in the human alone, and not in other animals, is due to enlargement of the cortex. Should this preponderance of the cortex over the medullary portion not occur in the human, that is, if the proportions remain like those of other animals, the brain fails to develop properly, or an entirely brainless monster is generated. The human brain, therefore, probably owes its superiority over the animal brain, to the adrenal cortex, in development anyhow. The growth of the brain cells, their number and complexity is thus controlled by the adrenal cortex.

Besides its action upon the sex cells and the brain cells, the internal secretion of the adrenal cortex acts upon the pigment cells of the skin, blunting their sensitiveness to light. In degeneration of the interior of the gland, which destroys the medulla, but not the cortex, the color of the skin is left unmodified. If, however, the cortex is invaded, as happens most often in the classical tuberculosis of the adrenals which drew the attention of the Englishman Addison to them, then a darkening of the skin, which may go on to a negroid bronzing, follows. That means an increased sensitiveness of the pigment cells of the skin to light. Skin color control may therefore be looked upon as an adrenal cortex function.

So much is known about the adrenal cortex. Upon the medulla, the interior gland of the gland, there has been lavished an amount of attention beside which the cortex is to be classed as a neglected wall-flower. Nearly everything that possibly could be determined about an internal secretion has in its case been settled or plausibly guessed at. The cells manufacturing the secretion, its exact chemistry and function, its action upon the blood, the liver and spleen, the heart and lungs, the brain and nervous system, have been minutely investigated, studied and charted. Its source in the food, its fate in the body, its place in the history of the individual and the species, its importance as a weapon in the struggle for existence, and the survival of the fittest have been made the subject of an astonishing number of researches, considering the short period of scarce three decades that intensive science has centered its barrage upon it.

In the first place, the medulla contains numerous nerve cells, belonging to the vegetative, also called the sympathetic nervous system. But these nerve cells are merely minor notes of the symphony. The motif is settled by a majority of large, granular cells, which stain a distinctive yellowish-brown when the gland is fixed in a solution of bichromate of potash. All chromium salts, in fact, stain the therefore labelled chromaffin cells. The characteristic staining power appears to be dependent upon, or correlated with, the presence of the internal secretion of the medulla of the adrenal, adrenalin. For the content of adrenalin, as calculated chemically, and the depth of stain as seen under the microscope, rise and fall together. Chromaffin reaction and adrenalin content go together. The poisonous skin glands of the toad have been found to give a marked chromaffin reaction, and to contain a large amount of adrenalin. Other masses of cells in the human body, especially along the course of the sympathetic nervous system, have been shown to give the reaction and to contain adrenalin.

The erratic Brown-Sequard pounded and hammered away for more than thirty years on the importance to life of the adrenal glands, since death occurred so quickly after their removal. But it was not until Schaefer, the Scotch physiologist, (who has done more than any other living man to stimulate study of the internal secretions) found that an extract of them, when injected into a vein, produced a remarkable though temporary rise of the blood pressure, that a real enthusiasm for its investigation was generated. As the upshot, a number of other significant properties besides the first of blood-pressure raising, have been put down to its credit. Chemical tests demonstrated that it originated in the medulla. The exact amount of it present in the medulla, in the blood issuing from the adrenals and in the circulation in general have been determined. The concentration in the blood is about one part in twenty million, while there is about a hundred thousand times as much stored in the gland as reserve. In infections and intoxications, after muscular exertion, and with profound emotions, there is a decrease of it in the gland and an increase in the blood. Pain and excitement, especially fear and rage, will bring about its discharge from the gland. With its entry into the blood, there is a tremendous heightening of the tone, a ***tensing***, of the nervous system. The nerve cells become more sensitive to stimuli, more sugar is poured into the blood from the liver, more red blood corpuscles are squeezed into the circulation from the blood lakes of the liver and spleen. There is a redistribution of the whole blood mass, a good deal of it being withdrawn from the internal viscera, and hurried to the skeleton muscles and the brain. The heart beats more strongly, the eye sees more clearly, the ear hears more distinctly, and the breathing is more rapid. The temperature rises, the hair of the head and the body becomes erect, the skin gets moist and greasy. It will help a fatigued muscle to regain its normal tone. In short, it has a reinforcing action upon the nutritive properties of the blood, the tone of the muscles, and the activity of the brain and the vegetative nerves.

Chemists set themselves the task of discovering just what was the substance possessed of such extraordinary and hitherto unimagined properties. The pure adrenalin was isolated, capable of evoking all the reactions of the impure adrenal extract mixtures. The final triumph was the preparation of it artificially in the laboratory, its synthesis. When a substance can be synthesized in the chemist's laboratory, it means that its composition has become thoroughly understood. Here at last was an example of those mysterious internal secretions, the existence of which had indeed been postulated and proven, but which had never actually been inspected by the eye of mortal man. To have it in a test-tube, indeed to possess it in large quantities in bottles, to be able to manipulate and examine it without fear of the co-action of admixed impurities, to see it with the eye, and to taste it with the tongue, was truly a marvel. The miracle aroused at once scores of researches.

THE GLAND OF COMBAT AND FIGHT

Considering its effects, one is reminded at once of the similarity to the expression of a primitive emotion like anger or fear. So, by turning a relation upside down, it was argued that if artificial adrenalin could produce all these effects of an emotion like fear, the emotion itself should produce an increase of the natural adrenalin in the blood. This was found to be the case. Cannon of Harvard has built up an entire theory of the adrenal as the gland of emergencies upon the basis of these effects. In the facing of crises the adrenal functions as the gland of combat. And indeed, as I have mentioned, the more combative and pugnacious an animal, the more adrenal it has, while the timid and meek and weak have less.

The Glands of Combat, the glands of emergency energy, the glands of preparedness,--such are the adrenal glands when viewed from the adrenalin standpoint. A picture of its activity in the evolutionary scheme of struggle and survival is something like the following: meeting an enemy, the animal is put in danger. It must fight or flee for its life. In either case, certain conditions must be fulfilled, if the body of the animal endangered is to be saved. To prevent injury to itself, and to do as much injury as possible to the foe--that becomes its immediate urge and necessity. Of the two animals, if in one the heart should begin to beat more strongly, the blood pressure to rise, the blood to flow more rapidly through the attacking instruments, the muscles, the teeth and claws, the brain and its eyes, while the other animal experiences none of these, the former will be the victor in fight or flight. Adrenalin may be looked upon as the invention for the mobilization at a moment's notice, or as we say, after generations of use, by instinct, of all these visceral and blood advantages in the struggle of combat or flight.

The nature of instinct, in its relation to the glands of internal secretion, is a problem for another chapter. But we may note that the James-Lange theory of an emotion regards it as a consciousness of the very changes in the organism adrenalin causes. Since adrenalin is the starter of the whole process, and since McDougal has defined emotion as the feeling aspect of an instinct, just as an instinct may be defined as the motor aspect of an emotion, the adrenals as emotion-genetic, and instinct-genetic, play a part in the most profound processes of the subconscious and unconscious.

THE MECHANISM OF FEAR

We may therefore visualize a mechanism of fear. An instant excess of adrenalin occurs in the blood of, say, a cat when it is alarmed by the sight of a dog. In that cat, at the image of its hereditary enemy, certain brain cells vibrate. A nerve tract, in use as the line for that particular message in a hundred thousand generations of cats, whirrs its yell to the medulla of the adrenal gland. Through the tiny, solitary veins of the glands, an infinitesimal quantity of the reserve adrenalin responds. And with what an effect! The blood, that primary medium of life, the precious fluid that is everything, must all, or nearly all, be sent to the firing line, the battle trenches, the brain and muscles, now or never. So the blood is drafted from the non-essential industries--from the skin where it serves normally to regulate the heat of the body--from the digestive organs, the stomach and intestine, which must forsooth stop now, since if the organism will die, their last effort of digestion has been done--from the liver and spleen, great chemical factories in normal times, but now of no moment. Besides, should they be wounded, it is better they should be bloodless, and so run the least chance of bleeding to death, or getting infected, for the more tissue there is around, the greater the danger of infection. So, like the skin, the liver which usually holds in its great lakes and vessels about a quarter of all the blood in the body, is almost drained and blanched. At the same time, its great storehouses of sugar open their sluices and pour into the blood, increasing its sugar content by about a third because the combustion of sugar is the easiest way of getting energy free in the cells, sugar being the most quickly burned up of all the foods, and so the great food of the muscles and the heart. The poisons of fatigue, acid products of the contraction of muscles, are antagonized and neutralized by substances formed in the course of the oxidation of the sugar. Adrenalin, too, is directly fatigue antagonist. It causes the blood to clot faster than under ordinary circumstances. It erects the hair of the animal, and dilates the pupils of the eyes. There is an increase of the apparent size, all of which are to intimidate the enemy, like an Indian's painting of his face blue and green. It also--but what else does it not do?

The story of adrenalin would have delighted the heart of Samuel Butler. His "Note Books," opulent as they are, would have been the richer in pages and pages with his comments on it. Contending as he did with the pompous, dogmatic mechanism worship of the new scientific clique of his time on the one hand, and the superstitions of the old theological caste on the other, he had to fight the hardest kind of guerrilla warfare in defense of the Purpose of Life. Adrenalin, that weapon of a gland tracing its ancestry back to the begetter of the brain itself, for brain and adrenal gland both have evolved from the small nerve ganglia of the invertebrates, would have backed up to the hilt his argument, which he had to elaborate on the indirect grounds of analogy and induction. Essential for defense, and for protection,-- an organ in which everything necessary for the stratagems of retreat, or the offensives of attack, are supplied ad libitum, while everything non-essential or detrimental to the matter of the moment is inhibited, arrested and suppressed--no more perfect sample of the design with which Life is drenched could be imagined by the most closeted of passionate idealists.

FAILURE OF THE ADRENALS

As the gland of acute stress and strain, the adrenals in modern life are called upon to function more heavily and frequently than in the past. As a matter of fact, the life of the beast of jungle and field, as well as of savage and barbarian, is just as full of emergencies and shocks as that of the average city man or woman. In the case of the latter, however, inhibitions, education, and the conditions of modern living, improper food, sedentary indoor confinement, and universal rack and noise, have undoubtedly made greater and greater demands upon the adrenal glands. Chemical quantitative studies have shown that by repeated stimulation, the adrenal glands may be exhausted of their reserve supply of secretion, which returns only insufficiently if not enough time is given for recuperation. There results a condition of temporary or chronic adrenal insufficiency, supposedly an insufficient functioning of the gland as a whole. In persons so afflicted there appears a fatigability, a sensitiveness to cold, cold hands and feet, which are sometimes mottled bluish-red, a loss of appetite and zest in life, and a mental instability characterized by an indecision, and a tendency to worry, a weepishness upon the slightest provocation.

A certain number of the temporary breakdowns or nervous prostrations, which seem to be growing more common or fashionable, may be sometimes traced to such a deficiency of normal response to the needs of everyday conflict by the adrenal gland. In some, mental and physical elasticity are totally lost, and even the slightest exertion in either field often causes so much weariness and exhaustion as to be prohibited. Depression and even melancholia are associated with the fear of not being able to accomplish good work hitherto easy and enjoyed. Sometimes they are obsessed with the thought that they have lost their nerve completely, and so dread to commit themselves in even the most trivial of situations. The vacillating frame of mind is so distressing at times as to arouse thoughts of suicide. When these symptoms concur in the type of personality whom I shall describe as the unstable adrenal-centered individual, there is evidence for explaining the process as the effect of an insufficiency of secretion by the adrenal gland.

Shock, collapse, heart failure and sudden death following abnormal emotion, like an attack of rage, or the terrors of a railroad accident, or bad news, or excessive exertion like running a long race or climbing a high mountain when in poor general health, as the phrase goes, or in the terminal stages of infections like epidemic influenza or Asiatic cholera, have been put down to an acute insufficiency of the adrenal gland. A lowered temperature, blood pressure, and blood vessel tone, exhibited in tests of the response of the skin to stroking, are present in all of these and point the same moral.

In the second half of the 19th century, an American physician, Beard, described Neurasthenia, a general disturbance of the body and mind, not properly classifiable as a disease, but serious enough to incapacitate or at least greatly limit the sufferer. The neurasthenic is to be recognized by the fact that the most painstaking objective examination of his organs reveals nothing the matter with them. Yet, according to his complaint, everything is the matter with him. He cannot sleep when he lies down, he cannot keep awake when he stands up. He cannot concentrate, but still he is pitifully worried about his life. The slightest irritant causes him to go off the handle. As he works himself up into his hysterical state as a reaction to a disagreeable person or problem, irregular blotches may appear on his face and neck. Generally, his hands and feet are clammy and perspiring, his face is abnormally flushed or pallid, the eyes are worried or starey, unwonted wandering sensations involving now this area of the body, or now that obsess him. As the blood pressure is too low for the age, the circulation is nearly always inadequate and palpitation of the heart is a frequent complaint. So frequent, that attention is often centered upon the heart, a diagnosis of heart disease is made, and the unfortunate is doomed for life--to brood over horrible possibilities. The brooding over themselves and their troubles is one of the distinctive features of the whole complex. Neurasthenia may masquerade as any organic disease. An individual with a soil for a neurasthenic reaction to life will become neurasthenic when confronted by any stone wall, including a serious ailment within himself.

Beard's Neurasthenia leaped at once into the limelight. It was seized upon and applauded in Europe as a good new name for an old condition, observed particularly in Americans abroad to rest from the fatigues of the get-rich-quick games of industrial speculators. In fact, the name of the American Disease was given to it. Various theories about the effects of climate, sunlight per square inch and unit of time, oxygen content of the air, and so on, were offered up upon the altar of scientific explanation. Sir Arbuthnot Lane, famous protagonist of Lane's intestinal kink, said that all Americans were neurasthenic. Neurasthenia became one of the most popular of diagnoses, and remains so today.

Neurasthenia, regarded as a reaction of people to the stress and strain of life, has without a doubt increased. The most casual of observers will tell you that the generation of the Great War is a neurasthenic generation. It takes its pleasures too intensely, its pains too seriously, its troubles too flippantly. But what is neurasthenia? Beard himself regarded it as a chronic fatigue and loss of tone of the nervous system, a literal interpretation of his term. That the conception, as far as it goes, is valid is proved by the fact that it is the neurasthenics who furnish the majority of the clientele of the cults, the Christian Scientists, the osteopaths and the chiropractors, and who are the subjects of the faith and miracle cures, like those of Lourdes. That is because their particular disease, or what appears to them to be their very own disease--and they certainly cherish their ailments--is but an expression of, a compensation for, indeed a consolation for, the underlying feelings of insufficiency or inferiority. Were there no moral code, were there no social system, nor the consequent inculcated conscience to be responsible to, there would be no such disguising symptom as the disease which preoccupies the consciousness. The feeling of insufficiency would be there, and would be recognized as in itself the disease. To the physiologist and the psychologist, the feeling of insufficiency is the disease, no matter how spectacular the overlaying phenomena--a cripple on crutches or a man blind and speechless. Shell shock is now acknowledged to belong to this group.

Now one of the outstanding effects of disease of the adrenal glands is the feelings of muscular and mental inefficiency. And as a matter of fact, a good number of observations conspire for the idea that a certain number of neurasthenics are suffering from insufficiency of the adrenal gland. The chronic state of the acute phenomenon, known as the nervous breakdown, really represents in them a breakdown of the reserves of the adrenals, and an elimination of their factor of safety. In the light of that conception, the great American disease--dementia americana--is seen to be adrenal disease--and the American life to be the adrenal life, often making too great demands upon that life, and so breaking down with it.

ADRENAL EXCESS

The converse of adrenal insufficiency, that of adrenal excess, also exists. In certain types of the middle-aged, a high blood pressure, accompanied by a great capacity for work, has been shown to be associated with hypertrophy of the cortex. In women, there is a degree of masculinity, as the adrenal in women makes for masculinity, neutralising more or less the specifically feminine influences of the internal secretions of the ovary. Such women possess a vigor and energy above the normal, and command responsible positions in society, not only among their own sex, but also among men. They are the ones who, in the present overturn of the traditional sex relationships, will become the professional politicians, bankers, captains of industry, and directors of affairs in general.

THE GONADS

(*Sexual, Puberty or Interstitial Glands*)

The gonads is the name applied to the generative or reproductive glands considered collectively. In the male, they are the testes; in the female, the ovaries. They are, therefore, sometimes called the sexual glands. As they possess definite canals for the removal of their gross secretion, the specific reproductive cells, ova or spermatozoa, to a surface of the body, they are first of all glands of external secretion. But they have been also found to hold secretory cells not concerned with the making of the reproductive corpuscles, but, as all the evidence indicates, with the manufacture of an internal secretion. These interstitial cells form the interstitial gland. A classic example of a gland of internal secretion lodged in the interstices of a gland of external secretion is thus furnished by the gonads.

ORIGIN OF SEX TRAITS

The history of sex goes back far in the scheme of life. The immortality of the ameba was at one time one of the indisputables of biology. Then some observations were made which threw doubt upon a long accepted fact, now declared a dogma. Lately, opinion has veered back to immortality. But in the case of a close relative of the ameba, the one-celled animal known as the paramecium, union with another paramecium, true conjugation, has been proved necessary to prevent death sooner or later. Sex here appears in its most primitive form, on the basis of exchange of necessary materials, between individuals to prevent death, their own having been, so to speak, worn out, in the course of metabolism.

Specifically different sexes come later, when mortality is a universal fate, as a means of rebirth and escape from death. Then the sexes develop their latest function, most prominent among the younger vertebrates, of acting as nature's most potent method of variation and differentiation. In the pursuit of the different, nature has exalted sex, and the intensity of the sex life. As far as the preservation of a species is concerned, and the reproduction of the individual, the asexual methods, budding, for example, would have done well enough. But when it comes to enacting a different individual apart from the effects of environment, sex stands out as the favored method of Life.

The development of the sexes and the sexual life brought a new element of conflict into the living world. Before the advent of the sexes the conflict was essentially for the means of existence, food alone. But with the sexual life came a conflict for sex pleasure, a competition among members of the same species for the same individual as their sex partners. The result was the introduction of a factor in evolution which Darwin examined so closely in the "Descent of Man."

The sex conflict has been the cause for the origin and the survival of certain physical and mental traits, helpful in sex attraction, sex combat, the growth of the embryo, and the nutrition and safety of the young of a species,--in short, the whole process of sexual selection. The proportions of the skeleton, the distribution of hair and fat, the construction of organs of attack and defense, the color of the skin, the cyclic processes of preparation for impregnation, the oestrus or heat period in animals, the menstrual period in the human being, the psychic reactions to danger and combat have all been thus determined. That man is bearded while woman is not,--that woman has potentially functional breasts while man has not,--the aggressive pugnacity of man contrasted with the more passive timidity of woman, have all been evolved in the sex struggle, surviving because most effective in that struggle. These so-called secondary sexual characteristics are an expression of the influence of the internal secretion of the gonads, or the interstitial glands. Some call them puberty glands, because their ripening initiates puberty.

We know that these interstitial glands, to stick to that name, (rather than to the name of the puberty glands, since they serve not only to induce puberty but to maintain maturity) are the actual primary dictators of the process by which male and female are distinguished, if not created. Castration was probably the first surgical operation carried out for experimental purposes, suggested no doubt by a curiosity concerning its effects. Trepanning of the skull, the geologic record indicates, was done even by the cave man. But as an experimental operation, castration seems to hold the primary position in the annals of surgery.

Its effects noted, the satisfaction of one of the lower human instincts, jealousy, popularised it. From the days of Semiramis, eunuchs have been commonplace figures of the East, their function definite: to guard the harems of the powerful. The age of Abdul Hamid witnessed no diminution of the barbaric tortures by which children are prepared for the profession. It is to the credit of England that in its dominions in the Orient the practice has been abolished. But it goes on even today. According to the best authorities, four out of five of these victims at the auto-da-fe of a vicious human instinct die immediately or soon after from exhaustion due to pain and infection. Not all of the ancient nations countenanced the brutal horror. The Hebrews placarded castration an unpardonable sin, making it a sin to castrate even animals. Nor was any man so mutilated permitted to worship in the house of the Lord (Deuteronomy xxiii, 11). Yet we have evidence that the latter Jewish kings employed foreign eunuchs in their harems, who often held the most important positions as ministers of the court.

Besides the eunuchs, another group of people have presented material for the study of the interstitial glands. These are the Skoptzi of Russia and the Lipowaner of Roumania. Among them castration is a religious ritual. Mankind has always been most brutal to itself in the name of the ideal. These sects were founded because in the eighteenth century an antipode of Joseph Smith and Brigham Young discovered this passage in Matthew xix, 12.

"For there are some eunuchs which were so born from their mother's womb, and there are some eunuchs which were made eunuchs of men: and there be eunuchs *which have made themselves eunuchs for the kingdom of heaven's sake*. He that is able to receive it, let him receive it."

He decided that he was inspired to spread the gospel of castration. A sect was founded who thought that surgery was the easiest way to enter the gates of Paradise, and they multiplied and fructified. The sect exists today, and some of the most interesting studies of the internal secretion of the interstitial glands have been made among them.

Related to acquired eunuchism is the condition of eunuchoidism, the eunuchs which were so born from their mother's womb. Baron Larey, the great surgeon of Napoleon's armies, was their first painter. He was the only altruist Bonaparte said he had ever met in his life. He portrayed a group of soldiers with peculiarly high-pitched voices, smooth and hairless skins, and atrophied generative organs. A somewhat similar picture is evolved in certain types of insufficiency of the pituitary gland. Features of the picture are exhibited with disturbances of the other internal secretory glands also, like the thymus.

But a host of experiments and data prove the interstitial glands to be the direct controllers of elementary sexuality and the specific sex traits of male and female. Beginning with Berthold back in the first half of the nineteenth century, who studied the fowl, a number of observations have been made on the effects of excision, translocation and transplantation of these glands.

The results of the experiments and observations can be summed up as follows: if the male individual is castrated before puberty, that is, before the advent of the sexual life, secondary sex qualities do not develop. In males, the generative organs do not grow, hair on the face does not appear, hair elsewhere on the body remains generally scanty, the voice continues as high-pitched as the child's, there is more or less muscle weakness, obesity, and mental sluggishness. In other words, we have an effeminate man, technically a eunuch. In the castrated female, the pelvis does not grow to the normal feminine size, the breasts do not swell as they should, more or less hair comes out on the face, the voice is low-pitched, and tends to be rather husky, the legs are longer, and again, the mentality is dulled. That is, a masculine sort of woman is produced.

In short, the castrated male takes on a feminine type, and the castrated female, a male type. In either case there is also an infantilism, a retention of the infantile mental traits, a lack of development of the adult mental attitudes and reactions. Now, if in the castrated male is transplanted an ovary, the positive characteristics of the female are evoked, such as enlarged mammary glands, and a tendency to secretion of milk. Experiments have also been reported in which a uterus was also placed in such an animal, with a means of entry, and pregnancy followed. If in the castrated female a testicle is planted, the masculine traits become much more marked and striking. A direct exchange of the male and female roles can thus be achieved. Castration after puberty cannot modify profoundly structures like the skeleton which are already completed. Yet it may unquestionably bring about definite retrogressive changes in the secondary sex characters: reduction or loss of virility, diminution of facial and body hair, and a general presenility or hastening of senility.

How remarkably these interstitial cells influence the entire structure and vitality of the organism is indicated by these facts. How much they have to do with sexual impulses, sexual excitement, and sexual desire, what the Freudians have popularized as the libido, and how subtly they act upon the coming and duration of adolescence and maturity, as well as sexual precocity and peversions, we shall consider in a later chapter. But it is enough now to remember that these interstitial glands are the primary dictators of the genital sense and flair of the individual. In any attempt at measurement of men and women, the quality and quantity of the internal secretion of the interstitial cells must be respected as a fundamental consideration. The womanly woman and the manly man, those ideals of the Victorians, which crumbled before the attack of the Ibsenites, Strindbergians and Shavians in the nineties, but which must be recognized as quite valid biologically, are the masterpieces of these interstitial cells when in their perfection. They are such solely because of the right concentration in the blood of the substances manufactured not only by these cells, but by all the glands of internal secretion. For it cannot be repeated and emphasized too often that the interstitial cells of the sex glands are most sensitive to all kinds of other influences, and, in particular, the other internal secretory organs. They may indeed be watched as an index scale or barometer of the general tone of the whole internal secretion system. Sex variations offer a variety of clues to variations, disturbances, predominances and abnormalities in all the components of the ductless gland association.

To take a single instance, the development of the long bones is dependent upon the handling of food lime by the body. Eunuchs and eunuchoids, that is, individuals with insufficient internal secretion of the interstitial cells, have longer bones and more fragile bones than the normal. Vice versa, those with an excess of the secretion have shorter and thicker bones. The earlier the onset of menstruation, which means puberty, the shorter the extremities, as the action of the internal secretion of the ovaries closes the story of the growth of the long bones.

The ovaries are a most important factor in the regulation of the power of the organism to keep lime in the bones. If they over-secrete in an excess which cannot be taken care of by the other glands of internal secretion, the body loses lime, a softening and curving of the bones occurs, and the most horrible deformities and tortures for the sufferer. Taking out the ovaries has cured some of the afflicted. Administration of the antagonizing gland extracts has helped others. An Italian, Bossi, in 1907, used adrenal gland curatively. More recently, a British student of the subject, Blair Bell, was given the direction of the treatment, at long range, of a number of cases in India, the land of chronic pregnancy with insufficient food, and consequent oversecretion of the ovaries, with the typical softening of the bones. At his suggestion pituitary was used successfully.

Some of the glands of internal secretion act as accelerators to the sex glands. Others act as retarding antagonists. Among the most important of the latter is

THE THYMUS

The thymus is the gland which dominates childhood. It appears to do so by inhibiting the activity of the testes or ovaries. Castration causes a persistent growth and retarded atrophy of the thymus. Removal of the thymus hastens the development of the gonads.

Situated in the chest, astride the windpipe, it descends and covers over the upper portion of the heart, overlapping the great vessels at the base of the heart. It is a brownish red mass, which when cut presents the spongy effect of a sweetbread. The more intimate view of detail revealed by the higher powers of the microscope shows conglomerations of the white cells of the blood known as lymphocytes. But scattered through the substance of the gland, between these lymphocytes, like the interstitial cells of the sex glands placed between the sex cells, are peculiarly staining cells in whorls. Of which there are many more in the thymus of embryonic and early postnatal life, known after their discoverer as Hassal's Corpuscles. They are believed by some to elaborate the specific internal secretion of the thymus. Present in all vertebrates, there seems to be more of it in the carnivora than in the herbivora, like the thyroid.

Concerning the exact function of the thymus, we are a good deal at sea. The latest opinion about the results of extirpation even in young and growing animals is that they are nil. Yet there is a certain justification for proclaiming the thymus the gland of childhood, the gland which keeps children childish and sometimes makes children out of grown-ups. There is a quantity of data for that proposition. In the first place, the curve of rise of growth of the gland seems to coincide with the period of childhood, the curve of its decline with the period of adolescence and the rise of the sex glands. In the past, it was accepted, that with puberty the thymus atrophied and was replaced by some sort of fatty tissue. Nowadays, it is held that secretion cells persist throughout life. When the extent of this persistence is too great, the gland being from five to ten times as large as the normal, a number of other features become prominent to make the extraordinary individual, the status lymphaticus, who amid the hazards of life will react in an extraordinary way. He will be taken up in the consideration of internal secretion personalities.

Then there are the varied and remarkable phenomena of thymus enlargement and hyperactivity in childhood itself. When an enlarged thymus is present in an infant, the initiation of breathing in the new-born, the introduction of the newcomer to the oxygen of the air, may be an exceedingly prolonged, difficult, matter. Such a baby is said to be born blue, and the breathing may be stridorous for days, becoming normal for a time, to be followed later by spells of trouble in breathing, breathlessness or breathlessness with blueness, and threatened extinction. Sometimes these spells come out of a clear sky in an apparently healthy child. That some poison, probably an oversecretion of the thymus, is responsible is shown by the relief obtainable by X-ray shrinkage of the gland, or the surgical removal of a part of it.

Moreover, the gland is influenced by and influences the factors of body weight and growth with an extreme readiness and lability. Deficient general undernutrition leads to rapid decline in its weight. Back in 1858, the pioneer student of the thymus, Friedleben, declared that the size and condition of the thymus is an index to be the state of nutrition of the body. Underfeeding for four weeks will reduce it to one thirtieth the normal. It seems to act as a storage and reserve organ, affording some protection against the limitation of growth by lack of food material. In exhausting or wasting disease, the weight of the gland sinks much more quickly than other glands. Scattered instances have been reported of children growing, putting on inches in height and expanding mentally, when thymus was fed to them, in whom every other measure previously tried had failed. A French study of over four hundred idiotic children with normal thyroids reported that over three fourths had no thymus at all. Everything points to the most direct and close relation between the gland and nutrition and growth, but with nothing tangibly definite like our knowledge of the thyroid and the pituitary.

There is evidence that the thymus is involved in the health and efficiency of muscle cells and muscularity. Certain tumors of the thymus, presumably destructive of the gland substance proper, and thus cutting off its secretion, are accompanied by a singular muscle weakness and atrophy of the muscle cells, entirely out of proportion to the general damage suffered by the other cells of the body when affected by the poison of a malignant growth. Also, the thymus has been discovered diseased in certain mysterious progressive muscular wastings. A remarkable fatigability of muscles, which appears after the slightest exertion, is a feature. The feeding of thymus has caused muscle cramps which apparently depends upon an increased excitability of the muscle nerve endings.

Feeding of thymus to some of the lower creatures of the animal kingdom will completely hold up differentiation. Take the unfolding of the specialized tissues and organs which transform the tadpole into the frog and the chrysalis into the butterfly. A tadpole kept supplied with enough thymus in a nutrient medium will swell into an extraordinary giant tadpole, but will not change into a frog. Recently, this experiment has been contradicted. Yet this effect corresponds to the conception of its importance in childhood as a retardant of precocity, physical and mental. Clinical observations emphasize that in childhood it is the chief brake upon the other glands of internal secretion which would hasten development and differentiation, checking them perhaps for a given time and so profoundly influencing growth.

THE PINEAL

The pineal is another gland which has been credited with similar abilities and a like holding-the-reins-tight-in-childhood function among the cells. Like the thymus, it has been supposed one of the distinctive organs of childhood and to die with it. Generations of anatomists solemnly asserted, repeating each other's mistakes with the aplomb of the historians who declare that history repeats itself, that the pineal body was a useless, wastefully space consuming vestige of a once important structure. That was the view in that century of grandly inaccurate assertions, the nineteenth. Not that they relegated it with that statement to the limbo of the dull and the uninteresting. Quite the contrary. They conferred upon it a distinguished romance and mystery by identifying it as the last heir and vestigial remnant of a third eye, situated in the back of the head, which may still be observed in certain reptiles. Imagine it! Somewhere, stuck away in a cranny of the floor of your head and mine, is this descendant of an organ that once sparkled and shone, wept and glared, took in the stars and hawks and eagles, and now is condemned to eternal darkness and an ineffectual sandiness. Today, we have not discarded that view of its history, but we know a little more regarding its composition and function.

What and where is the romantic object? It is a cone-shaped bit of tissue hidden away at the base of the brain in a tiny cave behind and above its larger colleague, the pituitary. Microscopic scrutiny reveals that it is made up in part of nerve cells containing a pigment similar to that present in the cells of the retina, thus clinching the argument for its ancient function as an eye. But the outstanding and specifically glandular cells are large secreting affairs, which too reach back to the tidewater days of our vertebrate ancestors, when Eurypterus and other Crustaceans were engrossed with the fundamental problems of brain versus belly. Besides these, there are the singular masses upon which has been fastened the unnecessarily opprobious epithet of brain sand. These, noted and commented upon from the earliest times, consist of collections of crystals of lime salts, sometimes small, lying about in discrete irregular masses, and sometimes grouped into larger mulberry-like concretions, varying much in size. These brain sand particles have become of practical importance in the detection of pineal disease because they, like all lime salts, will stop the X-rays, and so can be photographed.

For a long time, indeed up to scarcely more than a few decades or so ago, the pineal was believed to have no present function at all, or at least no ascertainable or accessible duty in the body economy. That it might perhaps be, in a sense, a gland of internal secretion was a despised theory. Then a classic case, the most extraordinary and curiosity-piquing sort of case, with symptoms involving the pineal gland, in a boy, was reported by the German neurologist, Von Hochwart. That boy provoked a little army of researches. He came to the clinic complaining about his eyes and other troubles which pointed pretty definitely to a brain tumor as the diagnosis to pigeon-hole him. Nothing extraordinary about him in that respect. But the story told by his parents was quite extraordinary, even to the jaded palate of the clinic professor and his assistants. They said that he was a little over five years old, a statement conclusively proved correct at his death. Up to the time at which his illness began, he had been quite normal in size, intelligence and interests. But with the onset of his misfortune, he had begun to grow, and rapidly until now he looked and corresponded in all measurements to a normal boy of twelve or thirteen. Hair developed all over his skin, most prominently and abundantly in the typically hairy places of adults. His voice became low-pitched, and most remarkable of all, his sexuality and mentality precocious. He became capable of true sexual life and is said to have asked many questions about the fate and condition of the soul after death. On one occasion he remarked reflectively: "It is odd how much better I feel when I let other children play with my toys than when I play with them myself." Other statements attributed to him imply the most astounding maturity of thought and mental process. Headaches finally came, and he died about four weeks later. The cause of the whole bizarre tragedy was found to be a tumor of the pineal gland.

As has happened before in medical history, no sooner was the one prodigy reported, than a score of others of the same ilk sprang into the limelight. Cases of precocious genital development, especially, some of them occurring as early as the second year of life, were linked with them. It is an interesting point to be noted that in these, as in those started by an overaction of the adrenal cortex, it is premature masculinity that is stimulated. The adrenal cortex must be classed as a gland of masculinity. The pineal possibly acts as a brake upon the adrenal cortex.

Very soon after the report of Von Hochwart's prodigy appeared, an experimental research on the pineal was begun in New York. The pineal glands of a number of young bullocks were obtained and used for feeding, to see whether an overaction of the internal secretion could be produced. Guinea pigs, kittens and rabbits were used. The experiments covered about two years in time. Of a dozen small kittens, the subjects outgrew the controls rapidly in activity, size, intelligence, and resistance to intercurrent disease. Of ten small rabbits, the controls weighed about a third less than the subjects, which were strikingly clean, active, fat and salacious.

Feeding of the gland was then extended to a particular class of defective children, children with well-shaped heads, normal eyes, symmetrically functioning limbs, excellent digestion, strong muscles and generally, normal, sometimes rapid growth. It is to them, particularly when mental normality has progressed up to the eighth, tenth or twelfth year and stopped, that the term "moron" has been applied. They have been a hopeless lot, belonging to the limbo of the incurables. Moreover, they, emphatically the physically normal ones, differ from one another enormously in the extent to which mental operations are possible. As all transitions and degrees exist, no definite classification and subdivision of them has been made. Yet ever since the cretin, once looked upon as an eternally damned defective, was transformed by thyroid feeding into an apparently normal being, there has been no dearth of effort to find the right kind of internal secretion to fit their desperate situations, but in vain. In defectives with definitely, organically damaged brains, no result of course was to be expected. In those of any class over fifteen, no response has been elicited by feeding pineal gland. In the others the results have been contradictory.

A set of observations have related the pineal to muscle function, inviting comparison of it with the thymus. There is a singular muscle shrinking and deforming disease, known as progressive muscular dystrophy, hitherto a complete and unsolved mystery. Newer studies of the pineal in this disease during life by means of the X-ray have shown it calcified, that is, buried in lime salts, which signifies put out of business. Recently thus another hint as to its function has been ferreted out.

The tadpole as a reagent to test out the growth effects of different glands of internal secretion has also been employed for the pineal. Ten-day-old tadpoles fed on pineal present a marked translucency of the skin due to a retraction of the skin pigment cells. Now without a doubt a number of as yet unknown growth and metabolic effects follow exposure of the body to the complete gamut of light rays. The interesting suggestion follows that the pineal influences the body by varying the degree of light ray reaction.

The pineal, the ghost of a once important third eye at the back of our heads, still harks back in its function to a regulation of our susceptibility to light, and its effect upon sex and brain. So it becomes one of the significant regulators of development, with an indirect hastening or retardation of puberty and maturity according as it works in excess, or too indolently. It appears thus the blood brother of the adrenal cortex which also influences the skin pigment and so susceptibility of the organism to light, brain growth and sex ripening. It is interesting that Descartes, in 1628, considered the pineal the seat of the soul.

THE PARATHYROIDS

Sometimes imbedded within the substance of the thyroid in the neck, sometimes placed directly behind it upon the windpipe, are four tiny glands, each about the size of a wheat seed, the parathyroids. For long they were swamped in the nearness of their great neighbor, and considered merely a variable part of it. There are some who contend that even today. But it has been proven that they are separate, individual glands, with a structure and function of their own, and a definite importance to the body economy.

On the animal family tree they appear early, contemporaneously with the thyroids. In the embryo they develop from about the same sites. And very often they look very much alike under the microscope, especially when the cells are in certain quiescent stage of secretion. Yet they are wholly independent in nature, activity and business.

First experimenters upon the effects of removal of the thyroid were confused by contradictory findings with different animals because in some they would take out the parathyroids at the same time without knowing it, and in others they would not. That possibility suggested, more careful dissectors accomplished the job of extirpating the thyroid while leaving the parathyroids intact and vice versa. In consequence some definite information about the parathyroids is available, even though their internal secretion has never been isolated, or its existence established as more than an inference.

When the parathyroids are removed, an astounding increase in the excitability of the nerves follow. It is as if the animal were thoroughly poisoned with strychnine. The slightest stimulus will make him jump, or throw him into a spasm. When the excitability of the nerves is measured by an electrical instrument it is found augmented by from five hundred to one thousand per cent. The reflexes, those automatic responses of brain and spinal cord to certain stimuli and situations, become enormously sensitive, so that merely letting the light into a darkened room will make the subject of the experiment go into a series of convulsions.

On the chemical side, an explanation for these nervous phenomena has been advanced. Lime in the blood and cells appears to be necessary in a number of ways. In the making of bone and teeth, in the coagulation of the blood, in the keeping of fluid within the blood vessels, and in maintaining the tone of the nerves, it plays a major role. Now the parathyroids, among all the glands of internal secretion, seem to act as the prime regulators of the amount of lime held within the blood and cells. For when the parathyroids have been completely and aseptically excised, without injuring any other organ, immediately the body begins to lose lime. Something has gone out of it that helped it to bind lime, and without that essential something, the internal secretion presumably of the parathyroids, the lime departs. As a conspicuous consequence the teeth fail to develop properly, particularly as to their enamel, for which lime is an essential constituent. Hair is lost, there is a general wasting, the nails get brittle, and the bones soften, and the animal dies. Supplying lime directly, particularly by direct injection into the blood, will relieve the symptoms.

In man, a condition of nervous over-excitability has been described as tetany. It occurs most often in the young, the pregnant, or in vomiting after operations. All sorts of tests have related the malady to the phenomena succeeding parathyroid deprivation, and they are now looked upon as aspects of it. Individuals have been reported suffering from an insufficiency of the internal secretion of parathyroids, with a sudden extreme depression, nervousness and restlessness, an inability to sleep or sit still, and a tremulous handwriting. Such reports round out the evidence for the importance of the parathyroids in an understanding of the factors which control growth, especially as regards lime utilization, for without lime properly handled no building of cells is possible. Also the parathyroids are necessary to a steadiness of muscle and nerve.

THE PANCREAS

The business of the parathyroids concerns the keeping of lime in the body. Another gland, the pancreas or sweetbreads, this time within the abdomen, a close neighbor of the solar plexus, alias the abdominal brain, is occupied with holding and hoarding sugar in the body, particularly in the liver, the great sugar warehouse. This matter of retaining sugar and controlling its output is one of the utmost significance for growth and metabolism, the resistance to infections, the response to emergency situations, and in general to the mobilization of energy for physical and mental purposes. For without sugar sufficiently at hand for the cells, no muscle work or nerve work, the essentials of the struggle for existence, are possible.

The pancreas is an organ with both an internal and external secretion. The external secretion, long known, evolved by the major portion of the gland, is poured into the small intestine to play the star in digestion. Scattered here and there among the definitely glandular cell groups creating the external secretion are smaller collections of cells, called the islets of Langerhans, which have been demonstrated to elaborate the internal secretion. There are about a million of these islands in each gland. The hormone has been called insuline. Unlike most of the glands with a double secretion in which the internal is absolutely independent, and so to speak, unconscious of the external, these two of the pancreas are often disturbed together, perhaps because trouble easily hits them both together.

Quite the most well-known disease due to disturbed internal secretory function of the pancreas is diabetes. An enormous amount of work has been spent upon the various aspects of it as a mystery. Hundreds of papers in a dozen languages upon the subject are in existence. In a nutshell, they have established pretty well that diabetes is a disease in which there is an excess of sugar in the blood and urine because of an insufficient amount of the secretion of the islands of Langerhans in the pancreas. Removal of the pancreas makes the body, essentially the liver, unable to retain sugar, as well as unable to burn up sugar for energy. The situation is comparable to a locomotive with its coal bins leaking, and the coal itself acting as if made of slate or some equally uncombustible or only partially combustible material.

The control of sugar mobilization from the liver, where it is stored as glycogen or animal starch, is divided between the pancreas and the adrenals, the pancreas acting as the brake, the adrenals as the accelerator of the mechanism. Adrenal and pancreas are therefore direct antagonists, the pans of the scale which represents sugar equilibrium in the organism. Diabetes may be regarded as a disturbance of the adrenal-pancreas balance, assisted by events which produce adrenal overwork like great or prolonged emotion, or by strain of the pancreas, effected by over-eating for example.

There are other minor glands of internal secretions. But those considered are by far the most important and the most recently explored. In a summary, one would classify them as follows:

Name	Secretion	Function
1. Thyroid	Thyroxin	Gland of energy production Controller of growth of specialized organs and tissues--brain and sex
2. Pituitary--		Gland of energy consumption and utilization--continued effort
anterior	Unknown	Growth of skeleton and supporting tissues

posterior	Pituitrin	Nerve cell and involuntary muscle cell, brain and sex tone
3. Adrenals		The Gland of Combat
cortex	Unknown	a. Brain growth--tone development of sex glands
medulla	Adrenalin	b. Energy for emergency situations
4. Pineal	Unknown	a. Brain and sex development b. Adolescence and puberty c. Light and maturity
5. Thymus	Unknown	Gland of Childhood
6. Interstitial glands of	Testes in male Ovaries in female	Glands of secondary Sex traits
7. Parathyroids	Unknown	a. Controllers of lime metabolism b. Excitability of muscle and nerve
8. Pancreas	Insuline	Controller of sugar metabolism

CHAPTER IV
THE GLANDS AS AN INTERLOCKING DIRECTORATE

Now in considering each gland of internal secretion as a separate entity, and labelling it with certain properties and actions, we of course commit the usual sin of the intellect: the sin of abstraction and isolation of its material. This crime of analysis the intellect commits every day in the search for truth. Before its dissection, it seems to have to dip the elusive article in a fixative, and bottle it in a vacuum.

Yet nothing in reality is more of a changing flux than the body in all of its parts and tissues and organs. And of all these, the glands of internal secretion stand out as the most susceptible to change. Made to react to stimuli of offense and defense, instantaneously responsive to situations involving energy exchanges and protective reflexes, they are never for any minute the same or alone. They never function separately. Each influences the other in a communicating chain. Let one be disturbed, and all the others will feel the impact of the disturbance and vibrate with it.

Any break in the somatic or psychic equilibrium, a blow or an infection, or a startling thing seen, or a worrisome thought felt, will start a process going. This will only wind up when every gland has been somehow touched, and a final equilibrium reestablished. The thyroid, maybe, was first excited, and then in turn the adrenals, with a boomerang reinforcing effect upon the thyroid, and at the same time a stimulating effect upon the pituitary. Each gland is thus influenced and influencing, agent and reagent in the complex adjustments of the organism.

ENDOCRINE CO-OPERATIONS

The body-mind is a perfect corporation. Not quite perfect, for continually there arise little insurgencies, inadequacies and frictions to which in time it will succumb. Yet, in the efficiency of its co-operations, and in the co-ordination of the needs and supplies of producer, middle man, and consumer, there is no one of the great organizations of the captains of industry which can for a moment approach it.

Of this corporation the glands of internal secretion are the directors. But the huge corporation, not to topple over with its own unwieldy size, must be composed of smaller units, each within itself a corporation, and governed by a directorate. There are, in the corporation-organism, different departments and bureaus, sub-divisions of function, which constitute the smaller corporations within the larger corporation. These subsidiary companies have their own glands of internal secretion as their directors.

Thus, the growth of the brain is presided over by the adrenal cortex, the thyroid, the thymus and the pituitary. They determine the size of the brain, the number of its cells, the complexity of its convolutions and the speed of its chemistry, which means the speed of thought and memory and imagination. As its directorate, therefore, they may be entitled. The disturbance of one of them means the disturbance of all of them, and a consequent deleterious effect upon the brain. Now take the burning up of sugar in the organism, the great material source of energy, which is controlled by the pancreas, the adrenals and the liver, the thyroid and the pituitary. Together they form the directorate of sugar metabolism. But, as is evident from a glance at the membership of the growth directorate, and comparing it with the directorate of sugar metabolism, there are some members who are present on both boards. An infection, an illness, an ailment, an exaltation or intoxication of such members will produce reverberations in both directorates. A disturbance of sugar metabolism might then cause a disturbance of growth. The advantages and disadvantages are before us of having, in the glands of internal secretion, an interlocking directorate, rulers over all the varied and manifold activities of the organism.

Behind the body, and behind the mind is this board of governors. Indeed, from the administrative and legislative points of view, the body-mind may be said to be governed by the House of Glands. It is the invisible committee behind the throne. Upon the throne is what? Man, the most baffling of complexities. Man who is not a mind, but owns a mind--Man who is not a body, but possesses a body, just as he might have a motor car, a fortune or a calamity. Back of all his daily activities, behind the life of body-mind is the mysterious unique individuality, the Ego, the Psyche or the Soul. Lately, a competitor with these ancient and honorable terms has come upon the scene as the Subconscious. In that darkened No Man's Land is determined a man's destiny. The endocrine association stands out as at least the most important physical determinant of the states and processes of the subconscious.

ANTAGONISMS AND CO-OPERATIONS

As within a corporation there are factions and cliques, influences that always work together, and forces that are always pulling in opposite directions, so within the interlocking directorate of the ductless glands there are antagonisms and inhibitions, co-operations and compensations. One gland will assist the action of another's secretion with its own, or will in turn be stimulated to secrete by it. Another will throw out its secretion in order to neutralize the effects produced. Or its own activity will be depressed or completely inhibited by it. Thus the pituitary arouses the interstitial glands and vice versa, whereas the pancreas and the thyroid are mutually inhibitory. Indeed, whole systems of glands may work in unison, or be pitted against each other in certain situations, especially when the organism is subjected to conflicting impulses with the clash of opposing instincts, like fear and anger. In general there is reciprocity and team work among the internal secretions.

A certain minimum amount of each must be present if life is to continue along the normal lines. Whether there is to be an excess of any one secretion above this minimum, or a deficiency below it, decides the fate of the individual. If there is deficiency of one, the other members of the directorate attempt to make up for what has been lost, and to carry on its work by an extra effort, to substitute. Or, released from the discipline of the deficient member, or the necessity for antagonizing it, they may be released from its stimulus to secrete, and produce less of their own specific secretion. A general reaction all along the line will accompany overaction, oversecretion, of one gland. Due to consequent stimulations and depressions of other glands, some may be excited by the event to overwork--some to assist--others, to act as antidote for--the excess secretion, while still others, relieved of a burden, do not have to supply as much of their quota under the circumstances and so shut down, or limit their output.

It is important to get clearly in mind these subtle inter-reactions of the different ductless glands. They may be antagonistic in their end effects because of the opposed functions of the nerves or organs stimulated. There are inhibitions and restraints produced when a gland will send out its secretions to stop another gland secreting. There are compensations resulting when because of insufficiency of a gland, others will endeavour, by manufacturing more of their own secretion, to compensate for the loss. There are mutual co-operations, partnerships, when a gland will oversecrete to assist another, or in response to another which is also oversecreting. There are losses of balance, so that when one gland ceases secreting, another will simultaneously or soon after. Normal secretion, oversecretion or undersecretion are thus adjusted, but leave a train of after effects.

So with loss or insufficiency of the thyroid, there may be pituitary overgrowth, because the pituitary may act as vicar for the thyroid. The thyroid and thymus are antagonistic, for the thyroid hastens differentiation, puberty and the coming of sexual maturity, while the thymus delays and retards them and prolongs the period of childhood. The thyroid and the pancreas are antagonists, for when the thyroid has been excised, the pancreas appear no longer necessary to act as a break upon the mechanism of sugar liberation into the blood from the liver. The thyroid stimulates the interstitial glands, for menstruation and pregnancy are impossible with no thyroid or an insufficient thyroid. Removal of the pituitary makes the thymus shrink because the restraining influence of the latter is no longer needed. But there is an enlargement of the thyroid to compensate. In castrates there is an increase in the size and number of the cells of the anterior pituitary, again a compensation or substitution effect. The pituitary and the adrenal cortex are mutually assistant, alike in their influence upon the tone of the brain and sex cells.

THE KINETIC SYSTEM

So there are combinations of glands to assist or restrain others, or to control a body function, or to determine the domination or abeyance of an instinct. One such has been named the kinetic system because it comes into play in situations which demand prompt adaptation without hesitancy, and a consequent immediate transformation of static or stored energy into kinetic or active energy. According to this conception the brain, the adrenals, the liver, the thyroid and the muscles together constitute a machine very much like an automobile. The self-starter of the machine is the brain, with storage battery (composed of stored past memories) and ignition combined. The thing seen without, or the idea felt within, act as the initial sparks, while the adrenals, as the carburetors, permit the freer flow of fuel, sugar, from the liver. The thyroid works as the accelerator, the original impulse finally landing upon muscles keyed up and supplied with food to meet the situation, be it that of removing a poison, removing an aggressor (attack) or removing the individual himself (running away). When one is exhausted by exertion and emotion, injury, intoxication or infection, it is these members of the kinetic system, the brain, the adrenals, thyroid and liver, which are exhausted. Exhaustion diminishes when the activity of the brain is diminished by anesthetics, and cured when it is abolished by sleep.

If the adrenal gland may be called the Gland of Emergency energy, the Kinetic System is entitled to the name of Council of Emergency Defense for the organism. The Kinetic Drive is the name that has been given to the whole system at work. It is one of the best examples we have of inter-glandular co-operations and reactions in reply to the threat of danger or the hint of pleasure.

THE CHECK AND DRIVE SYSTEM

Another instance of the complexity of these inter-glandular reactions is furnished by the thyroid and the adrenals. The thyroid and the adrenals are mutually stimulating--when the thyroid oversecretes, the adrenal dittos, and vice versa. Yet they have directly opposed effects upon the economy--because they act upon antagonistic portions of the involuntary or vegetative nervous system, the system which is independent of the will. Before proceeding further, it is worth while sketching this division of the nervous system.

In the construction of a motor car from the point of view of absolute control of it at every moment, the first thought of the mechanic is an adequate *brake* and an efficient *regulator* of speed, instruments antagonistic, but necessary to work simultaneously or alternately. The involuntary or vegetative nervous system is built upon the same principle. It supplies every organ in the body beyond the control of the will (that is to say, the brain) with two sets of filaments which have opposing functions. One group of filaments in general increases or activates the function of the organ to which it is distributed. The other group of filaments, when tingling, inhibits or prohibits that function. They are like the two buttons on the wall which regulate the supply of electricity to incandescent bulbs, one switching on the current, the other switching it off. It has been agreed to call the stimulative or activating portion the autonomic or drive system. To its antagonist has been left the older name of the sympathetic or check system. It is because they do not both act upon these two components of the vegetative nervous system, but only upon one, that the thyroid and adrenal though in themselves complementary, come to exert opposite effects. For the internal secretion of the thyroid has a selective affinity for the autonomic or activating system, while that of the adrenals has a selective affinity for the sympathetic or inhibiting system.

In the stomach, for instance, extracts of the adrenal glands have been proved to intensify the function of the sympathetic or check system in different degrees, so that there is a lessening of the amount and acidity of the gastric fluid. On the other hand, thyroid extracts will intensify the action of the autonomic or drive system, so that the amount and acidity of the digestive juice is increased.

The stomach cell may, therefore, be regarded as a test-reagent for the different internal secretions, as they affect the check and drive systems.

These constitute an automatic device for regulating the activities of every organ. Three factors enter into the mechanism. One is the amount of the circulating internal secretions. Another is the organic and functional integrity of the nerve filaments comprising the check and drive systems. The third consists of the number and vitality and limitations of the terminal receiving cells acted upon by the nerve filaments, which in their turn have been acted upon by the internal secretions. Upon every organ, including the mind, through the brain, a stimulus from without or within will act according to its ability to influence one or others of these factors.

Normally, the check and drive systems are properly balanced. But under stress and strain the balance is upset. Indeed, the Kinetic Drive may be defined as a mechanism contrived in the course of evolution as the normal, healthy mode for meeting stress and strain. The Kinetic chain of organs, brain, adrenals, liver, thyroid and muscles, began working together in desperate situations for their possessor ages ago. Successful in helping him to survive, they have survived as a functional unit.

It was probably evolved in the Post-Tertiary Era, about twenty million years ago, when the coming of the carnivores introduced direct body-to-body conflicts, and their concomitants, a quick and versatile nervous system. During the Tertiary epoch the earth basked in the heat of a tropical sun nearly everywhere on its surface. The luxuriant vegetation of the torrid zone flourished and swarmed, for the temperature all over was what it is today at the equator. Gigantic vegetarians were the animals, creatures like the dinosaurs, enormous, gargoylean monsters, of an incredible size and strength, but clumsy and grotesque, with small brains and little intelligence. For what need was there for brain and intelligence when food lay about so abundantly at hand for them to gorge themselves. As there was no competition for food, there were no enemies.

Then as the earth evolved and grew cooler, vegetation failed, the ancestors of the present carnivora appeared, the fathers of the wolf and tiger, light, lithe and pugnacious, with senses acute and ferocious weapons of attack, who set out to destroy everybody. They destroyed pretty nearly all of the huge leaf-eating species, and only the more plastic and smaller ones, who were more keen-sensed and swift-footed (of whom the deer and antelope, horse and ox are the descendants), escaped. The smallest either took to the air to become the bat, or, like the forerunners of the squirrel and ape, took to the trees.

It was the coming of the carnivores, therefore, that accelerated the development of brain matter, and started the process which created man. But in the millions and millions of years of conflicts, instincts grew into being that sank deep into bone and marrow. The most fundamental reflexes, those immediate responses to irritation or danger, were laid down, and among them the drive and check system. When the animal had decided to fight its enemy or was forced to fight, or determined to prey, then was the time for the drive system to do its utmost to speed up everything that would help in the fight, while the check system came into play to hinder whatever would interfere or burden in the fray. First the drive mechanism must have been hit upon, and then the value of the check devices must have been found in fear and flight, and especially in hiding and simulation of death, when even breathing had to be inhibited. Until finally there developed, for everyday use, a complete check and drive nerve machinery for every organ, to be used according to the exigencies of the moment, with the thyroid as the primary stimulant and controller of the drive system and the adrenal as the primary dictator over the check system.

THE HARMONY OF THE HORMONES

All the glands, in fact, work in unison, with a distribution of the balance of power that diplomatists might envy. In the co-ordinating synchronism, the vegetative nervous system plays the part of an agent that acts as well as is acted upon. The chemical interaction of the internal secretions is not the only way in which they influence each other. For, as the case of the thyroid and the adrenal so well shows, secretions which, when directly interacting, are mutually reinforcing, when affecting nerves, may become clashing opponents.

The Kinetic Chain is about as good a case as there is of the glands of internal secretion co-operating. The Check and Drive systems, with the adrenals and thyroid opposed, are one of the best instances of their antagonisms. Besides, there are a number of other relationships between them that might be cited. They all bear with more or less pressure, positive or negative, upon the sex glands which will be considered in its place. If one wished to consider all the glands in their pro and anti relations, a separate volume would be required.

THE VEGETATIVE APPARATUS

The combination of the internal secretions and the vegetative system has been spoken of as the vegetative or autonomic apparatus. The vegetative apparatus is the oldest part of the nervous system. And some acquaintance with its constitution is necessary to any understanding of the possibilities of control of human nature.

For modern thought does not regard the brain as the organ of mind at all, but as one unit of a complex synthesis, of which mind is the product, and the vegetative apparatus is the major component. That involves the blasting of the last current superstition of the traditional psychology, the dogma that the brain is the exclusive seat of mind.

That an animal is a vast concourse of cells is one of the accepted fundamentals of biology. What is not so generally taken into consideration is that the assemblage is formed by the agglutinations of millions of years, and that it is hence composed of parts of different ages and pedigrees, some exceedingly ancient and hoary, some middle-aged, and some relatively new and recent. In the invertebrates, who date further back in the history of the planet than any vertebrate, the nervous system consists of discrete patches of nerve cells, the ganglions composing the ganglionic system of which the vegetative or autonomic nervous system of man is the direct descendant and representative. The brain and central nervous system are definitely later acquisitions, imposed upon the original stratum of the check and drive machine.

The primitive chassis of the mechanism, so to speak, is the so-called vegetative nervous system. Grouped with that system are the primeval breathing, feeding and reproducing inventions, the viscera boxed up in the chest and abdomen. The third partner is the glands of internal secretion, which act upon the viscera both directly and indirectly through the check and drive effect upon the vegetative nerves. The glands are like tuning keys, by which certain strings in the instrument may be tightened, so that its vibratory activity is increased, or they may be loosened, the vibrations decreased, the activity lessened. Tuning up the motors is a constant process in the organism. Finally, there are the large nerve masses at the base of the brain known as the basal ganglia, which contain the nerve centers for the co-ordination of the other three. All these together constitute the oldest family of the corporate organism. Beside them, the brain and the face and the prehensile organs are mere parvenus.

THE OLDEST PART OF THE MIND

Granted, then, that this vegetative apparatus is the most deeply rooted core of our being. What warrant is there for the grandiloquence of the phrase: the Oldest part of the Mind? There is, indeed, room for rhetoric, even poetry, here. For all the evidence points to it as the rightful occupant of the throne upon which Shelley placed his Brownie as the Soul of the Soul. Or to put it in another way, we think and feel primarily with the vegetative apparatus, with our muscles, especially the involuntary, with our viscera, and particularly with our internal secretions. Whenever there is thought and feeling, there is movement, commotion, precedent and concomitant, among these. They are the oldest seats of feeling, thought and will and continue to function as such.

Just what evidence is there for this conception? In the first place, there is the fascinating story of the origin of vertebrates from invertebrates of the sea scorpion or spider type. Then there is a whole group of data which demonstrate that the primitive wishes which make up the content of a baby consciousness are determined, settled by states of relaxation or tension in different segments or areas of the vegetative apparatus. According to this, the brain enters as only one of the characters in the play of consciousness. It is just the organ of awareness by the organism of itself as an integer which must adjust itself to the specific condition within the disturbed vegetative apparatus. Consequently the brain emerges not as the master tissue, but as merely the servant of the vegetative apparatus.

Consciousness is a circuit. Swinging around in it are the wish-feelings generated by the vegetative dynamo. From each viscus, from the stomach and intestine, from the kidneys and bladder, from the liver and spleen, from the blood-vessels, from all the glands of external and internal secretion, there flow along the vegetative nerves, to and from the brain, energies of various qualities and intensities. All the members of the vegetative apparatus are more or less active, and so all our wishes are all more or less active. All our working hours we are aware of hunger, satiety or indifference, of a desire to empty the intestine or bladder, or of a lack of necessity of doing so, of a state of tranquillity of the blood-vessels and sweat glands, or of a perturbation of them, of a varying tensity of even the muscles that are, as we say, under the control of the will, of the state, in fact, of all the elements of the vegetative complex. The stream of feeling which constitutes the undertow of consciousness originates outside of the brain altogether, and is composed of currents arising from viscera, muscles, blood-vessels and glands.

Now the component currents are of different sizes and positions and variable degrees of warmth. That is another way of saying that whether or not a current is to become the center of the stream, or to approach it, or whether it is to be hot, cold, or tepid, depends upon the degree of activity of the various parts of the vegetative apparatus. A convenient name for this is ***tonus***. Tonus can be experimentally watched and measured. Thus hunger, the most primitive of the wish-feelings, has been found to be simultaneous with certain characteristic contractions of the stomach. Stop those contractions, and you stop the hunger. The contractions begin slowly and weakly, and no awareness of them occurs in the mind. As they grow stronger, consciousness becomes a sensation rather like an itch somewhere in the upper abdomen, and accompanied sometimes by a sense of general weakness. The vegetative activity going on as a current almost on the outside of the stream of feeling has swelled and warmed, and so forced itself, in a manner of speaking, into the center of the stream. Or if you will, the rest of the stream has to arrange itself around it as the center. A similar mechanism for the tonus of the other members of the vegetative system, and how they determine consciousness and behaviour is understandable. It has been shown that when the bladder tone and the intestinal tone are of a definitely measurable size, one has the desire to empty them. The same applies to the sex glands. The pressure within a viscus is dependent upon the ratio between the amount of contraction of the involuntary muscle in its walls, the external pressure, and the quantity of its distending contents, the internal pressure. The resultant quotient, the internal pressure divided by the external pressure, measures the intravisceral pressure. The primitive wish-feelings are the direct expressions of the various intravisceral pressures, or tones. The primitive soul is an awareness of the fused primitive wish-feelings of themselves as a whole, and of the struggle between them for recognition, isolation, and, as we say, satisfaction. This satisfaction consists in a degradation of the highest intravisceral pressure to a point at which some other intravisceral pressure becomes higher and therefore predominant.

PHYSICS OF THE WISH

Mind, consciousness, may then be portrayed as an ocean comprised of mobile current layers, complexes built up around the awareness of different intravisceral pressures. A shifting hierarchy of such pressures form the points of focusing of consciousness that result in conduct. Behaviour may be defined as the resultant of the organism's pressure against the environment's counter pressure until there is a sufficient reduction of the specifically exciting intravisceral pressure. Just as water flows to its own level, so will conduct flow to reduce intravisceral pressure to its own level. A physics of the soul comes into prospect, in which a mathematical analysis will state the process quantitatively in terms of some common unit of pressure.

Not only conduct, but also character, because it is past conduct repeated, associated, and fixed, will be so statable. For intravisceral tonus or pressure is not simply or only an acute or passing affair. There is for it a persistent or average figure, the so-called normal for it, below which or above which the acute situation will bring it. **Character** is a ***matter then of standards in the vegetative system***. Character, indeed, is an alloy of the different standard intravisceral pressures of the organism, a fusion created by the resistance or counter pressure of the obstacles in the environment. Character, in short, is the grand intravisceral barometer of a personality.

Thus the comfortable, healthy, happy, well-balanced, progressive, constructive, virile personality is one in whom there is a continuously harmonious reduction of the intravisceral pressures in the environment called society. For in a gregarious creature, like man, fellow beings are the most powerful determinants of negative and positive vegetative pressures. Not so well rounded are other types existing because of inferiorities or excesses of the standard visceral tone. There is, for instance, the sexually cold type, comfortable by creating for itself an anaphrodisiac environment composed of pressures that can be fitted into its own. Or there may be an insufficiency of standard pressure in the alimentary tract, and we have the ascetic, mal-nourished, striving, uplifting type. Different types will be made by the permutations and combinations of factors that determine the intravisceral pressure and the environmental, i.e., social resistances or counter pressures.

INTERNAL SECRETIONS DETERMINANTS OF VEGETATIVE PRESSURES

Now of all the different factors which determine the tones, that is to say, the internal pressures, of the various parts of the vegetative apparatus (including all structures not controlled by the will in the term), the internal secretions or hormones are by far the most important. This significance is conferred upon them because it is by their activities primarily that these pressures are produced, regulated, lowered and heightened; in short, controlled. We have seen how the thyroid and adrenal hold the reins of the drive or check systems in the vegetative apparatus. Together with the other ductless glands, they decide the advance or halt, forward or retreat, tension or relaxation, charge and discharge, of the visceral--involuntary muscle-- blood vessel combination which is at the core of life. Here again they emerge as the directorate.

Carlson, the Chicago physiologist, who probably knows more about being hungry than any other man on the planet, once demonstrated that the injection of an ounce or two of the blood, which means the internal secretion mixture, of a starving animal, into one not starving increased the signs of hunger and the accompanying hunger contractions of the stomach. There can be no doubt that hunger is the expression of a certain specific concentration of internal secretion or secretions in the blood. When the quantity, in the cycles of metabolism, becomes sufficiently great, it stimulates the stomach to contract in a way which augments the pressure within it to a point at which the feeling of hungriness, and the wish to satisfy it, or to get rid of it, becomes imperative, and the dominant of consciousness.

Without doubt the sexual cravings are likewise so determined. Sex libido is an expression of a certain concentration, a definite amount peculiar to the individual, of the substance manufactured by the interstitial cells, circulating in the blood. It arouses its effects probably by (1) increasing the amount of reproductive material in the sex glands in a direct chemically stimulating effect upon the germinative cells, and so raising the internal pressure within them, (2) stimulating the involuntary muscles within the walls and the canals of the sex glands, and so, by augmenting the tenseness of the muscles, elevating the total intravisceral pressure, (3) by a direct chemical and indirect nervous effect upon the brain, the muscles, the heart, as well as the other glands of internal secretion stimulating the organism as a whole. Though the isolation in pure form of the substance or substances involved has never been scientifically achieved, their inference is entirely justified. It is indeed the only comprehensible mechanism conceivable that will fit all the known facts about the matter. And even though the assertions of Brown-Sequard were only the exaggerations of a semi-charlatan, it is certain that some day in the near future the particular substance, that he claimed he had discovered, will be handed about in bottles for the inspection of the curious.

Besides thyroxin, adrenalin, and the libido-producing secretion of the interstitial cells, the substance produced by the paired glandlets, situated behind the thyroid, the parathyroids, have a profound influence upon the vegetative apparatus and the vegetative nervous system. These direct the lime exchanges within the cells of the organisms, including the nerve cells. It has been shown that lime is, relatively, a sedative to cells. It raises the threshold or strength of stimulus necessary to evoke a reaction. Removing the parathyroids means removing the lime barrier, for with their deficiency there is a change in, and then an escape, from the blood, of the lime, by way of the kidneys. The result is sometimes an enormous increase in the excitability of all the cells, and especially of the vegetative apparatus. What that means for the individual whose comfort depends upon a stability of the intravisceral tones and pressures may be readily imagined.

The pancreas likewise acts as a sedative to the vegetative apparatus. In particular, this applies to the sugar mechanism in the liver under the discipline of the check and drive organization. The adrenal and the pancreas are the direct antagonists in the struggle for control of sugar. Removal of the adrenals will cause a decrease in the amount of sugar in the blood, while removal of the pancreas will produce an increase. Excess of sugar in the blood may thus be concomitant with changes of character considered incorrigible.

In different locales of the vegetative apparatus, as indeed of the body in general, the directorate seems to be handed over to a committee of control, generally made up of two members working in opposing directions. Such a division of power in the general directorate is analogous to the small holding corporations which divide functions in, for example, the United States Steel Corporation. The relative ratios of tonus in these smaller internal secretion balances are of the utmost significance as causes of differences in the vegetative apparatus, which are the basis of differences in structure, power, and character between individuals.

THE GENERAL LAWS OF THE DIRECTORATE

Our knowledge of the glands of internal secretions as an interlocking directorate presiding over all the functions of the organism is still exceedingly meagre. As yet, we seem to be knocking at the portals of the chemistry of the imponderable. There are holes in the bronze doors, and we glimpse the unfathomable distances of unexplored regions. But we do see something, and we do glimpse a beginning. Already the outlines of a differential anatomy, and a different physiology and a differential psychology, which will explain to us the unique in the constitution, the temperament and character of an individual, emerge. It is worth while, before proceeding to the details, so valuable to a society which would become rational, to summarize the general principles emerging, expressing the directing powers of the ductless glands over the individual. *They may be regarded as the present postulates of a new science of the whys and wherefores separating and setting apart, as so recognizably distinct, those peregrinating chemical mixtures: men and women*.

1. The life of every individual, in every stage, is dominated largely by his glands of internal secretion. That is, they, as a complex internal messenger and director system, control organ and function, conduct and character. The orderliness of human life, in the sequential march of its episodes, crises, successes and failures, depends, to a large extent, upon their interactions with each other and with the environment.

2. One or several of the glands possesses a controlling or superior influence above that of the others in the physiology of the individual and so becomes the central gland of his life, its dominant, indeed, so far as it casts a deciding vote or veto, in its everyday existence and incidents as well as in its high points, the climaxes and emergencies.

3. These glandular preponderances are at the basis of personality, creating genius and dullard, weakling and giant, Cavalier and Puritan. All human traits may be

analyzed in terms of them because they are expressions of them.

4. Specific types of personality may be directly associated with particular glandular prominences, so that we have the thyroid-centered types, the pituitary-centered types, the adrenal-centered types, etc. These are the classic Three, the prototypes in their purity most easily described and recognized.

5. Combinations of these, as well as of other glands--with joint predominance--occur and indeed form the majority of populations. The phenomena of varieties in species are thus explained.

6. Internal secretion traits are inherited, and variations in heredity are essentially the structural representation of the resultant of a parallelogram of forces exerted by each of the parental prepotent glands. If they are of the same type, they may reinforce each other: if not, inhibitions and compensations will come into play. Mendelian laws may apply.

7. The process of evolution, as the play of natural selection upon these variations, becomes comprehensible from a new standpoint.

8. Certain diseases, and disease tendencies, both acute and constitutional, as well as traits of temperament and character, and predetermined reactions to certain recurring situations in life, are rooted in the glandular soils that compose the stuff of the individual.

9. The subconscious, of which the vegetative apparatus is the physical basis, leads back to the internal secretions for the profoundest springs of its secrets. We shall see how and why.

10. Given the internal secretory composition, so to speak, of an individual--his endocrine formula--and so his intravisceral pressures, one may predict, within limits, his physical and psychic make-up, the general lines of his life, diseases, tastes, idiosyncrasies and habits.

11. Within limits, if the previous history of an individual is known, his physical appearance may be approximately described, and his future outlined.

12. Conversely, given the physical and psychic composition of an individual, and his past history, one may deduce the internal secretion type to which he belongs.

Examples:

A. One Thyroid-centered Type has
   Bright eyes
   Good clean teeth
   Symmetrical features
   Moist flushed skin
   Temperamental attitude toward life
   Tendency to heart, intestinal and nervous disease

B. One Pituitary-centered Type
   Abnormally large or small size
   Musical--acute sense of rhythm
   Asymmetrical features
   Tendency to cyclic or periodic diseases

C. One Adrenal-centered Type
   Hairy
   Dark
   Masculinity marked
   Tendency to diphtheria and hernia

These are some of the master types. They have their variants depending upon the influences of the other glands, especially the interstitial cells of the sex glands.

ANTE-NATAL DEVELOPMENT

In their ensemble, the glands of internal secretion wield a determining influence upon the development of the individual from his very inception. If his various powers may be conceived of as an orchestra, they may be said to conduct it from the very beginning of its movements, and to cease only with its termination. From the moment when the spermatozoon penetrates and fecundates the ovum, the fate of the future being is settled by their disposition. The seal of his destiny is soaked with their substance.

POST-NATAL DEVELOPMENT

Every particle of protoplasm, every granule of the impregnated ovum carries the representatives of the parental ductless glands. As a consequence, they transmit chemically, with no figure of speech involved, the peculiar familial, racial and national characters from progenitors to offspring. They confer upon the child a number of the properties commonly recognized as inherited. All those features which distinguish Caucasian from Mongolian, Scandinavian from Italian, Italian from Jew are determined by them.

In short, at every step of his life, in every relation and association, in every expression of the inner forces that control his being, the normal individual is influenced by his internal secretions. Let us now see how.

CHAPTER V
HOW THE GLANDS INFLUENCE THE NORMAL BODY

The origin of the remarkable differences between individuals that distinguish species, varieties and families, has long been one of the chief puzzles of biology. It may indeed be called the leading puzzle, which led Darwin on to the collection of the data that culminated in the "Origin of Species." The why of the Unique is the fundamental problem of those who would understand life.

An explanation is an attempt at a consistent and persistent, sometimes an obstinate clarity of mind. A vast number of observations gathered by laboratory experimentalists as well as by those naturalists of the abnormal, physicians in active practice, prove that the construction of the individual both during development before maturity, and maintenance during maturity, his constitution, in short, is directed by the endocrine glands. It is possible now to present an explanation of the individuality of the individual.

To assert that variation is responsible for the individual, that it is the mechanism which isolates him as a being like none other of his fellows, not even his parents, brothers, and sisters, is merely to beg the question. What is variation? The internal secretion theory of the process offers, for the first time, an explanation that is coherent and comprehensive, based upon concrete and detailed observations. It provides an adequate interpretation of the numberless hereditary gradations and transitions, blendings and mixtures. It suggests a control of heredity in the future.

THE PURE TYPES

In the pure types, only one gland, either by being present in great excess above the average, or by being pretty well below the average, comes to exercise the dominating influence upon the traits of the organism. As the strongest link in the chain, or as the weakest, it rules. The others must accommodate themselves to it. Among them as commanders of growth, development and normal function, it holds the balance of power. In every emergency it stands out by its strength or by its weakness. It thus creates its own type of man or woman, with attributes and characteristics peculiar to itself. These pure types, as we have seen, are mainly the thyroid, the pituitary, and the adrenal-centered.

Each with the signs peculiar to it can be identified among the faces that pass one in the street. And they differ so markedly among themselves that they provide a new and accurate means of classifying varieties among the races of the species: man. The thyroid type differs as much from the adrenal type as does a greyhound from a bull-dog. The greyhound has a certain size, form, character and capacity. The bull-dog has similar qualities which are yet quite different. Each is built for a particular career. Among human beings, the pure thyroid type is easily distinguished from the pure adrenal type, and both of these from the pure pituitary type. Each is stamped with a significant figure, height, skin, hair, temperament, ambition, social reactions and predisposition to certain diseases.

THE MIXED TYPES

Among the mixed types, the lines of distinction are less clear, and so they are more difficult to classify. The mixed types may be said to be hyphenated. In them, two or even three of the internal secretory glands conflict for predominance. The combined action makes for a resultant modification in the primary glandular markings and effects. A hyphenated classification thus becomes inevitable. Especially is this so if the two glands are mutually antagonistic and inhibitory. A compromise effect is then necessitated. Or an individual may be dominated by one gland at one period of his life and by another at a later period. One of the glands, the thyroid, for example, will show, by the traces it has left upon the earliest developing features, that it was in control at the very earliest dates of his history, while other signs will disclose the more recent influence of the adrenal or of the pituitary. The combination becomes classifiable as the thyroid-pituitary type, or as the thyroid-adrenal type.

That the external features as well as the chronic diseases of human beings are controlled by some common factor has long been suspected. Inquiries into morbid phenomena with a hereditary trend yielded information that has paved the way for the internal secretion theory. It has long been known that certain diseases effect only certain individuals of a definite constitution. Apoplexy, diabetes, arteriosclerosis, Bright's disease, are met with almost exclusively in what the older clinicians talked about as the apopleptic type. On the other hand, they said, anemias, tuberculosis, hemophilias, scrofulas occurred more among the lymphatic type. But they had no idea whatever of the true functional basis of the two different types. The truth as we of today view it is that these two types represent different textures of human beings, fabricated of different internal secretions. They are really two different breeds of the species Homo Sapiens. The materials being different, the color and feel of them is different, and the resistance to wear and tear is different.

ENDOCRINE ANALYSIS

The modes of classification glimpsed at are certainly exceedingly broad and sweeping. It is well enough to establish types and classes. But beneath them are sheltered the infinite possibilities of permutations and combinations, which explain the countless variety and complexity of form and function. Every individual born among the vertebrates, for example, must have a certain definite amount and percentage of pituitary gland, anterior and posterior, pineal, thyroid, parathyroid, thymus, adrenal, pancreas, interstitial and so on. Now if, to state it in terms of percentages, for the sake of argument, the pituitary is 25, the pineal 10, the thyroid 36, the parathyroids 15, the thymus 29, the adrenals 60, the pancreas 49, the interstitials 72 (the gland when acting maximally to be graded as 100), we see at once how different such an individual must be from one who has, say, pituitary 84, pineal 39, thyroid 26, parathyroid 42, adrenals 96, pancreas 22 and interstitials 89. One obtains at once from the contrasts of such figures some idea of the possibilities. As each point plus or minus must count to produce some difference in the individual, the results are manifest. Varying within the numerical limits imposed by genus, species, variety and family (which limits are probably responsible for the persistence of the particular genus, species, variety, or family) the individual becomes an individual because of the relative values of the percentages in his blood and tissues of these different internal secretions. We thus begin to gain an insight into the patterns according to which men, women and animals are woven.

We are, as yet, far from an exact endocrine analysis of the individual. But we know that the endocrines rule over growth and nutrition, a vast dominion which incorporates every organ and every tissue. By enhancing or retarding the nutritional changes, the growth of the organ or tissue is favored or restricted. The size and shape of an individual, as a whole, as well as of the specialized cell masses composing him, as hands and feet, the nose and ears, and so on, are therefore controlled by them. Whether an organism is to be tall or short, lean or corpulent, graceful or awkward, is decided by their interactions. These, like human covenants, vary with the different reactions of the parties to the contract. And so a great deal depends upon whether they work harmoniously or discordantly, and upon which does the most work and which the least.

Undersecretion and Oversecretion

It is when a gland, either in the course of development, or because of the influence of starvation, shock, injury, poisoning or infection, begins to undersecrete or oversecrete that its effects upon growth and nutrition become grossly manifest. A veritable transfiguration of the individual may occur, the black magic of which may perplex him for a lifetime. A man, made eunuchoid by an accident or by mumps, will observe in himself astonishing changes in his constitutional make-up, mentality and sexuality. He would be more astounded to learn that beneath the appearances, the changes, so alarming him, there are profound alterations in the rate at which he is taking in oxygen, burning up sugar, accumulating carbon dioxide and excreting waste byproducts through the kidneys, which are responsible for them.

The differences between the normal and abnormal are only a matter of degree. And so, to be sure, are differences between types. But it is hard to realize that the striking distinctions between the thyroid type and the pituitary, comparable, as said, to the differences between a greyhound and a bull-dog, are dependent solely upon quantitative variations in the general and local speeds of metabolism, among the cells.

DIVISION OF LABOR

Besides the antagonisms and co-operations between them, there are certain lines along which the glands, in their effects, specialize. The thyroid, for instance, is concerned specially with the regulation of the shape, form and finish of an organ. The pituitary shines at the periods of developmental crises, determining them and modifying them. It exerts the greatest influence upon the time of eruption of the teeth, both the temporary and the permanent, the onset of puberty, the recurrence of menstruation in women, and the time of occurrence of labor. The interstitial glands distribute the basis of the powers and limitations of masculinity and femininity. Abnormalities of these glands also affect the individual all along the line, in all of his aspects. So affected he may apparently change into a wholly different being. He may change in size, in the shape of his head, feet and hands, as well as in his habits, aptitudes and dispositions. So he may find it necessary to purchase an entirely different size of hat, more commodious clothes, and newly fitting gloves and shoes. At the same time, his family, relatives and friends, discover that the erstwhile generous, frank, neat and punctual and liked, has become stingy and suspicious and slovenly and hated. And all because a gland has begun to undersecrete or to oversecrete. The transformation will be slight or marked, depending entirely upon the extent of impairment, positive or negative, of the gland involved.

But it is not only in the shaping of the normal individual's architecture that the internal secretions dominate. Over that subtle something known in all languages as vitality, expressive of the intensity of feeling, thought and reactions in cells, they rule supreme. Gay vivacity and grim determination, the temperament of a Louis XIV, and the soul of a Cromwell, are the crystallizations of these chemical substances acting upon the brain.

INTERNAL SECRETION VARIETIES

There is no better way of illustrating the influence of the internal secretions upon the normal than the analysis of the variation of traits with variations in glandular predominances. The general build of an individual, his skeletal type, the proportion between the size of his arms and that of his legs, as well as that between his trunk and his lower extremities, whether he is to be tall, lanky and loutish, or short, squat and dumpy, are to be considered. Different facial types are the expressions of underlying endocrine differences. The head and skull offer a number of clues to the controlling secretions in the blood and tissues. Whether the forehead is to be broad or narrow, the distance between the eyes, the character of the eyebrows, the shape and size and appearance of the eyes themselves, the mould of the nose and jaws and the peculiarities of the teeth, are all so determined. The skin, in its color, texture, the quantity and distribution of its fatty and other constituents, eruptions and weather reactions, is influenced. Also the mucous membranes, the color and lustre and structure of the hair, as well as its general distribution and development, are hieroglyphics of the endocrine processes below the surface. Whether the muscles are massive or sparse, atrophied or hypertrophied, soft or hard, easily fatigable or not, bespeak conditions in the glandular chain. In short, we must regard the individual as an immensely complicated pattern of designs traced by the hormones as the primary etchers of his development. Though it must be admitted that the number of unknown and unsolved relations in the pattern are still enormously great, enough has been established to make possible a rough working analysis of the particular, unique organism placed before us for examination as Mr. Smith, Mrs. Jones, or Miss Smith-Jones.

WHAT IS THE NORMAL?

Anthropologists, from the beginning of anthropology, have battled in vain for a satisfactory inclusive definition, or, at least, description of the normal. With the introduction of the biometric method, the goal at last appeared within sight. A cocked hat curve expressing the distribution and range of the normal looks formidable. The attainable turned out a mirage, for the curves constructable by the measurement of traits of a population only proved the truth of the old axiom that all transitions and variations between extremes exist. The Problem of the Normal seemed more elusive than ever. And the best that could be done for the elucidation of its mystery, was to apply and observe the law of averages.

From the endocrine standpoint, the reason for this becomes clear. The biometric method concerned itself with externals, with, as it were, symptoms. Since these external signs are but manifestations of the inner chemical reactions, of which the internal secretions are the determining reagents, or factors, with permutations and combinations possible in all directions, the diversity and variability of each individual and his traits stands explained and understandable. The normal, as the perfect or nearly perfect balance of forces in the organism, at any given moment, emerges as a more definite and real concept than that which would abstract it from a curve of variations. Moreover, since the directive forces within the organism are pre-eminently the internal secretions, the normal becomes definable as their harmonious balancing or equilibrium, a state which tends not to undo (as the abnormal does) but to prolong itself.

The potential combinations and compensations, antagonisms and counteractions, attainable within the endocrine glands as an interlocking directorate, point the cause for the elusive quality of the normal. Tall men and short men, blonde women and dumpy women, lanky hatchet-faced people, stout moon-faced people, Falstaff and Queen Elizabeth, George Washington and Abraham Lincoln, Disraeli and Walt Whitman, Caesar and Alexander, as well as Mr. Smith and Miss Jones come within the range of the normal. There are all kinds and conditions and sorts of men and women, and all kinds and sorts and conditions of the normal, because an incalculable number of harmonious relations and interactions between the endocrines are possible, and do actually occur. The standard of the normal must obviously not be a single standard, but a series of standards, depending upon which glands predominate, and how the others adapt themselves to its predominance. Adrenal-centered types, thyroid-centered types, pituitary-centered types, thymus-centered types, as well as hyphenated compounds of these, such as the pituitary-adrenal types, exist as normals. They can be conceived of as normal types because they exist as normal types.

THE SKELETAL TYPES

Now men, for as long as we have any knowledge of their thoughts and classifications and attitudes, have been accustomed to first think of one another, to classify and size one another as tall or short, slender or broad, thin or corpulent. The biological necessity, indeed, instinct of the one animal to relate the other animal to aggressive or harmless agencies in his surroundings, accounts for this. Relatively, of course, for all these modes of description imply offensive or defensive possibilities of the stimulus for the recorder in relation to himself. The interest in stature is fundamental, and has persisted in the most civilized, nations. The relationship of height and weight, as well as of length and breadth, to other physical traits, have formed the subject of scientific study. There is, for instance, the classification of Bean, who divided mankind generally into two types, those of a medium size, stocky long legs and arms, large hands and feet, short trunk, and face large in comparison to the head (the meso-onto-morphs) and those who were either tall and slender, or small and delicate, with the smaller face, eyes close together, long, high, narrow nose, and trunk longer as compared with the extremities (the hyper-onto-morphs). Bean showed, too, that the hypers (to use a short word to contrast with the mesos) were present to the extent of almost a hundred per cent in a series of tuberculosis, and about ninety per cent in a series of central nervous system disease. All of which is exceedingly interesting and suggestive, but throws no light upon the underlying mechanisms of statures.

STATURE AND GROWTH

Stature is essentially determined by the growth of the long bones. They are the pace-makers, and the muscles and soft tissues follow the pace they set. Now the primary determinant, catalyst or sensitizer of the growth of the long bones is the anterior pituitary. All statures should therefore be first scrutinized from the point of view of the pituitary. Individuals over six feet tall or under five feet five inches should be looked upon as having a pituitary trend. This pituitary trend may be primary, due to its own undergrowth or overgrowth, or it may be due to lack of inhibition from the sex glands such as occurs in eunuchs and eunuchoids, or excessive or premature inhibition from them as happens in certain salacious dwarfs.

The long bones grow at a point of junction between the bone proper and an overlying layer of gristle or cartilage, known as the zone of ossification. It is upon this zone of ossification that the various growth influences appear to focus and concentrate their efforts, among them the internal secretions. After growth has been finished, that is, after adolescence, these zones of ossification close, so that growth is no longer possible unless they become reactivated. Upon the zone of ossification must act the pituitary, and indirectly the thyroid, the interstitial cells, the thymus and the adrenals. Individuals oversized or undersized either belong to the pituitary type, or if hyphenated, have the pituitary as one of the dominants in their composition. The necessities of child-bearing determine a greater angle between trunk and lower extremities in the female. Underactivity of the pituitary, for instance, will prevent the development of the normal angle. The ratio in length of the upper limbs to the lower is a fairly constant relationship for each sex normally Deviations occur with a break somewhere in the chain of cooperation of the internal secretions controlling the growth of bone.

HANDS, FINGERS AND TOES

The size and shape and general configuration of the hands, fingers and toes are details that tell an endocrine tale. Students of hands naturally have grouped them as the long slender and the short, broad, the bony and the well-filled out, the tapering fingers and the stumpy. The character of a hand is determined anatomically by the length and breadth of the bones, the amount and distribution of fat, and the thickness and elasticity of the skin. Over these, the essential control lies in the pituitary and the thyroid. So we find that pituitary types have, when there is oversecretion, large bony, gross hands, spade-shaped, or when there is undersecretion, hands that are plump, with peculiarly tapering fleshy fingers. The hyperthyroid has long slender fingers, the subthyroid pudgy, coarse, ugly foreshortened hands, often cold, and bluish.

FACIAL TYPES

An artist will see in a face the past history of generations, a narrative of the adventures of the blood, a record of tears and smiles, wrinkles and dimples, the victories and defeats of buried drudgery and romance. These signatures which the Faculty of Life have scribbled or engraved over it as upon a diploma, bespeak for him spiritual moments. To the student of the internal secretions the lines, expressions, attitudes are important for they tell of the state of tensions and strains in the vegetative apparatus with which they are inseparably connected. It is when one comes to the consideration of the face as a complex of brows, eyes, nose, lips and jaws that he becomes most interested. For in the modeling and tone of every one of the features each of the endocrine glands has something to say. In consequence there has been described the hyperpituitary face, and the hyperthyroid face, the subthyroid face and the subpituitary face, the adrenal face, the eunuchoid face and the ovarian face and also the thymic.

To bring to mind an immediate complete image of the hyperthyroid face, one should think of Shelley. The oval shape of it, with the delicate modeling of all the features, the wide, high brow, the large, vivacious, prominent eyes with the glint of a divine fire in them and the sensitive lips all belong to the classical picture. Generally flushed over the cheek-bones, there is undoubtedly a certain effeminate effect associated with it. At least, it is the least animal and brutish of the faces of man.

On the other hand, the subthyroid face is that of the cretin and cretinoid idiot, in a mild degree. So characteristic that we recognize the portrait in the descriptions of Pliny in early Roman tunes and of Marco Polo in his Asiatic travels. Coarseness, dullness, pudginess are its keynotes. Irregular features, tendency to wide separation of the eyes and pug nose, sallow, puffy complexion, waxy thickened nose and eyelids, deep-set, listless, lacklustre eyebrows, and thick prominent lips comprise the catalogue of the physiognomy. On the whole, the sort of face one passes in the street as stupid and common. But there are a number of fascinating and marvelous varieties of the stupid and common.

The adrenal face is most often dark or freckled. It tends to be irregularly broadish. It is hairy, one is struck forcibly. There is a low hair line, which makes the brow appear rather low, and there is a good deal of hair over the cheek bones. The adrenal type is round headed.

The face of the hyperpituitary is striking and pretty sharply defined. It is long and narrow, with a tendency to prominence of the bony parts. Square, protruding jaw, high, thin, straight nose, emphasized eyebrows, and marked cheek-bones, comprise the leading points in its composition. On the other hand, the subpituitary is more rounded and trends toward the full moon effect, the chin recedes, the cheek-bones are buried under fat, the nose spreads more and is flatter. In its general expression, there is a complacence and tranquillity which is often mistaken for sleepiness, and often actually is dullness.

The eunuchoid face is usually fat with puffy eyelids. The skin is smooth and cool, marble-like often, poor in pigment and color. Sometimes it is sallow, wrinkled and senile in a man in his early twenties. At others, it is distinctly feminine in its hairlessness, and the delicate texture of the skin, as well as in the clean-cut patterning of the features. Every gradient between premature senility and sex inversion is encountered.

The thymic face frequently stamps its possessor at sight. Its owner has a smooth, soft skin, with little or no hair, and a dead white or "peaches-and-cream" complexion. One wonders, when unacquainted with the type, who the man's barber is, or where he learned to shave himself so well. It may be curiously velvety to the touch and swept by a faint sheen. Among children occur the most exquisite samples of the kind designated as the angelic child. The face is finely moulded and beautifully proportioned, features artistically chiselled, eyes blue or brown with long lashes, cheeks transparent with rapid, fleeting variations in coloring, thin lips, and oval chin. In the adult, the chin is receding, and the mouth seems underdeveloped in one variety.

THE TEETH

As closely connected with the internal secretions as are the bones of the face and the skull are the teeth. Tooth formation is essentially a modified bone formation. And as the bones of the face are influenced, so are the teeth influenced. But as each tooth is a miniature organ, inspectable by the eye as a unit, the action of the ductless glands is more obviously reflected for the observer to read. By their teeth shall ye know them. Upon the whole history of the evolution of each tooth, in the growth of the dental follicle and its walls, the fruition of the dentinal germ, the making of the enamel organ, the dental pulp, the cementum and the peridental membrane, the endocrines leave their mark.

There are certain general statements about the teeth and the internal secretions that can be made. The teeth of the thyroid types are pearly, glistening, small and regular; in other words, the teeth to which poets have devoted sonnets. The pituitary types have teeth that are large and square and irregular, with prominence of the middle incisors, and a marked separation or crowding of them. The interstitial types have small irregular upper teeth, with turned, stumpy or missing lateral incisors. The thymus types have youthful, milky white teeth that are thin and translucent, and scalloped or crescentic at the grinding edge. The teeth of the adrenal type are all well-developed, tend to have a yellowish color, with a reddish tinge to the grinding surfaces.

The degree and regularity of development of the middle upper cutting, biting teeth, as distinguished from the grinding molars, the middle and lateral incisors, and the canines offer further guides to the endocrine constitution analysis. The size of the central incisors seems to be directly proportional to the degree of pituitary predominance. On the other hand, the size and regularity of the lateral incisors seem proportional to the influence of the interstitial cells. When these are inferior in the make-up of an individual, the lateral incisors are nearly always distorted. The size of the canines appears to be a measure of adrenal activity. Long sharply pointed canines mean well-functioning adrenal gland equipment to start in with, inherited from a bellicose progenitor.

No individual peculiarities of the teeth are accidental. Just as the absence of hair on the face in a man or a moustache effect in a woman stand for some definite stress or strain in the mechanics of interaction of the internal secretions, so likewise do variations in dentition, as to the time of eruption of the teeth, their position and quality, and their resistance to decay.

Proper balance between the thymus and pituitary will permit the eruption of the teeth within the normal time limits, both the milk teeth and the permanent teeth. When there is equilibrium between the pituitary and the gonads, the teeth will be regular in shape and position. Carious teeth, in children and adults, sometimes indicate endocrine imbalance. Thyroid and adrenal balance determines the resistance to decay of the molars. Early decay of the molars in children is significant of insufficiency of the thyroid. When the first permanent molar, which should appear in the upper arch in its usual position between the sixth or eighth years, does not, there has been a prenatal disturbance of the pituitary, according to Chayes and others. Rapid decay of the teeth in childhood should always call attention to the parathyroids.

In pregnancy, the teeth suffer particularly because of disturbances of the endocrines. The saying, "A tooth for every child," is said to have its equivalent in every language. The bicuspids and second permanent molars erupt around puberty, when profound readjustments are going on among the glands of internal secretion. They consequently suffer with their abnormalities or divergences from type. The teeth thus furnish a good deal of information concerning the distribution of the balance of power among the hormones.

THE SKIN

The skin is influenced in its color, moisture, hairiness, texture, fat content and disease vulnerability by the endocrines. The question of color is very interesting, for it is probably the expression of the blending action of the different internal secretions. Davenport, the American student of heredity and eugenics, has shown that neither white nor black skins are either perfectly white or perfectly black, but are mixtures in various proportions of black, yellow, red and white. The exact percentages of the pigments in each particular skin, can be determined by means of a rotating disc. Thus a white person's skin may have the following composition:

Black 8% Red 50%

Yellow 9% White 33%

The composition of the skin of a very black negro may be:

Black 68% Red 26%

Yellow 2% White 7%

Now the fact that in Addison's disease in which the adrenals are destroyed there occurs a coincident increase in the black in the skin, and other evidence pointing to adrenal implication in dark complexioned white people, as well as in those possessing pigmented spots, seems to indicate the adrenals as controllers of the black and white factors. Davenport has concluded that there are two double factors for black pigmentation in the full-blooded negro which are separately inheritable. The determinants of the red and yellow have still to be worked out.

The moistness of the skin, as perspiration, depends upon the number and activity of the sweat glands. It varies with the water content of the body, the state of the vegetative nervous system, and the body temperature. Thus the skin of the hyperthyroid and the subadrenal is soft and moist, because of their antagonistic effects upon the sympathetic system. The subthyroid and the hyperadrenal have dry and harsh skins for the same reason, if no other glands intervene. However, in both of the latter, if there is a persistent thymus, the skin will retain the bland quality of adolescence.

There is a curious variation among the different internal secretion types in the reaction of the skin to stroking. When the skin, especially the skin over the shoulders, the breasts and the abdomen, is stroked with some blunt object, the blood vessels react either by a greater filling up or emptying of themselves. The latter occurs most regularly in the subadrenal types, the former in the hyperthyroid. Both forms of reaction run parallel to the different check or drive effects of the vegetative apparatus. With too much drive, that is, too much thyroid, there is the flushing reaction; with too little check, that is, with too little adrenal, there is the whitening. These differences probably explain the emotional reactions of the face. In anger, for example, some people become a dead white, others a fiery red. Whether one will do one or the other may depend upon the relative predominance of the thyroid or of adrenal in the individual.

In the distribution of fat beneath and throughout the skin all of the endocrine glands appear to have a voice. The typically hyperthyroid and hyperpituitary individuals tend to be thin, as well also as those who have well-functioning or excessively functional interstitial cells. In all of these the administration of the respective internal secretions increases the burning up of material in the body, and all of them have a higher rate of tissue combustion than their confreres, with a subthyroid or subpituitary keynote in their cell chemistry, or with insufficient interstitial cell action. Generally the latter have a very dry skin, the former a moist skin. With delayed involution of the pineal, obesity results.

The elasticity of the skin is another quality that varies with the concentration in the blood of the internal secretions. Elasticity of the skin, its recoil upon being stretched like a rubber band, may be taken as a measure of the activity of all the endocrine glands. For, as can be noticed especially upon the back of the hand, the older a man grows, the less elastic becomes the skin. In older people, raising the skin upon the back of the hand will cause it to stand up as a ridge for a few seconds and then slowly to return to the level of the surrounding skin. Whereas in a youthful person it will quickly snap back into place. This quality of elasticity of the skin is due to the presence in it of the so-called yellow elastic fibres, cell products, with a resilience greater than anything devised by man. The preservation of the resilience is a function of the internal secretions. Thus, after loss of the thyroid, the ridging effect characteristic of senility can be produced in one young as measured by his years. It has been said that a man is as old as his arteries, and also that as he is as old as his skin. It might better be said that he is as old as his elastic tissue, young when he is rich in it, old when poor and losing it. And as elastic tissue and internal secretions stand in the relation of created and creators, or at least preserved and preservers, a man may be said to be as old, that is as young, fresh and active as his ductless glands.

THE HAIR

There is no characteristic of the human body, except perhaps the teeth, more influenced in its quality, texture, amount and distribution than the hair. And again, each of the glands of internal secretion plays a part, but most importantly the thyroid, the suprarenal cortex and the interstitial sex glands. All contribute their specific effect, and the blend, the sum of the additions and subtractions constituting their influences, appears as a specific trait of the individual, a trait so significant as to be used by the professionals absorbed in the study of man, the anthropologists, as a criterion of racial classifications.

Some acquaintance with the history of the normal growth of hair is necessary to its understanding. There develops during the life of the fetus within the womb a curious sort of wooly hair everywhere over the entire body (excepting the palms and soles which remain hairless throughout life), remarkably soft and fluttery--the lanugo. At about the eighth month of intra-uterine existence, a good deal of this lanugo is lost, to be replaced on the head and eyebrows by a crop of thick, coarse, pigmented real hair. So it happens that at birth the infant's hair is a queerly ir-regular growth, a mixture of what is left of the general lanugo development, and the localized patches of the more human hair. Until puberty this children's hair re-mains the same, although at times, particularly after dentition, and after infectious diseases which undoubtedly alter the relations of the internal secretions, changes of color and texture occur. Then, with sexual ripening, there appear in males the so-called terminal hairs, over the cheeks and lips and chin, and, in both sexes, in the folds under the shoulders and over the lower abdomen, the hair which might be distinguished as the sex hair in contradistinction to the juvenile hair of the head, the extremities and the back.

Now the smoothness of the face in children is connected with the activity of the thymus and pineal glands. Among individuals in whom the juvenile thymus persists after puberty, no growth of hair occurs on the face, and in precocious invo-lution or destruction of the pineal, hair appears on the face and in other terminal regions in children of six or less, a symptom classical in the child who suffered from a tumor of the pineal, and discussed immortality with his physicians. It is probable that these thymus and pineal effects are indirect through their action upon the sex glands. For in the types with persistent juvenile thymus there occurs a maldevel-opment of the sex glands, while in those with early pineal recession the sex glands bloom simultanously with the appearance of adolescent hair and mental traits. The hastening of sexual hair by tumors of the adrenal gland may also be put down to a release from restraint of the interstitial sex cells.

There are certain spheres in the hair geography of the body, over which partic-ular glands may be said to rule or to possess a mandate. The hair of the head seems to be primarily under the control of the thyroid. Thus in cretins reconstructed by thyroid feeding, the straight, rather animal hair becomes lustrous and fine, silken and curly. In the thyroid deficiency of adults, a prominent phenomenon often is the falling out of the hair in handfuls. Baldness is frequently associated with a progres-sive decrease of the concentration of thyroid in the blood. At the same time, there tends to be a thinning of the eyebrows, especially of the outer third.

The hair of the face in males, and the other terminal hairs in both males and females, is regulated by the sex glands primarily. In the female, the ovary, that is to say, the interstitial cells of the ovary, inhibit the growth of hair upon the face. In destructive disease of the ovaries, as well as in other affections of it, hair in the form of moustache, beard and whiskers may appear in female. That is why in women after the grand sex change of life, the menopause, hair often grows in the typically male regions because of loss of the inhibiting influence of the ovarian internal secretion upon them. After castration of the ovaries, the same may result. Removal of the male sex glands, or disturbances of them, will interfere with the proper development of the normal facial hair. Of the hair of the chest, the abdomen and the back, the adrenals seem to be the controllers. Adrenal types have hairy chests in males, and hair on the back in females. They have also a good deal of hair upon the abdomen. The hair on the extremities varies a good deal with the pituitary. People with hair upon hands, arms and legs, alone, are generally pituitary, or have a striking pituitary streak in their make-up.

When the adrenals increase in size in childhood, a remarkable triad follows--general hairiness, adiposity and sexual precocity. One fact should be noted. When the adrenals evoke precocity, and an early awakening of the secondary sex characteristics, it is a masculine precocity, and an approximation to the masculine even in females. There is a definite trend toward an increase of the male in the individual's composition at the expense of the female. We shall have to consider this in greater detail when we analyze the internal secretion basis of masculinity and femininity. In general, the degree of general hairiness is an index to the amount of adrenal influence upon the organism. All the endocrines which affect the hair growth also act upon the sebaceous glands which oil the skin.

THE EYES

Eyes present clues to internal secretion constitutions dependent upon influences of architecture and function. The thyroid eye is typical. It is large, brilliant and protruding. The individual is "pop-eyed." On the other hand, subthyroidized eyes tend to be sunken and lustreless. The eyes of a pituitary type are either set markedly apart, or close together, with the hair at the root of the nose so prominent as to constitute a separate bridge known as the nasal brow. The size of the pupil, and its humidity, which have so much to do with the expression of the eye, vary directly with the activities of the driving and checking divisions of the vegetative system, and are a pretty good index as to which, at the time of observation, is predominant. When the check system is in control, the pupils are large and dilated. When its antagonist and rival, the drive system, is on top, the pupils are small and contracted. The reactions of the pupils when charged by strong emotion, like fear or anger, likewise turn upon the status of check or drive internal secretions in the economy of the organism at the time the exciting agent presents itself.

MUSCLES

It would seem, at first sight, that organs like muscles, mechanical instruments for the manipulation of the organism in space, would be more or less independent of the subtler processes of internal chemistry of the blood and tissues. But no assumption would be more beside the mark. Just as much as the bones and viscera, the teeth and the hair, they show grossly how they are being influenced by all the endocrine glands. So thyroid types generally have a skeleton sparsely covered with a muscular mantle. Pituitary types have large well-developed muscles. The pineal gland has some definite relation to muscle chemistry not yet probed. Thus, it has been shown that when the pineal has been completely destroyed prematurely by lime deposits in it, there is concomitant a wasting of muscles in places. This waste is sometimes replaced by fat. Pictures and images in wood and stone of these muscle freaks dating from the fifteenth, sixteenth, and seventeenth century are in existence. Then there is the extraordinary fatigability of the muscles which occurs in the thymus types, who nevertheless have large well-rounded muscles, a paradox of contradiction between anatomy and physiology. Such a type, for instance, may be picked out by a football coach for an important position in a line-up, simply on the tremendous impressiveness of the muscle make-up, only to see him bowled over and out in the first scrimmage. The tone of muscles, the quality of resisting firmness or yielding softness, is essentially determined by the adrenal glands, especially in time of stress and strain.

Brown-Sequard was the first to show that extracts of sex glands could increase the capacity for muscular work. Whether this was a direct effect upon the muscles, or indirect through the nerves or other endocrines, no one can say. Certainly the carriage of an individual, outer symptom of the inner tonus among his muscles and tendons, may be said to be as distinctively an endocrine affair as the color of his skin. And like its variations, variations of their tone, development, reactivity, fatigability, and endurance may be traced to corresponding states of overaction, or underaction, and odd combinations of the different hormones. Much remains to be learned about them and the manner of their control. Such an affliction as flatfoot, dependent upon a laxity of the ligaments in one who seems perfectly healthy and strong, may lead the analyst back to a thymus-centered personality. That is but one example.

Since, too, muscle attitudes, muscle tensions and muscle relaxations play so large a part in the production of fundamental mental states: the attitudes, moods, memories and will reactions, the vegetative apparatus enters, to play its part as a determinant.

SEX

Over no domain of the body have the endocrines a more absolute mandatory than over that of the whole complex of sex. Both as regards the primary reproductive organs, their size and shape, and the character of their implantation, malformations and anomalies, as well as the physical and mental traits lumped as the secondary sexual, puberty, maturity, and senility, voice changes and erotic trends, virility and femininity, the internal secretions are dictators at every step. So significant are these, that even a rough summary of the discoveries and the outlook in the field involves some consideration of the details.

CHAPTER VI
THE MECHANICS OF THE MASCULINE AND THE FEMININE

I t needs a poet to chant the epic of sex. The mystery of it puzzled the minds of the earliest Sumerian thinkers. As a source of deepest excitement, it generated the most revolting ceremonies, bizarre customs, astounding cruelties and incomprehensible stupidities of the race. Men and women, as soon as they have done with their usual business of keeping themselves free of disagreeable sensations, hunger, cold, fear of enemies, betake themselves to it as a primary interest all over the world. The most advanced psychologists of the day link the sex impulse with the windings and twistings of all human activity.

Yet the Homer of sex through the ages is still to come. But at all times the mystery evoked speculation and attempt at explanation. Acting upon their theories as to the nature and function of sex, men have, ever since the passing of the primeval matriarchates, segregated women, equalized them, worshipped them, or enslaved them. Opinions have varied from ancient national aphorisms to the effect that women have no souls to the most ultramodern utterances of biologist-publicists that the differences between men and women are the differences between two species. There are other epigrams, vast sweeping generalities, extant concerning the nature of sex, and women particularly. All partake of the complexity of truth and therefore own a certain validity. Still, since as a matter of fact, these items have been based upon superficial observations colored by the tradition and verbiage of the milieu, they are valuable more as human documents, as material for the psychologist, than as scientifically obtained data, able to stand unblinking before the rays of the critical searchlights.

SCIENCE VS. ART

Not that all the vast accumulation needs to be thrown pell-mell, higgledy-piggledy into the discard. The love lyrics of the poet, the magic of the emotions of Shelley and Poe, for instance, with their marvelous music and exquisite intonings of feeling, furnish us with important information. They are the facts of the sex life, as much as the song of the nightingale, or the mocking laughter of the cuckoo pursued by its mate. So Sappho and Elizabeth Browning, to take only two samples, have contributed some of the feminine reaction. The erotic motive in literature has but paralleled the erotic motive in life, with all of its vagaries, delusions, confusions, ecstasies and suffering.

We have had concerning sex not knowledge, but a series of attitudes, the attitude of virtue, the attitude of pruriency, the attitude of good taste, the attitude of the theoretic libertine, the attitude of the satyr's vulgarity. All these poses, of course, have supplied not an iota to an understanding of the foundations of the problems of sex, biologically considered. Thus, a masculine master has coined that immortal phrase, the Eternal Feminine. And in a matriarchate we should undoubtedly hear of the Eternal Masculine. Each leaves one as unenlightened as the other. A rough and ready code of life attributes certain grossly characteristic qualities of mind and body to each sex. This is supposed to be enough for common sense. Beyond that the mystery has been wrapped in cotton wool. That perhaps explains the enormous popularity of contemporary pornographic and so-called sex literature.

There are bound up with sex feeling and sex knowledge many customs, beliefs and habits, many legal statutes and social institutions, in the complex that is called sentiment, to which science looms as the sacrilegious ogre who devours romance. Without spending space upon the ravages of the sentimental idealist, certainly responsible for as much human disaster as the brutal realist, it is manifest that a revolution in sex standards and relations is inevitable as soon as the new doctrines filter down as matters of fact to the levels of the common intelligence. And surely, nothing else could be wished for in the world desired by all of us, the world ruled by intelligence, and intelligent good will.

SEX CHEMISTRY

A few general statements may be put down outright as material to go upon before we proceed to details.

1. Femininity and masculinity have a definite chemical basis in the reactions of the internal secretions of which they are the expression. That is to say, that just as a precipitate of chalk is formed when one throws some carbonate of soda into lime water, so the masculine and the feminine are to be looked upon as precipitates and crystallizations of a long series of linked chemical reactions in the fluids of the body, in which the internal secretions play a determining part.

2. Femininity and masculinity are expressions of the interplay of all the internal secretions. It used to be said by smart cats and accepted by the tabby cats, that a woman was a woman because of her ovaries alone. It is being said by some great discoverers of the day that man is a man because of his testes alone. Neither of these dogmas is true. There are individuals with ovaries who show every deviation from the feminine and there are individuals with testes who exhibit every variation from the masculine. The other endocrine glands are of equal importance.

3. There is no absolute masculine or absolute feminine. The ideals of the Manly Man and the Womanly Woman were erected by the blind ignorance of the nineteenth century illusionists, and a line drawn to cleave them. But indeed biologically there exists every transition between the masculine and the feminine. The explanation of these different sex types consists in the different admixtures of the internal secretions possible and actual. When we speak of the feminine we really mean the predominantly feminine. And when we speak of the masculine, we mean the mainly masculine. Between, all sorts of transitions are possible and occur.

Man in relation to the internal secretions we have considered in reviewing the interstitial cells. To him, we shall return later. Let us turn now to that fascinating subject of the ages, Woman. What produces and maintains the Feminine?

THE CAUSE OF SEX

To all appearances, that inscrutable simplest of living things, the fertilized ovum, beginning of the human, starts bisexual, double sexed, both masculine and feminine, or perhaps neither masculine nor feminine. Then a form develops. Then within that form a patch of cells arise which the microscopist recognizes as the forerunners of the male or the female reproductive cells. Then some more development. And at birth, sex is definitely settled, as far as the reproductive organs are concerned.

Our knowledge here, as everywhere, is still fragmentary. Statistical reviews seem to show that in times of stress, war, famine, pestilence, more boys are born than girls. But that is neither here nor there. It sheds no further light on the subject. Monosexuality is a distinction of the human species: the sexes are pretty clearly differentiated. In some animals, such as some worms, there is a bisexuality of the individual. There are present the reproductive organs of both sexes, capable of impregnating other individuals as well as of being impregnated. In some of these, even self-impregnation may occur. This is the condition of hermaphroditism.

But the higher up one goes in the scale of evolution, the greater becomes the distinction between the sexes. Anatomic hermaphroditism becomes a rare anomaly. Life appears to have perfected this trick of separate sexes, sex specialization, in short, for the sake of the efficiency which goes with specialization.

When a germ cell divides, its nuclear material breaks up into segments known as chromosomes. Now it has been found, for example in the case of the common squash bug, anasa tristis, that there are 22 chromosomes in the female, and 21 in the male. In the female two of these are visibly different from the rest, while in the male there is one odd one, the remaining 20 being like the corresponding 20 of the female. Before the germ cell becomes fit to mix with a germ cell of opposite sex, in the process of fertilization, it must lose one half of these. So the number of chromosomes for the species is kept the same or constant. This is the process of maturation. In the process, when the chromosome number is halved among the females, 11 go into each mature egg. But among the males, the odd chromosome, also known as the X-chromosome, can perforce go only into half of the sperm cells, leaving the others without it. So the sperm are formed in equal numbers of 10 and 11 chromosomes respectively.

When fertilization occurs, and the sperm cell fuses with the egg, the following may take place: (1) a ten chromosome sperm may unite with the eleven chromosome egg, and produce a twenty-one chromosome individual or (2) an eleven chromosome sperm may unite with an eleven chromosome egg producing a twenty-two chromosome individual. It has been found that the twenty-two chromosome individual invariably develops into a female, and the twenty-one into a male. Therefore, femaleness is a positive quality, dependent upon the action of the X-chromosome, and maleness an absence of femaleness, due to lack of the extra, odd chromosome. In man, two X-chromosomes have been discovered, half the sperm containing 12, and the other half containing only 10 chromosomes. The number of chromosomes in human cells consequently is 22 in the male and 24 in the female.

The X-chromosome is the bearer of sex destiny. There still remains the work to be done on the actual control of sex by man, apart from its natural determination. For the time being, let the feminists glory in the fact that they have two more chromosomes to each cell than their opponents. Certainly there can be no talk here of a natural inferiority of women.

THE SECONDARY OR ENDOCRINE SEX TRAITS

Yet the matter is after all not so simple as this would make it out to be. All that can be safely laid down is that the character of the reproductive organs is determined by the extra chromosomes. And though these reproductive organs have a good deal to do with the masculine or feminine quality of the organism as a whole, through their internal secretions, they are not alone. All the other internal secretions have their say in the final outcome, determining what may be called the dominant sex quality, but leaving inherent the latent soil of the other sex. This may become active and dominant in its turn, under certain conditions of stimulation, abnormality, or disease, dependent upon a rearrangement of status and influence among the ductless glands. Bisexuality preceded monosexuality in the animal pedigree, and co-exists with it even at the highest points of the genealogical tree.

While from the standpoint of the species, the criterion of the sex classification of its members will depend upon their capacity to fertilize or to be fertilized, a quality that may, therefore, be spoken of as the primary sex character, a number of other traits have been evolved by sexual selection, the secondary sex traits. They have come to be just as important, to the individual, as far as his or her consciousness of sex attitudes and reactions to it are concerned. The terms primary and secondary sex characteristics, though inapt, must be allowed to stand.

These accessory sex-serving traits undoubtedly survived because of their usefulness in external adornment for attracting attention in courtship, in the metabolic requirements of sex combat and the sex act, and in the necessities of caring for the young, until well-grown. The rooster's comb and spurs, the male frog's claspers, the stag's antlers, and so on, are familiarly and obviously so useful. Besides there are fundamental differences in inner physiology. The human male consumes more oxygen than the female per minute, since he has more red corpuscles in his blood.

In some caterpillars the blood is yellow in the males and green in the females. W.I. Thomas has devoted an essay of some fifty pages to a review of the organic differences between man and woman. The ordinary criteria, employed every day by the man in the street to distinguish man from woman may be arranged as follows:

Man	*Woman*
Hair on face	Hairless face
Skin coarse and lean	Skin fine and plump
Muscles powerful	Relatively weak
Bones heavy	Bones light
Aggressive--bass voice	Reserved--treble voice

THE ROLE OF THE OVARIES

While the primary sex characters, as such, are present and distinguishable from birth, quite the opposite holds for the secondary sex traits. During childhood they are in abeyance or at least pretty sharply suppressed. Girls and boys who are permitted to dress alike, to play the same games and among whom no consciousness of sex is encouraged are often difficult to tell apart. The boys will be boys, and most of the girls tom-boys.

With puberty comes a marked change of attitude toward the other sex. Puberty is the time of ripening of the specific germ cells. It is then the ovaries begin to secrete ova ripe for fertilization, and the testes begin to secrete sperm ready to fertilize. Before this can happen an event announced in the female by the onset of menstruation, two conditions must be fulfilled in the endocrine history of the individual. There must be a certain atrophy and retrogression of the thymus gland, and there must likewise be a similar atrophy and retirement of the pineal gland. Both of these involutions of the glands of childhood must occur before the normal hypertrophy and development of the sex glands and their secretions can start. Besides, there must be a minimum activity of the thyroid, adrenal and pituitary glands. Without them, below a certain minimum, the reproductive organs and their secretions will remain infantile, causing a persistent infantilism or delay of puberty.

Formerly there was ascribed to the ovaries, in a lump and without qualifica-

tion, an absolute despotism over the specifically feminine functions of menstruation, gestation, parturition, and lactation. Nowadays, we see its domain as a limited
monarchy, if not indeed as one sovereign state of a republic, a member equal but
not superior to the others of a board of directors. Its true business comes down to
two particular roles: first, the production of ova, and, second, the secretion of a hormone or hormones. Over the other functions once supposed its monopoly, all the
ductless glands rule.

What concerns us now is its internal secretion or secretions. One of them is
known as lutein and it has never been chemically isolated in its pure form. The existence of lutein, like the existence of electricity, is an inference, something we are
sure is there because of its effects. It originates in a remarkable part of the ovary, the
corpus luteum. Besides, there are the products of the interstitial cells, the creations
of a special layer of cells around the ovum, the membrana granulosa. They produce
a substance tonic to the uterus.

When the ovaries are removed, there occurs an atrophy of the womb muscle,
due to loss of this tonic substance. This atrophy, accompanied by an abolition of the
normal periodic uterine contraction, makes conditions unfavorable to pregnancy. It
has been claimed that the secretion of the corpus luteum is necessary for the complete progress of a pregnancy. Cases are on record, however, of ovaries taken out
soon after the onset of pregnancy, without interference with the gestation.

Castration is comparable in every way with the menopause or the time of cessation of sexual life, a process that might be called self-castration. It produces certain general constitutional effects. Adiposity often develops, undoubtedly associated with underfunction of the thyroid and pituitary glands. The woman breathes
less oxygen per minute and burns up less food and tissue. There is some disturbance
of the lime balance with an increased excitability of the vegetative nervous system.
Concomitant is the release of some brake upon the blood pressure mechanisms, so
that a family tendency to high blood pressure will flare up. Some women are rendered unstable by the process, others are completely transformed, and still others
adapt themselves, with little or no discomfort, to the new situation. The response
to the revolution in the cell-republic of the castrate by the other endocrines, the
thyroid, the pituitary, and the adrenals, determines which it is to be.

For normally, with feminine puberty, there is an increased activity of the thyroid, the posterior pituitary and the adrenal medulla. These changes indeed constitute the formula of normal feminization. In the male, the ripening of the testes is accompanied or perhaps preceded by augmented function of the adrenal cortex and the anterior pituitary. This difference in biochemistry accounts for the contrast between the sexes in the skin, hair, fat, cartilage (voice) and bone changes. Ovary and adrenal medulla and posterior pituitary and thyroid predominance constitute the feminine formula. Testis and adrenal cortex and anterior pituitary predominance comprise the masculine endocrine directorate.

THE REACTIONS OF THE OTHER GLANDS

As in so many other aspects, the facts about the various influences exerted by the endocrine glands upon the reproductive system are complicated and disjointed. A chink of light has been let in upon a dark cave, and slowly the chink will widen. But the gross effects are clear.

Around the ovary and the uterus, the endocrines gyrate as the planets around the sun. The ovary is the organ for the preservation and maturation of the germ plasm, that treasure which the body is built but to cherish and hand on as a sacred heirloom. The ova, the female egg cells, are the fundamental concern of the ovary. Secondarily, it secretes its messengers to keep the rest of the body, and particularly the other endocrines, in touch with the necessities of the adventures of these ova. It is thus enabled to bend every force and power at its command to the service of the reproductive instinct.

In learning their role so well in the course of evolution, the thyroid, the pituitary and the suprarenal have become indispensable stimulants (in various degrees peculiar to the individual), to the primary function of the ovary. As a consequence, to hold the sex stimulating glands in check, there had to appear others, restraining them and so preventing sex precocity. These are the thymus and pineal. So closely are they all related that insufficient action of the thyroid, pituitary or adrenals may cause atrophy of the ovaries and uterus, with abolition of genital function. If the sex glands themselves fail, as occurs usually in most women sometime in the forties, the thyroid-pituitary-adrenal association must readjust itself to the new development. The adaptation evokes the phenomena of the transition to a new life, the climacteric.

THE SIGNIFICANCE OF PUBERTY

Tracing the development of sex life there is a certain order of events in a normal history. Before puberty, the ova have lain asleep, as it were, in a cocoon state. Now with puberty they awaken. And with them all those profound mechanisms and inventions that have to do with their nutrition up to ripening. Then revolve the cycles that are translated as menstruation, the propulsion, fertilization and implantation of the ova in the uterus,--the full development of the fetus,--its birth, and feeding after birth--all of which are ductless gland controlled.

Samuel Butler once noted that:

"All our limbs and sensual organs, in fact, our whole body and life, are but an accretion round and a fostering of the spermatozoa. They are the real "He." A man's eyes, ears, tongue, nose, legs and arms are but so many organs and tools that minister to the protection, education, increased intelligence and multiplication of the spermatozoa, so that our whole life is in reality a series of complex efforts in respect of these, conscious or unconscious according to their comparative commonness. They are the central fact in our existence, the point towards which all effort is directed."

Nothing could be said more truly of Woman, and the ova she carries. All that transpires during pubescence is symptomatic of the underlying tidal stir in the cells. The uterus becomes gorged with blood periodically, to provide an enriched soil for the perhaps to be fertilized ovum to plant itself. The breasts grow, and fat is deposited in particular places as reserve material for the making of milk. The qualities which are to appeal to the eye and ear and even nostrils of the male appear. Instincts dawn, an independence of spirit germinates, emulsified with a curious shyness and coyness and a desperate loneliness and secrecy. And all because there have been let loose in the blood from the glands of internal secretion the chemical substances that set going the clockwork of sequential incidents elaborated and repeated through countless aeons of time.

FEMININE PRECOCITY

Ordinarily, in the north temperate climate, puberty begins about the fourteenth year, but may begin anywhere from the tenth to the sixteenth. Feeding and environment indirectly, the state of the internal secretions as a whole directly, determine this. In girls, those definite signs, menstruation and the growth of the breasts, before the age of ten, mean premature awakening of the ovaries and a concomitant co-reaction of the other endocrines, creating the ensemble of maturity.

In females, the primary stimulus, the initial spark of femininity, must originate in the ovary. There are other forms of precocity in the female, dependent upon stimulations of other glands, but these forms are masculinisms, a masculinization of the personality, and not a true awakening of the feminine constitution. So one must distinguish sharply between a precocity by masculinization and precocity of premature feminization. The latter always implies the touch of the fairy's wand upon the sleeping ovaries. Sexual precocity in boys may be produced by a premature over-activity not only of the specific reproductive organs: the testes, but also by an early excess of secretion on the part of the cortex of the adrenal gland or the pituitary gland, or by a too early involution of the pineal or thymus. When such abnormalities of adrenal, pituitary, thymus or pineal occur in girls, it is the masculine streak in the hastening of growth that is made manifest. All this emphasizes the relative bisexuality of every normal, no matter how pronounced, when superficially viewed, his or her form of predominating sex may be. Under the right conditions recession of the most marked virility or femininity becomes conceivable, and occurs.

THE SECRET OF THE MASCULINE

Masculinization having entered upon the scene, one may well ask: what truly (which means chemically) lies behind all these differences and divergences between male and female? What is the secret of the variable internal secretion admixtures? You can tell us that the recipes are different, the ingredients different, the results different as a Nesselrode pudding is from, say, a rice pudding. But what is the inner mechanism of the process? Since the masculine and the feminine are but expressions of certain relative capacities and potentialities, some single principle must run through the making of both.

Recognizing of course the qualifications inherent in so broad a statement the answer is: the handling of the lime salts. Life originated, or at least lived and worked for long ages in sea water. During these eras the salts of the sea have come to play a dominant role in its being. The lime salts, because of their peculiar properties of dissolving or precipitating themselves according to electrical conditions in their medium, have come to occupy a central position in all the processes of growth, metabolism and sex differentiation. So it is that masculinity may be described as a stable, constant state in the organism of lime salts, and the feminine as an unstable, variable state of lime salts. The male skeleton contrasts with the female as the stronger, larger, heavier and straighter because it is an expression of a greater capacity to utilize, store and keep lime in the system. Women throughout their reproductive period are liable to rapid and pendulum-like fluctuations of their lime content.

Menstruation, pregnancy, lactation, all draw upon the stores of lime, sometimes depleting them to the point of softening of the bones and wrecking the whole skeleton. The endocrines control the transport, and course, combinations and permutations in the history of lime's progress among the cells, and are in turn themselves affected by it. Man is relatively free of these liabilities, and so remains man by his freedom from the recurrent crises involving the lime salt reserve which constitute the essence of the life story of woman.

THE SEX INDEX

It follows from these considerations that when it becomes necessary to size the sex composition of a man or woman, a measurement becomes establishable which may be spoken of as the sex index. To be able to say of Mr. Llewylln Jones that he is sixty per cent masculine and forty per cent feminine, or of Mrs. Worthington that she is seventy per cent feminine and thirty per cent masculine would be of the utmost value under all kinds of circumstances. Unfortunately, lacking as we do the exact figures of an advanced blood chemistry (yet in its most infantile infancy) a direct indexing of the sort is impossible. But it is certainly conceivable, along the lines of measurement suggested by the Binet tests and others, that a scale of evaluation of the secondary sex traits may be elaborated, which would turn out as valuable in understanding the frictions of the individual, and more concretely, that aspect of it to which pathologists of the mind are tracing so much needless misery and suffering: maladjusted sexuality, expressed and suppressed. Nothing will contribute more to harmonious adjustment for these sufferers than recognition of the fact that we are all, more or less, partial hermaphrodites.

THE FUNCTIONAL HERMAPHRODITE

The complete or total hermaphrodite we define as the individual who possesses the reproductive organs of the male and the female, both testes and ovaries. So rare is such a combination in man that for a long time its occurrence was doubted, descriptions of it regarded as myth. However, undoubted cases are on record, examined by the most careful of observers, of ovo-testis or mixed reproductive organs. Strangely enough, the history of these cases, shows that at one time the masculine set, and at another the feminine set, will hold sway over the sex traits and functions. Blending does not happen.

Rare though the true hermaphrodite may be, the partial hermaphrodite is relatively frequent. The mixed ensemble of the directly contrasting type, such as the concomitance of testes with feminine secondary sex traits, or of ovaries with masculine sex traits, have been described from time immemorial as freaks. Occurring even more frequently is the mixed sex ensemble, in which the type of reproductive organs and of secondary sex traits run roughly parallel, emulsified with certain traits of the opposite sex. Physical features of one sex, instincts and mental attitudes of the other co-exist in the same individual by reason of an excess in one direction or a deficiency in another of the internal secretions. The degree of masculine trend in a woman is a crude measure of adrenal domination, the degree of feminine deviation in a man is roughly proportional to the amount of pituitary influences in his make-up.

Whether one or the other sex tendency will dominate depends upon the quantity of sex hormone divergence from the ideal normal. But also determinant are the environment stimuli provoking excessive or deficient secretory reactions from the other endocrines involved, through the vegetative nervous system. Such especially are the associates of the mixed sex individual. Ordinarily the combative male and the submissive female are differentiated by contrasts of skin and hair, fat and bone structure. The combative male is built as a fighting machine, the submissive female as an organism of attractive grace and beauty for impregnation and parturition. When one sees the fragile woman aggressive, the masculinoid woman submissive, one may infer an education of experience that has brought the usually recessive glands into the foreground, and by their hyperactivity imposed a bisexuality of function upon a unisexual anatomic structure. A man apparently as formidable as a tyrannosaurus, may be ruled by his wife for the same reason. These combinations of a single organic sexuality with a functional bisexuality, based upon internal secretion disturbances, are frequent, and merit the name of functional hermaphrodites or mixed sex types.

MIXED SEX AND THE FAMILY

The psychology of the family in its relation to the endocrine traits of its members is something that still remains to be thoroughly worked out as a problem of tremendous importance. Particularly are the reactions of the mixed sex types to be carefully considered. For, since the family is fundamentally a sex institution, devised to satisfy the sex needs, all the way from companionship to parenthood, it is apparent that the mixed sex types will be tried the hardest by its inexorable conditions. It is in relation to the mother (or nurse) first, the father next, and other associates in proportion to their proximity, that the primary endocrine-vegetative mechanisms, the germs of the growing soul, become established. These are superimposed upon the hereditary instinct apparatus.

Fear, rage and love reactions develop first in association with the suckling reflex, and the accompaniments, the mother's smile and voice, the color of her hair, eyes and skin, her breasts and odors. Each time the babe reacts to a pleasant or unpleasant stimulus, there is an outpouring of certain internal secretions, a cessation of others, a tingling of certain vegetative nerves and organs, a hushing of others. The ensemble of reactions tends to be repeated around the same stimulus, until the whole becomes automatic. One may observe the same process in the lower animals. Offer a piece of meat to a dog and his mouth waters. Ring a bell before offering the meat. Repeat this a number of times, and after a while the mere ringing of the bell, without the presence of the meat, will cause his mouth to water. This associated vegetative secretion reflex is the most fundamental to grasp in an understanding of the deepest strata of personality.

Now there are, besides the associated vegetative-endocrine reactions, certain inborn automatic processes in the vegetative system and in the internal secretion system, which work automatically to produce increased intravisceral pressures. The reduction of these pressures below the point of their intrusion upon consciousness, their relief, as we say, also form the centers of constellations around feelings of satisfaction or love. Such, for example, are the voiding of excretions. Sooner or later, these automatic reactions, and the associated reflexes formed around the mother, father and other associates, come into conflict. Inhibitions or prohibitions of the automatic act at certain times or moments are imposed by somebody. And so there occurs a pitting of the automatic mechanism against the associated reflex. Conflict with adjustment by suppression must occur. Thus a sense of self as active wisher (for the automatically pleasant experience), and punishable suppressor (of the same in favor of the acquired associated reflex) develops.

So far, so good. Compromise by regulation from above, from the brain, of the automatic reactions follows, as training. No absolute repression is forced, no absolute encouragement is indorsed. Harmonious equilibrium, or normality, continues. But now there come upon the scene the unconscious fears.

In the paleontology of character, these fears are the deepest strata, the eocene era, so to speak, of the soul. They are the hardest to get at and the most silent, as well as the most dominant of the influences which guide conduct. In Sir Walter Raleigh's words:

"Passions are best likened to streams and floods.   The shallows murmur, the deeps are dumb."

During the first period of childhood, up to five or six, the primary fears group themselves around the taboos and secrets of its life.

Though we have every reason for believing that the sex glands are acting in some way upon the organism during this time, nothing definite is known. Yet, as the numerous studies of the subconscious recently made prove, sex curiosity like the other curiosities, flowers. More than about the automatic visceral reactions, these curiosities evoke the repressive imperatives of the associates, the mother and father especially. These repressive influences may be and often are the effects of ignorance, prudishness, vulgarity, or homosexuality, or the sex perversions that are known as sadism and masochism. But by the necessities of the case, the sex wishes become overlayed by reflexes associated with the mother and father and close associates as love. This might be termed the oligocene. As the circle of acquaintance widens, other loved objects usher in the miocene phases of the development. With these become interspersed various hates and detestations, deliberately cultivated and accepted by the consciousness. So we have a cross-slice of the personality in the first five or six years of childhood.

But now, with the onset of the second dentition, a subtle change begins in the endocrine equations of the body. The second dentition itself is an expression of a certain internal secretion wave passing through the cells, an increase of action of some hormones, a decrease of others. And a consciousness of physical sexuality appears, while the outlines of character, hitherto mere tracings, become firmer, heavier, quasi-indelible lines. That there is some activity on the part of the internal secretions of the sex glands, the ovaries and testes, can be demonstrated by accurately charting the behaviour of a boy or girl after this time. It will be found that there is a cyclic variation of health and conduct, more or less marked of course in each case. A cold may appear periodically at the end of each month, an increase of irritability and waywardness may be observed, or, on the contrary, a decrease of the regular restless playfulness. The ghost of sex begins to haunt the scene.

Now all kinds of possibilities of conflict emerge. The child is still a bisexual, growing into a mixed sex type, depending upon the nature and amount of its internal secretions. The influencing adult of the family, the most important of the external factors encouraging or depressing the tendencies of the child, possesses a fairly fixed ideal of monosexuality which he or she, generally quite unconsciously, seeks to impose upon it. A doting feminine mother will make her son as much as possible like her husband: if she dislikes her husband, as much as possible like her father or grandfather. A masculinized mother will tend to make a sex object out of the son, however, which means his feminization. But, on the internal secretion side, the boy may be definitely masculine. That is, after adolescence he would be strongly masculine, *if the vegetative-endocrine mechanisms created by the mother's personality had not slipped into the inside track*, so to speak. As a consequence, continual subconscious conflict between the two sets of sex reaction will, sooner or later, disturb, perhaps disrupt and ruin his life.

So an infant may start life with a fairly balanced endocrine equipment, with its wake of a normal life (barring accidents and infections), and yet he may end as an inferior, insane, criminal, or failure directly because of establishment of conflict between himself as one sort of sex type, and his obligatory associates of another sort of mixed sex type. This applies also to the mother-daughter, the father-son, and the father-daughter relationship.

Male and female created He them, is a bald misstatement of the facts. Male and female emerge as final by-products of endocrine heredity, environmental treatment and adaptation. Often the male-female, the female-male, persist anatomically, or are forced to persist functionally. Society, constructed upon the Biblical dogmas of man as a fallen angel, and absolute sex, is responsible for much misery and suffering meted out to the functional hermaphrodite, as we shall see later in an analysis of the endocrine character of Oscar Wilde. The privileges and powers of sex relationship, marriage and parenthood, should be safeguarded for the mixed sex type, the man or woman with the variable sex index. For there are no tragedies in life more pitiful than those in which an aggressive masculinely built type is forced to assume a submissive, receptive, passive, feminine role and vice versa, the tragedy of compelled homosexuality, because of wrong associates.

MASOCHISM AND SADISM

The functional hermaphrodite enables us, too, to understand the phenomena of masochism and sadism, to a certain extent, on the chemical side. The masculine personality, the combination of masculine, e.g., adrenal cortex and gonad internal secretion predominance, is built for aggression. The feminine personality, the union of feminine, e.g. thyroid and ovarian superiority, is constructed for submission. Reverse the possibilities, or confuse them, as occurs in the functional hermaphrodite, and the attitudes become reversed or perverted. So a masculinoid personality in woman will make for sadism, a feminoid personality in a man for masochism. Variants and refinements of these perversions will often be found in the functional hermaphrodite who must satisfy two doubly flowing streams of visceral pressure within himself. Persistence of the thymus or pineal gland tends to a prolongation of the infantile and child types, that will be taken advantage of.

CHAPTER VII
THE RHYTHMS OF SEX

If one permits a drop of ink to fall into a glass of water, amazing figures and shapes, bizarre and chameleon, are born as the blue swirls and whirls through the resisting medium. Unseen forces and currents, tides and pressures, set up a seething and flowing, pulling and twisting of the drop of ink until it becomes a strange wraith created out of the molecules. A temporary individuality lives in the water.

So likewise the forces of sex, essentially the forces of the internal secretions, mould and sculpt and mould again the woman out of the flesh and blood. Adolescence--puberty--menstruation: the maid,--pregnancy--labor--lactation: the matron, thirty years of ups and downs of these processes around the idea of love or suppressed love, against an aesthetic background of some sort--and finally the loss of the stress and strain of sex, the menopause. All the landmarks of the life of woman, in their entirety, are erected and dominated by the tides and currents, the phases of concentration and dilution, of the different internal secretions in the endocrine mixture which is the blood.

Marvelous are all the manifestations of the reproductive necessity. Considering that reproduction was at first merely a form of growth, a discontinuous kind of growth, that seized upon sex as a splendid means to escape death, the chemical methods evolved arouse a sense of awe. A baby is born with her or his glands practically as fixed for her or him as the color of the eyes. Thymus and pineal keep him a child, keep him unsexed. Then at puberty, a new current is added to the calmly flowing river, and behold! a turmoil. Ovaries or testes actively functioning erupt upon the calm spectacle, and the girl is transfigured into the maid, the boy into the youth. After the ovaries, the corpus luteum: after the corpus luteum, the placenta:

after the placenta, the mammary glands: after that the cycle begins again until the ovaries are exhausted and the chain is broken. Besides, all the other glands of internal secretion beat in rhythm, fluctuate in their activities, may divide prematurely the tides or dam them completely.

Innumerable varieties and combinations of interglandular action supply us with the limitless types of adolescent girls. Some endocrine cooperatives that make one girl stable and settled, will make others unstable and unsettled. Alicia may be hyperthyroid, and so excitable, nervous, restless, and subject to palpitation of heart and sleeplessness. Bettina may have too much post-pituitary, and so will menstruate early, tend to be short, blush easily, be sentimentally suggestive and sexually accessible. Christina may be adrenal cortex centred and so masculinoid: courageous, sporty, mannish in her tastes, aggressive toward her companions. Dorothea may have a balanced thyroid and pituitary and so lead the class as good-looking, studious, bright, serene and mature. Florence, who has rather more thyroid than her pituitary can balance, will be bright but flighty, gay but moody, energetic, but not as persevering. And so on and so on.

Environment, habit-formation, training, education serve only to bring out the internal secretion make-up of the girl, or to suppress and distort and so spoil her. Adolescence will be peaceful, calm, semi-conscious, or disturbing, revolutionary and obsessive according to the reaction of the other endocrines to the rise of the ovaries. Harmony, and so continued happiness of the mind and body, means that they have been welcomed into the fold. Disharmony, ailments, unhappiness, difficulties, mean that they are being treated as intruders, or are acting as marauders. The after life, sexually the period of maturity, barring accidents, diseases, and shocks, will bear the same character. The kind of adolescence provides the clue to the kind of maturity, for both are effects of the same endocrine factors.

THE SEX GLAND CHAIN

Furthermore, the activities of a normal woman involve a series of sex glands. Since there function, in addition to the ovaries, the glands of the uterus, the breasts or mammary glands, and the placental gland (the secreting cells of the tissue which comes out as the after-birth). Each of these contributes directly to the reproductive life of the individual. To call the ova the sex glands is to confer upon them a name which really belongs to a chain of glands.

All of the members of the sex chain, including those of the thyroid, the adrenal and the pituitary, are necessary to the functions of menstruation, impregnation, settlement of fertilized ovum in the wall of the uterus, labor and lactation. A disturbance of one of them will set up disturbances all along the line, and a resonance of distress or compensation upon the part of all of them. As an interlocking directorate over the sexual functions of the female, they are members one of the other. So what helps or hurts one, helps or hurts all.

THE CYCLE OF MENSTRUATION

Essentially, the ovary is a collection of follicles, nests of cells, acting as safe deposit vaults for the ova that are to become candidates for fertilization. At birth, there are some 30,000 to 200,000 of these, of which a good many atrophy during childhood so that there are no more than about 30,000 left at puberty. Of the 30,000, only an elite 400 actually mature between the ages of fifteen and forty-five. About every twenty-eight days, one of the follicles swells, becomes filled with liquid, pushes or is pushed to the surface of the ovary, there to rupture and expel into the abdominal cavity the tiny ripe ovum. The rest of the torn follicle makes itself over into a peculiar yellowish body, the true corpus luteum, should pregnancy occur. If pregnancy and the consequent placenta do not occur, it shrinks and turns into a scar, the false corpus luteum. The true corpus luteum resembles closely the adrenal cortex in make-up and staining reactions. It seems as if, once successful impregnation has been achieved, the feminine organism adrenalizes itself, makes itself more masculine and less feminine, inhibiting the posterior pituitary and the adrenal medulla, as well as the ovaries. Besides, the corpus luteum stimulates the thyroid to prepare for the heavy demands to be made upon it during pregnancy.

Before menstruation, there is a stage of preparation, a stir and twittering of the endocrines, the premenstrual state. Currents of communication flow between the different glands, messages and replies pass to and fro. When these are properly balanced, so that all goes well, the consciousness of the woman will be disturbed by no knowledge of them. In some women abnormal sensations appear, a sense of fullness in the breasts, or of weight in the back or pelvis, or pain in the head. The last is probably due to swelling of the pituitary beyond the capacity of its bony container. In a good many women, nervous and mental phenomena herald the expected menstruation because of a complete upset of the balance between the internal secretions, with resulting disturbance of the nervous system. Irritability, depression, excitability, melancholia, exaltations, restlessness, hysteria, loss of self-control, or even more marked mental aberrations may appear. Following them, and roughly paralleling them, may come various abnormalities of menstruation itself. The character, extent and duration of these furnish us the best clues to the endocrine stability or instability of the particular feminine organism.

Menstruation is simply the uterus saying: well, not this time. As the destined ovum within its nest, the follicle, grows, its fluid affects the interstitial cells to send their specific stuff into the blood. There it circulates, hits this gland and that, makes some more active, others less, transforms the chemistry of the cells, and engorges the mucous membranes, most of all those of the nose and of the uterus. It is all to welcome the mature ovum and its possible impregnation, to prepare a site for its landing and settlement, blood and food for its nutrition, safety for its development. But it is not to be. No sperm at hand, or effective enough to penetrate that wandering ovum. Love's labour's lost. All must return to the so-called normal, really the intermenstrual state. The womb must surrender some of that blood, the glands return to their routine, and a sex diastole of the whole organism succeeds. Until again, another follicle swells, another ovum matures, and the premenstrual state of sex high tide cycles back.

Seven to ten days before menstruation we know that sex high tide is beginning for that is when the blood pressure goes up. As this rise of blood pressure is probably controlled by the posterior pituitary, we have a clue to the reason for the rhythmic variations in the rate of production of its secretion by the ovary. For, since menstruation is so closely connected with the phases of the moon and the tides, the rhythmicity of the posterior pituitary may be traced to the days when the pineal was an eye at the top of the head, and in direct relation with the pituitary.

Menstruation has been said to be a miniature labor. It is not that as much as it is a miniature abortion. It is an effort of nature still-born. But nature is quite used to its disappointments and returns placidly to the daily grind. The four phases of a woman's twenty-eight day cycle succeed each other as the premenstrual, the menstrual, the postmenstrual and the intermenstrual, with the precision of pistons moving in a motor, when no interfering factor as disease, profound emotion or climate disturbances are present, affecting the endocrines.

The sequence of events appears to be about as follows: The amount of post-pituitary secretion reaches a certain concentration. This in turn stimulates the thyroid and adrenal medulla. They in turn activate the ovarian cells, which congest the uterine glands and lining membrane. The follicle bursts, the ovum is discharged and wanders, the uterus waits and wonders. Nothing happens, the curtain is lowered, the scenery is removed, the actors revert to civilian clothes. That is the story of menstruation, the central phenomenon of woman's pre-pregnancy life. One sees it clearly as a play of an internal secretion syndicate.

THE PREMENSTRUAL MOLIMINA

The premenstrual molimina is the traditional title accorded symptoms, sensations, feelings, observations of women in the premenstrual phase. In the light of endocrine analysis, they become exceedingly important indicators of the underlying constitution of the individual concerned. Indeed, the premenstrual period furnishes a direct clue to the dominating internal secretion in a woman. Moreover, these premenstrual phenomena are the shadows cast by coming events. For they mimic and prophesy the events of the last crisis of feminine sex life, the cessation of ovulation which goes by the name of menopause, gonadopause, or change of sex life. The premenstrual phenomena provide a positive film, so to speak, of the latent negative picture of the endocrine system of the girl or woman.

Thus, there is the sub-pituitary or pituitary insufficient type, in whom the excessive swelling of the gland causes headache, and a dull, heavy, tired feeling, a definite depression. Drowsiness, sleepishness, indifference to surroundings, general sluggishness of thought, feeling and reaction, a phlegmatic frilosity, all go with it. It is due to an overweighing of the pituitary, controller of good brain tone, and alive wakefulness, by the demands of the organism.

On the other hand, the hyperthyroid type of woman reacts with an exaggeration of her tendency. When the posterior pituitary begins to secrete more in her its stimulation of the thyroid is enough to tip it over the normal line. Such a woman in the premenstrual phase becomes irritable and restless, does not know what to do with herself, cannot concentrate on conversation, occupation or any single activity, may become excited to the point of mania. Hot, tremulous, sleepless, or sleeping badly, she has a much harder time of it than her pituitary sister.

These samples of premenstrual internal secretion reaction are the extremes of a vast number and variety of types. There are women in an unstable quasi-premenstrual state for the greater part of their lives. Sometimes an infectious disease or a psychic blow will put a woman into this class. The significance of these cyclic changes has been tremendously increased by the recent formal admission of women to participation in public activities on a plane of equality with men.

Evidence exists that in man, too, there is some cyclic rhythmicity of his endocrines, which sets up a fluctuation in his physical and mental efficiency. The curves of these variations have still to be plotted, and will doubtless contribute no little to our knowledge of the control of human nature. One unexpurgated fact stands out: the reproductive mechanism of woman has rendered her whole internal secretion system, and so her nervous system, all her organs, her mind, definitely and sharply more tidal in their currents, more zigzag in their phases, more angular in their ups and downs of function, and so less predictable, reliable and dependable.

THE MASCULINOID WOMAN

The masculinoid woman, as a functional hermaphrodite, exists first as a congenital entity, with an inborn distribution of endocrine predominances that make for masculinity. There are also numerous acquired forms. The infections of childhood, measles, scarlet fever, diphtheria, and above all mumps, may so damage the hormone system that an inversion of sex type follows. However, the stimulative and depressive effects of environment are even more significant. The effects of environment in producing changes in an organism, the changes the biologist sums up as adaptation, can be tracked in many instances to responsive reactions of the glands of internal secretion to demands made upon them by changed external conditions. So a cold climate, which necessitates a more voluminous hair covering for an animal, will evoke a hypertrophy of the adrenal cortex. Secondarily other effects appear as by-products of the adaptation. The adrenal cortex makes for pugnacity, temper, animal courage, irritability and anger reactions. So a hairy animal will, in general (unless other endocrines come in to defeat the primary effect), be more pugnacious, courageous, irritable and combative. The same applies to woman. An environment which tends to encourage the masculine traits in her, to arouse repeatedly her pugnacity and combative decisions in the more rapid give and take of the masculine world, will rouse the adrenal cortex to greater activity, and so make her face hirsute, her attitudes aggressive, and perhaps render her sterile. Concomitantly there may be a disturbance of menstruation.

The presence or absence of sterility, natural or enforced, always present, or say appearing after the birth of one child, must all be donated a prominent place in studying the endocrine make-up of a woman. When there is not enough ovarian secretion, the ovum may not be able to burst through the ovary, a necessity before it may begin its travels to the uterus. Next, the propulsive action of the genital ducts may be insufficient because of defective corpus luteum. Or the uterus may not have received enough posterior pituitary or thyroid to make it fit soil for the ovum to plant itself in. Or there may be too much of these, which cause the uterus to massage itself daily by gentle contractions and so keep it well-toned. Excessive massage will throw the ovum out. All these are factors in the sterility problem, with its psychic resonances affecting the maternal instinct.

THE MATERNAL INSTINCT

There have been created high odes to an unknown god, sensuous lyrics of love, apostrophes and addresses to every human passion. But no poet, to my knowledge, has risen to the heights of the maternal instinct. Some contemporary clap-trap about sentimentalism will perhaps decry and ridicule the demand for an apotheosis of it. There are some who deny its existence, and assert that maternity is forced upon every woman. Reduced to its elements, such nonsense turns out the absurd pose of the theorist desperate to epater le bourgeois or to cover up hidden defects in his or her make-up.

Without the maternal instinct, without the hope of immortality through somatic or spiritual posterity, we should all, who were sane enough, have to condemn ourselves to the futilities of hedonism. So that the criminal who was condemned to roll a huge boulder up a hill, only to see it roll down again, would have to thank his lucky stars for his lighter punishment. The future, tomorrow, the Kingdom of Heaven on Earth, or if you will, the Republic of Supermen, means to all of us what the child means to the madonna. The cynical epicurean careerists and careeristinas, and the depraved degenerates of a comfort-lusting civilization may have suffered an absolute atrophy and castration of that instinct. But they are pathologic specimens, and we are not for the moment concerned with them.

The Freudians have set up a great hullaballoo about creative activities as sublimations of the sex instinct, or as they would have it, the libido. That is their obsession, the confusion of the sex instinct, the instinct for sex life and satisfaction in the relation of the male to the female, with the maternal instinct. The paternal instinct bears the same relation to the maternal, as the breasts of the male do to those of the female, i.e., a functional hermaphrodite trait. The maternal instinct is the instinct to create, provide and care for offspring.

The mother expresses the deep craving of protoplasm for immortality. What drives her is the instinct of Life to preserve itself unto eternity in infinite space and time. That separates it sharply from the temporary needs of the sex instinct. The artist, the man of science or letters, the statesman, craftsman and maker of every sort is instigated by the maternal instinct. He creates for his own pleasure, to be sure. But it is in its essence the pleasure of the bird making its nest.

It is necessary, therefore, to distinguish between the sex instinct and the maternal instinct. For different glands of internal secretion have been found responsible for them. A distinct difference in the quality and amount of the two instincts may be observed in the same person. A strong maternal instinct may be seen again and again to dominate a woman with but little or no sex urge or passion. Numerous physiologically frigid women have lived successful and happy married lives because of contented maternity. Other women, with normal or exaggerated sex instinct who welcome and stimulate the sex life, may have no wish for children, no functioning maternal instinct at all, and if sterile, will accept their fate with indifference or even exultation. These variations occur because of a difference in chemical source and determination of the two instincts. While the ovary, stimulated by the thyroid and the adrenal medulla, is the chief determinant of the sex instinct, to the posterior pituitary must be credited the chief hormone of the maternal instinct. The interactions of the two glands, the ovary and the posterior pituitary, modified by accessory influences, determine the relative intensity of the two instincts. In a sense, the two glands may be said to be antagonistic and yet one stimulates and complements the other.

THE TRANSFIGURATIONS OF CHILD-BEARING

Though what happens at puberty, what happens all through life through the agencies of the endocrines is amazing enough, what occurs during the period of child-bearing is perhaps the most amazing of all. As emphasized, pregnancy is the time, among the internal secretions, of a great uprooting and stirring, of fundamental and cataclysmic changes in the most intimate chemistry of the cells. It is as if a dictator, inspired by his country's danger, its enemies at the gates of its capitol, were to draft and mobilize everyone, man woman and child from everyday activities to the necessities of defense. Or rather it is as if there appeared within the heart of our civilization a common purpose and intelligence, now so palpably lacking, which magnetized and drew to itself all the streams of individual self-aggrandizing effort. Imagine that possibility and how it would change the face of the earth and the entire basic constitution of human life and society. So do the profound tides of the hormones, centering around the new creature being made in the womb, transfigure the face and constitution of the child-bearing woman.

During pregnancy, in consequence, the integrity of every structure of the body is tested. A stern, relentless accountant goes over the cells, counts up their reserves, establishes a balance, credits and debits according to the demands of the growing parasite within them. Follow changes in the skin, the bones, the nervous system and the mind. That is, all the glands, subtle recorders, transmitters, producers of the vibrations of change are influenced. But the most influential are the most affected, as the most dominant personalities in a community are most disturbed by a revolution.

In Sinclair Lewis' "Main Street," the best novel ever made about America as a nation of villagers, the heroine, Carol Kennicott, has this to say to someone sentimentalizing about maternity.

"I do not look lovely, Mrs. Bogar. My complexion is rotten, and my hair is coming out, and I look like a potato bag, and I think my arches are falling,... and the whole business is a confounded nuisance of a biological process."

The exploration of the internal secretions has brought us an explanation and an understanding of why child-bearing is a nuisance. We know now that if Carol Kennicott's complexion became rotten and her hair fell out, it was because her thyroid was not adequate to the demands of pregnancy, and that if her arches were falling, and her figure acquiring a potato bag dumpiness, it was because her pituitary was insufficient. In all probability she was a thymus-centered type, which accounts for much of the material that goes to make up the novel.

Different endocrine types react characteristically toward the situations of pregnancy. The adrenal type may not be able to respond with the necessary enlargement of its cortex which is normal for the needs of gestation. So pigmentations, darkenings and discolorations of the skin, especially of the face, the traditional chloasma develops. The hyperthyroid type may become sharply exaggerated, almost to the point of mania and psychosis. The subthyroid will suffer an emphasis of her defect, and pass on, because of pregnancy, to the truly diseased state of myxedema, the state of dull, slow, stupid, semi-animal semi-idiocy. The pituitary type becomes more masculinized. The face becomes more triangular and coarser, the chin and cheek-bones more pronounced, and there is a growth of all the bones, so that she is seen to grow visibly in height and breadth, and in the size of the hands and feet. Concomitantly, there is a changed, a more matured and steadier outlook upon life, all due to stimulation of the anterior pituitary, controller of growth, physical and mental.

In general, the major endocrines, the pituitary, the adrenals, and the thyroid should hypertrophy and hyperfunction during pregnancy. Should they not, should adverse mechanical circumstances or chemical malfunction prevent, dire effects may follow. A woman with the closed-in type of pituitary, shut up in a small non-expansile sella turcica, will suffer the most violent headaches, will become fat, will frequently abort. One whose thyroid cannot rise to the demands of gestation, because of previous disease (like typhoid or measles) which injured her thyroid excessively, may be poisoned by the new elements introduced into the blood by the growing fetus, as it is the job par excellence of the thyroid to render innocuous these poisons. Of adrenal insufficiency, failure of the adrenals to hypertrophy sufficiently in pregnancy, little is known. Possibly the corpus luteum, the endocrine formed of the torn egg nest in the ovary, makes up for any deficiency in this respect. For there is the most curious resemblance imaginable between the cells of the adrenal cortex and those of the corpus luteum, some day to be completely explained.

THE PLACENTAL GLAND

The placenta, an organ and gland of internal secretion newly formed in the uterus, when the fertilized ovum successfully imbeds itself within it, must be considered in any analysis of the transfigurations of child-bearing. Born with the pregnancy, its life is terminated with the pregnancy, for it is expelled in labor as the after-birth. Its importance and function as a gland of internal secretion has become known only recently. Many still doubt and question the accordance of that rank to it. But feeding experiments with it, in various endocrine disturbances in human beings, have proved its right to the title.

The placenta is created by the fusion of the topmost enlarged cells of the uterine surface and the most advanced cells constituting the vanguard of the growing and multiplying ovum. These front line invaders interact with the cells in contact with them to make a new organ which serves as lung, stomach and kidney for the embryo, since it is the medium of exchange of oxygen, foodstuffs and waste products between the blood of the mother and the blood of the embryo. Ultimately it acts, too, as a gland of internal secretion, influencing the internal secretions of the mother, and also those of the embryo.

Settlement of the fertilized ovum in the womb introduces into the system new secretions, new substances which are partly male in origin, since the ovum contains within it the substance of the male sperm which has penetrated it. This masculine element causes a rearrangement of the balance of power between the endocrines towards the side of masculinity. They push down the pan of the scale to inhibit the post-pituitary. So menstruation, the menstrual wave which follows the increasing tide of post-pituitary secretion, is postponed. For ten lunar months, not another ovum breaks through the covering of the ovary, and the uterus is left undisturbed. The placental secretion plays a most important role as brake upon the post-pituitary, the most active of the feminizing uterus-disturbing endocrines. Until at last something happens that puts the placenta out of commission in this function of restraint, and the long bottled up post-pituitary secretion explodes the crisis apparent as the process of labor.

A condition of self-poisoning often occurs in pregnancy, with symptoms orchestrating from mild notes like nausea and vomiting to the high keys of convulsions and insanities. They represent what happens when an unbalanced endocrine system is attacked by the placenta. Depending upon where in the internal secretion chain the weak point, the Achilles' heel spot, will be found, the nature of the reaction will vary. And even after labor, after the explosive crisis, so much of the reserve endocrine materials may be consumed, that an actual mania or a chronic weakness may come in its wake.

Yet the placental secretion must not be looked upon as something wholly evil in its potentialities. Without enough of it to hold the uterus stimulating endocrines, particularly the post-pituitary, in check, still-birth results. If there is enough, and not too much of it, the woman will not feel ill at all, or perhaps only transiently, but will be possessed of a curious feeling of drowsy content and passive, relaxed happiness. Let there be relatively too much of it, too little of the other glands, and the grosser transfigurations and ailments of the child-bearing period follow.

THE MAMMARY GLANDS

Once pregnancy is terminated by labor, the placenta is expelled from the body as the after-birth. The placenta removed, a new arrangement of the balance of power among the endocrines becomes necessary. But a new-comer appears upon the scene to take up the function left vacant by the absent placenta. This new-comer is the secretion of the activated breasts, the mammary glands. They make for a persistence of the state of equilibrium among the endocrines attained during pregnancy.

The mammary glands are typical glands of external secretion. They make the milk and pour it out of the breasts through little canals into the mouth of the suckling. Yet evidence forces us to conclude that they are also glands of internal secretion, that their internal secretion substitutes to a certain extent for the loss of that of the placenta but not quite.

What seems to happen in fact, is this: the corpus luteum secretion stimulates the dormant cells of the mammary glands, formed during puberty, but latent until the advent of pregnancy. We know that injection of corpus luteum will cause an hypertrophy of the breasts. The same effect is produced regularly during the menstrual period, with a consciousness of swelling of the breasts. Their atrophy at the menopause coincides with the shrinkage of the ovaries that takes place at that period. Activity of the breasts parallels indeed more or less the activity of the corpus luteum.

With the prolonged activity of the corpus luteum during pregnancy, prolonged stimulation of the breasts occurs. The secretion of the post-pituitary would now cause the change from the internal cell secretion to milk. But it is inhibited from so doing by the placenta. When the placenta is removed, after labor, the post-pituitary can act, and a free flow of milk is established. However, to counterbalance this, and to prevent the post-pituitary from overacting, the breasts secrete a hormone with an action like that of placenta, but not so strong, which tends to inhibit the ovary. So is put off the imposition of a pregnancy upon a period of lactation, obviously bad for mother, infant, and embryo. We have here an exquisite sample of the checks and compensations which make for a self-balancing of the whole endocrine system.

CRITICAL AGES

The Dangerous Age is a phrase coined by a Scandinavian writer as a more dramatic euphemism for the time of life when sex function ceases, the climacteric. As a matter of fact, the age of adolescence is just as much of a dangerous age as the age of deliquescence. The only difference between them is that the dangers of the one have been hushed up, the dangers of the other well boomed and advertised. Both are dangerous to the individual, because both are periods of instability and readjustment of the cells, particularly the brain cells, to a deranged endocrine system and blood chemistry.

Moral attitudes differ at the two ages, not so much as an effect of experience, as expressions of different visceral pressures produced by newly dominant internal secretions. So in Eugene O'Neil's play, "Diff'rent," we see the woman Emma Crosby as she is in her youth, when her ovaries have budded and bloomed for only a few years, and her other endocrine influences are still dormant. She breaks off her engagement to Captain Caleb Williams on the eve of her wedding because she is informed of the episodes of a sex affair he was involved in on his last voyage, under circumstances not discreditable to him. The next act shows her thirty years later when, as an elderly spinster, she is passing through the climacteric, and is in the state of sexual hyperesthesia some women are afflicted with before the menopause. It is as if the ovaries and the accessory sex internal secretions erupt into a sort of final geyser before they are exhausted. So the captain, ever faithful, finds her, and discovers to his horror that she is a thousand times more like other women than he has ever been like other men. Because of his ignorance of the underlying chemical basis for the transfiguration, tragedy follows. Critics may cackle about a sex starved woman, who has repressed her natural desires, and hail the play as a contribution to the Freudian clinics. As a matter of fact, it is a study of libido variation, with endocrine variation, at two stages of the inner chemical life of a woman.

The chain of events at the menopause, the acme and then ebb of the sex tide, may be summed up something like this:

The ovaries cease producing their eggs and so shrivel as a storage battery atrophies when it dries up. An important member of the endocrine board of directors thus drops out, and so a rearrangement of gland activities, a new regime, becomes necessary. If a balance of power is established quickly and equitably, very little happens. Quickly the woman passes on to the next plane of her existence. But if some endocrine proves recalcitrant, and takes advantage of the situation to make itself dominant, trouble and maladjustment, and their psychic echoes, come. Anterior pituitary control will mean a relative masculinization, with hair on the face and aggressive attitudes. Post-pituitary most often refuses to settle down, and expressing its ambition as headaches, flushes, obesity and hysteria, may cause extreme misery and unhappiness to its possessor. Sooner or later, if the harmonious equilibrium of the normal life is to be revived, all the glands must regress, thyroid, pituitary and adrenals.

With the waning of the ovarian function, the thyroid type will also exhibit its particular flare. If there is thyroid excess the woman will be excitable and irritable, the thyroid deficient will be depressed and dull, the thyroid unstable (that is swinging between excess and deficiency) will have a cyclic up and down alternation of mood and temperament. The adrenal centered will have a high blood pressure and masculinoid traits, the adrenal inferior will have a low blood pressure and suffer from a constant weakness and fatigability. So each form of reaction to the critical ages is individualized according to the predominating glandular influence in the constitution of the woman. When the womb has atrophied, and the breasts have shrunk, the typical tan complexion, and the angular masculinoid figure, face and psyche follow, and the transfiguration has been completed.

Man has his critical age of sex cell deterioration as well as woman. The age period swings between forty-five and fifty-five. Here enters upon the scene that organ of external and internal secretion, the prostate, the most important of the accessory sex glands in the male. Experiments with its extract upon growing tadpoles have demonstrated it to have the same differentiating effects as thyroid, but without the poisoning effects. Furthermore, the microscope reveals cyclic changes in its cells comparable to the menstrual phenomena of the uterus. Indeed it is accepted as the homologue or male representative of the uterus. Small and undeveloped during childhood, its growth at puberty parallels that of the other reproductive organs. Its secretion has been shown to be necessary to the vitality of the sperm cells. The regression of the prostate, its retirement from the field of sex competition, is the central episode of the male climacteric. Accompanying its shrinking are prominent an irritable weakness, despondency, and melancholia, which may emerge at any time if there is disease or disturbance of it. The influence of the prostate upon man's mental condition, and its contribution to the sex index, still remains to be investigated in detail.

SEX CRISES

At the periods of interstitial cell hyperactivity, when a wave of radicalism in the blood sweeps through the tissues, the other endocrines are tested, and their latent stability or instability is made manifest. Even before puberty, cyclic variations of health and conduct may be observed in boys and girls which undoubtedly depend upon currents among the internal secretions. Children, who, in the best of circumstances, habitually are attacked by a wanderlust and run away from home, or suffer from fits of naughtiness, are samples of such endocrine lability. Children specialists have found that at about the end of the second year their charges begin to individuate. In a certain percentage, sex traits appear pretty early. But the fact of the matter is that it is rather the minority of girls who spontaneously exhibit the traditional stigmata of the natural girl. The doll-cherishing, housekeeping imitator of mother is another story.

At puberty arise the most exquisite cases of life crisis dependent upon hormonic crisis. The boy becomes restless, irritable and quick-tempered when his thyroid and adrenals respond to the call of the interstitial cells. If they do not, he will become dull, heavy, lazy and listless. The girl correspondingly is transformed into a vivacious, gay, nervous and apprehensive butterfly, or a sedate, dreamy, bashful, or even morose moth. It is interesting to note that poise, mental equilibrium, is not established until physical growth ceases, marked by a cessation of growth of the long bones known as ossification of the epiphyses. Poise seems to be controlled by the ante-pituitary. The growth of the long bones is also dominated by the ante-pituitary. It would seem as if, its secretion dedicated to the one function, could not be available for the other. So it happens that those in whom growth ceases early (probably because of an earlier and more vigorous invasion of the internal secretion system by the interstitial cell product), develop mental maturity more rapidly and possess more of it than those in whom growth continues. The acumen and salacity of certain dwarfs is proverbial. The puberty phenomena teach that sex crises of every sort are dependent fundamentally upon fluctuations, periodic or aperiodic, of the sex index, as we have defined it.

THE DETERMINING FACTORS OF SEX LIFE

The material summarized in the preceding paragraphs furnish some slight inkling of the vast dominion of Sex, in all its relations, somatic and spiritual, over which the glands of internal secretions rule. The founder of modern pathology, Virchow, said that woman is woman because of her ovaries. He meant that woman is a woman, the sort of woman she specifically is, because of her internal secretions. But no divine decree has laid down a line of cleavage between man and woman. There are fundamental constitutional differences between man and woman. But it is just as true that man is man because of *his* internal secretions.

We have seen that the concepts of Man and Woman are the end-points of a curve including variations of every possible combination that are embraced in the construction of a sex index. This sex index is not an absolute constant, although its range of fluctuation is pretty well fixed at birth. It varies from day to day, year to year, depending upon the influences that have been brought to bear upon it. But it determines the character of the three planes of sex: the endocrine, the vegetative, and the psychic. The endocrine is concerned with the fundamental chemistry of sex, the internal secretions, which determine the chemical reactions that provide the free energy for the sex process. Upon the vegetative plane occur those transformations, tensions, and relaxations, in the viscera, which are controlled in part by the endocrines and in part by the experiences of the individual as registered in his subconscious. Upon the psychic, conscious planes appear the echoes and reflections of the occurrences upon the other two planes, as well as reactions arising in the brain from the necessity of the organism reacting as a whole to isolated episodes. Accompanying is a self-awareness of the organism as a unit. The three planes are not like separate plates of glass one raised above the other, the usual idea picture of planes. They are nebulae, swirling into each other, influencing and being influenced continually. The reactions among these three complexes of sex create the milieu for the variations and aberrations of tendency, character and conduct which stamp his unique quality upon the individual. Sex morale is likewise so influenced. The fundamentals of sex ethics will, in due time, be revised in accordance with these conceptions.

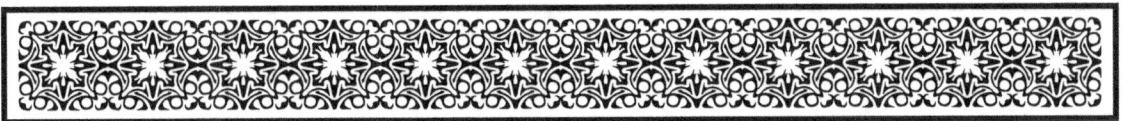

CHAPTER VIII
HOW THE GLANDS INFLUENCE THE MIND

It is impossible to review here in detail all the facts accumulated concerning the influence of the internal secretions upon all the processes of mind, intellectual and emotional. A volume would not suffice for their adequate consideration. Reflexes, instincts, habits, tendencies and emotions are involved in their machinery. The development and normal functioning of the intellect, the pure reason as Kant called it, are controlled by them. Brain, without them in solution, without enough of them in that wonderful solution, the blood, sleeps or remains dormant like the butterfly in the cocoon. The cretin, who has not enough thyroid or no thyroid, is an imbecile because of his deficiency. Supply him with thyroid from outside sources, feed him animal thyroid, be it of the sheep, the pig, or the goat, and behold a miracle! he is restored to the level of at least the relatively normal intelligence.

Acuteness of perception, memory, logical thought, imagination, conception, emotional expression or inhibition and the entire content of consciousness are influenced by the internal secretions. The most ultramicroscopic activities of the molecules and atoms in the highest nerve cells and nerve tissues are dominated. The speed of their chemistry and their associations, and thus the speed of thought, are regulated. Iodine has been shown to increase the electric conductivity of the brain that is, the rate at which electrons will fly through it. The thyroid may then be regarded as manipulating the amount of iodine brought to play upon the brain cells at a particular moment of danger or exaltation. Adrenalin increases the electric conductivity of the brain. Nerve impulses, and with them sensations and ideas, travel faster or flow more quickly through iodinized or adrenalinized brain cells. In dangerous situations we think more rapidly and keenly, for in emergencies the blood floods the brain with extra thyroid and adrenal secretions.

THE BODY-MIND COMPLEX

Mind, still regarded by most of mankind as something distinct and apart from the body, is thus exhibited as but part and parcel of it. A deaf, dumb, and blind animal, deprived of tongue, and olfactory mucous membrane, without sensations from the outside world can grow no mind, in the sense of intelligence. The sense organs of the body mediate the primary mind stuff. Without internal secretions and a vegetative system there could be no soul, in the sense of complex emotion. Nor those combinations of thought and emotion which synthesize attitudes, sentiments and character. The internal secretions and the vegetative system mediate the primary soul stuff. Mind is thus emulsified with body as a matter of cold literal fact. The soul was once a subtlety of metaphysics. Now when mind appears soaked in matter saturated with chemicals like the hormones, therefore woven out of material threads, the independent entity created out of intangible spirit flies like a ghost at dawn.

View the outlook. Mind, the slippery phantom, now becomes controllable for the purposes of everyday life, because we can put our fingers upon, touch, handle and change these material factors, the internal secretions and the vegetative system. Through them we may affect the very quality of the nerve tissue. The future of the race, the future of human nature, depends upon the knowledge to be born of the researches into the vast possibilities of this idea. Man, the Adventurer, the prey of Chance and Luck, will then become, indeed now becomes, the Captain of Fate and Destiny.

It is, of itself, a revolution in the intellect, to conceive of instincts and emotions, suggestibility and contra-suggestibility, initiative and imitation, volitions and inhibitions as chemical matters. In all their relations, mutually reacting effects and defects, excesses and deficiencies, the internal secretions set up psychic echoes and reflections. When morbid and their equilibrium dislocated, we may even have phobias and neuroses.

A man's nature is essentially his endocrine nature. Primarily, when he is born, he represents a particular inherited combination of different glands of internal secretion. They, constituting the inventory of his vital stock in trade, start him in life. Afterwards, food, the routine of his existence, the accidents of experience, education, disease and misfortune, in short, environment, modify him because they modify his ductless glands and his vegetative apparatus, as well as his brain, depressing some parts, and stimulating others, and so rearranging the system. In particular will he be transformed as the gland is affected which is the centre of the system to which the others adapt and accommodate themselves. The inertia of the system is very great, almost absolute, and always tends to return. If he has children, he hands on his constellation of endocrines, in spite of mishaps, not at all or only slightly transformed. Sometimes, however, the experiential transformation has been sufficiently deep, and shaken the very constitution of his germ-plasm. So family dispositions and traits, national and racial temperaments, are propagated, maintained and varied.

THE SEX INSTINCTS

Hormone reactions, as we have seen, initiate the complicated forces, processes and expressions of sex. The dictum of the founder of modern pathology, Virchow, that Woman was in effect an appendix to the ovaries, has long been taken to apply to her psychic traits as well as somatic. Her mind, like her skin, her hair and her pelvis, is a product of the ovarian endocrines. But these determinations are by no means her monopoly. Man is likewise a creation of the chemical wheels within wheels and springs within springs that are his glands of internal secretion. That he is not so obviously an appendix to his testes is due to two reasons. First, the male sex hormones have not the instability nor cyclic rhythmicity of the female. Secondly, and perhaps consequently, his sex instincts have become overlayered with other more labile instincts, with habits and customs and necessities that appear to oust the sex instinct into an altogether decentralized position. Moreover, it is the function of the female to be the excitor in the sex process: her subconscious, thoroughly aware of the fact, sees to it that the sex instinct stands starkly central and dominating in her life.

The moods of love, like the more stereotyped manifestations of sex, are dependent upon a proper supply to the blood of the internal secretions of the reproductive organs, the gonadal endocrines. If the testes are removed from frogs, it is found that the clasp-reflex, symptom of sex desire, is abolished. If, after an interval of several days, the testes' extract is injected into the frog, the reflex reappears for a few days. The hormone provoking this sex reflex is present in the testes only during the breeding season. In birds, the seasonal nesting and migrating instincts may be eliminated by interfering with their ovaries. At the same tine there is a change in their plumage toward the male type. Similarly, the males, when their sex endocrines are cut off, will change their psychic nature as well as physically. Besides owning his flag-waving comb, his spurs and brighter feathers, the rooster struts to attract the female, and fights aggressively with his sex competitors. When he is made a capon, he loses his spurs and comb and distinctive plumage, and in addition becomes retiring and submissive, in short, a pseudo-hen in his instincts as well as in appearance. If the genital glands are extirpated from a male before puberty, the wattles remain small, pale and bloodless, no active, amorous or combative instinct emerges. The creature maintains a demure silence, and may even be sought by a virile male. So we may see homosexuality of a kind in the lowest animals. On the other hand, hens deprived of ovaries tend to metamorphose in the male direction, even to acquire the male spurs, and to display the male attitudes.

All through the animal world, in the springtime, when the pituitary awakens or increases its secretion, and so stimulates the sex glands to augmented activity, emotions of sex and their expression are provoked by the inner stirring. When the nightingale warbles passionately and the mocking bird gurgles provokingly, when the robin fills its scarlet breast and the starling floats in ecstasy through the perfumed air, when the pigeon coyly woos its mate, and the butterfly flirts with the dazzling multicolors of its wings, when all the marvelous devices of sex attraction in nature, selection and courting, mating and reproducing are pondered, who but must wonder at the infinite possibilities of reaction of the sex hormones? All is for love, and all is because of the love in the blood that is manufactured unconsciously by a few hidden cells.

EXPRESSIONISM AND EXHIBITIONISM

We need a detailed examination of the various forms of expression art has differentiated into, in its relation to exhibitionism and as effects of the circulating libido-producing substance of the gonads. Sex exhibition differs in man and woman because of the differently combined internal secretions that are their substrates. The male's attitude, aggressive pursuit, is instigated by the compound adrenal and gonad endocrines. The female's various emulsions of coyness and display are motivated by posterior pituitary and gonad hormones in alliance.

It is a dogma to state that the internal secretions of sex do not begin to function until after puberty. Some children manifest exhibitionism with a certain independence of environment. Before adolescence a good many girls act like tom-boys, and are distinguishable externally from boys only by their clothes. But others display signs of sex differentiation that are to be traced back to an awakening interstitial gonad action. Some boys have no interest whatever in sex. Others will show an intense curiosity spontaneously, a curiosity which perhaps may be explained as a larval precocity, dependent upon the minimum of sex hormone production by the gonads. Close observation of the correlation of somatic and psychic development in extreme examples of these children corroborates this view. Jonathan Hutchinson has described full-busted children of London already boasting of their affairs. Indeed, as education and environment affect the body (in so far as they influence it as a whole) by exciting or inhibiting the glands of internal secretion, sex-arousing stimuli from without must be considered to evoke their effects as stimulants of the latent puberty glands.

At puberty, when the sex glands bloom, and the complex of the sex instincts is activated, exhibitionism manifests itself in a host of guises and disguises. Femininity in a woman, the womanly woman, or the eternal feminine, may indeed be defined by the degree of somatic and psychic exhibitionism she presents. A woman who has a delicate skin, lovely complexion, well-formed breasts and menstruates freely will be found to have the typical feminine outlook on life, aspirations and reactions to stimuli, which, in spite of the protests of our feminists, do constitute the biologic feminine mind. Large, vascular, balanced ovaries are the well-springs of her life and personality. On the other hand, the woman who menstruates poorly or not at all is coarse-featured, flat-breasted, heavily built, angular in her outlines, will also be often aggressive, dominating, even enterprising and pioneering, in short, masculinoid. She is what she is because she possesses small, shrivelled, poorly functioning ovaries. Between these two types all sorts of transitions exist, according as the other endocrines participate in the constitutional make-up. But no better examples could be given, off-hand, of the determining stamp of the internal secretions upon mind, character and conduct.

INSTINCT AND BEHAVIOUR

The sex instinct, analyzed as an endocrine mechanism, provides the clue to the understanding of all instinct and behaviour. If the post-pituitary regulates the maternal instinct, then its correlates: sympathy, social impulses, and religious feeling, must be also influenced, and so is furnished another example of a chemical control of instinctive behaviour. McDougall, once of Oxford, now of Harvard, introduced into psychology the idea of the simple instinct as a unit of behaviour, regarding the most complex conduct as a compounding of instincts. The instinct itself he analyzed into three elements: a specific stimulus-sensation, an emotion following, all ending in a particular course of muscular reaction. Translated into endocrine terms, what happens may be pictured as a series of chemical events.

When the activity of a ductless gland rises above a certain minimum, its hormones in the blood sensitize, as a photographic plate is sensitized, a group of brain cells, to respond to a message from the outside world, with a definite line of conduct. There is a registration by the brain cells of the presence of the specific stimulus. Then there is communication by them with the endocrine organs. As a result, some of them are moved to further secretion, and others are paralyzed or weakened. In consequence of changes of concentration in the blood of the various internal secretions, tensions, movements and tumescences, as well as relaxations, inhibitions and detumescences, occur throughout the vegetative system--the blood vessels, the viscera, the nerves and the muscles. Each wires to the brain news of the change in it. In addition, the brain cells themselves are excited or depressed by the new hormones bathing them. In their final fusion, the commingling vegetative sensations constitute the emotion evolved in the functioning of the instinct.

To lower the new tensions throughout the vegetative system to the normal range, the instinctive action is carried out. This superficially is regarded as the essence of the instinct. As a matter of fact, it is only the endpoint of a process, the resultant of a drive to restore equilibrium within the organism. It may all happen in less time than it takes to tell about it.

The play of an instinct may therefore be analyzed into four processes. They succeed one another as sensation--endocrine stimulation--tension within the vegetative system--conduct to relieve tension. The dash is the symbol of a cause and effect relationship.

This equation for an instinct, based upon an analysis of the working of the sex instinct, is the model for the analysis of all instincts, and therefore of all the compounded instincts that all human behaviour may be resolved into. Conduct, that fascinator of the common gossip and the great novelist alike, normal and abnormal, social and asocial, in all their complexities, even unto the third and fourth generation, the Freudian complexes, is governed therefore by the same laws that determine the movements of the stars and the eruptions of volcanoes. The most interesting factor in the instinct equation is the endocrine, because that is the one that is most purely chemical.

ENDOCRINE CHARGING OF WISHES

It is *the* distinction of modern psychology that it has established the wish (craving, need, desire, libido) as the moving force in any psychic process. The position of the wish in psychology as the force within and behind the instinct may be compared to that of energy in physics, when it was elevated to a central position in the explanation of physical processes in the nineteenth century. The concept of the *charged* wish has illuminated all the hidden recesses and rendered audible all the subdued murmurings of the mind. The truly novel in the content of the idea is the recognition of the fact that the wish is charged. Now it could never be charged in a vacuum. That means that a wish could never be born in the brain alone. For the brain has no power to charge itself with energy--it can only store and transmit. If a wish is potential energy that must be transformed into kinetic, it must have a source. That source is the vegetative system. Without the vegetative system, the great complex of viscera in the abdomen and chest, blood and its vessels, endocrines, muscles and nerves, the brain would remain but an intricate cold storage plant of memories, associations of past experiences. It would need no change and initiate no effort. But when the wish enters upon the scene, it is as if a dead storage battery has been refreshed with new current. Enriched with billions of electrons there is a stir and a movement, dynamic mind. But the dynamo is the more ancient possession of the animal, the vegetative apparatus. In short, what must always be remembered is that a wish is never cerebral, but always sub-cerebral, visceral, in its origins.

The sub-cerebral makes the cerebral. Activities in the nervous system below the brain and especially the vegetative system, force upon it its function of the active verb. It has to be, to do, and to suffer, and then to manipulate the environment to satiate the insatiable viscera, insatiable because the local chemistry is continually raising the tension of one or the other of them. A physics of human behaviour becomes possible with the aid of these concepts of endocrine regulation of intravisceral pressure, and intervisceral equilibrium, an intramuscular pressure and an intermuscular equilibrium, with the brain as the shifting fulcrum of the system.

The sensation of hunger, as we have seen, serves as good an exemplar as any of this mechanism of the wish. Hunger is preceded and accompanied by contractions of the stomach of increasing intensity. Those contractions must be brought about by a substance acting upon the nerve endings in the wall of the stomach. As it closes down upon itself, waves pass up and down. With each wave, the pressure within it rises. The exact amount of the pressure may be accurately measured by means of a small balloon swallowed and then inflated. When the pressure rises above a certain figure, the sensation of hunger breaks into the consciousness of the individual. We infer that certain sensory impulses sent up to the brain attain a strength that finally forces itself into the conscious field of feeling. The sensation of hunger varies from individual to individual because of variation in the reaction throughout the vegetative system. Most often it is a sense of movement or even an itch in the upper abdomen. Let some cause produce a weakening or cessation of the movements of the stomach--as fear and anger--and the sensation of hunger disappears coincidently with the drop in the pressure within it. As the mathematicians would say, the wish is a function of the pressure, and so of the concentration of substance behind the pressure.

We have in hunger the wish reduced to the lowest terms, the most primitive form of it. Yet we may resolve all wishes, even the most idealistic, into the same terms. As the vegetative system becomes habituated by repeated experience to react in the same way to the same stimulus, permutations and combinations of wishes become possible until at length the inscrutable complexities of the behaviour of civilized man are evolved. We have to thank Von Bechterew, the greatest of Russian physiologists, for these fundamental principles, so important for the understanding of the control of human life and conduct.

The associated reflex, aboriginal ancestor of the involved train of associations that constitute the highest thought, conduct and character, is the unit of the system. Recall the classic example cited. If a piece of meat is shown to a dog, his mouth waters. If now you proceed to ring a bell before offering the meat, his mouth will water only when he sees or smells the meat. If, however, the ringing of the bell precedes the meat a sufficient number of reactions, a time comes when merely the sound of the bell will cause salivation, without the presence of the meat. So it is with the associated reactions of the internal secretions. A stimulus originally indifferent to the endocrines may, by association, the laws of which are many, come to act like a spark to the endocrine-instinct mechanism. Hence we can account for the subtle play of instinct throughout all thinking.

Even objects resembling the specific excitant of an instinct only remotely, or in some one quality, may start its mechanism and a host of associations bound up with it. Thus the maternal instinct may be excited by the sight of a baby. But because a baby is small and delicate, anything small and fine, a tiny book, a toy, a miniature, may arouse it. The object is then said to be appealing. The doctrine of association of instinctive and so of endocrine reactions enables us to understand the feeling--tone that at any moment pervades consciousness as well as its content.

Choices, the psychology of selection of food, color, friends, mates, amusements also become explicable rationally. For conflicts among the different components of the vegetative system are continuous and inevitable. If the pressure within a viscus has been heightened, and persists, that is, is not disturbed by some other associated factor or instinct, conduct results to lower the pressure to what it was before the instigator of the tension appeared. But if another instinct is sparked, or another associated factor comes into play, another focus of increased pressure within the vegetative system is created, with another stream of energy flowing to the brain and demanding an outlet. This clash of instincts, the struggle between different foci of the vegetative system competing for the possession of the brain, is a common everyday process in conduct. Which will win means which will will. And so we have an energetic basis for volition.

Which will win appears to depend primarily upon the kind of endocrines that predominate in the make-up of the individual, secondarily with his education. For it is the endocrines that are really in conflict when there is a struggle between two instincts. And if one endocrine system conquers, it must be either because it is inherently stronger, its secretion potential, that is, the amount of secretion it can put forth as a maximum, is greater (so explaining the term dominant)--or because a past experience has conditioned it to respond, although the opposing endocrine system does not. Fear and anger, respectively bound up with the activities of the adrenal medulla and cortex, we shall see, provide as good exemplars as any of this process.

The response of the ductless glands to situations varies with their congenital *capacity*, and acquired *susceptibility*. Capacity is a question of internal chemistry, modifiable by injury, disease, accident, shock, exhaustion. Susceptibility depends upon the play of the forces focusing upon them that may be summed up as associations. In the ability of one endocrine system to inhibit another we have the germ of the unconscious. Hence the modus operandi of the repressions and suppressions, compensations and dissociations, which may unite to integrate or refuse to integrate, and so disintegrate and deteriorate a personality.

As the personality develops, the vegetative system becomes susceptible to the manifold associates of family, school, church and society, art, science and religion, and last but not least sex. All the different nuances of personality are expressions of a particular relationship, transitory or permanent, between the endocrines and the viscera and muscles. Conversely, behaviour shows what a person actually is chemically; that is, what endocrine and vegetative factors predominate in his make-up.

FEAR, ANGER, AND COURAGE

Fear and anger are the oldest and so the most deep-rooted of the instincts. An ameba, contracting at the touch of some unpleasant object, feels fear in its most primitive form. And anger, the destructive passion, must have appeared early upon the scene of life. Certainly these two instincts were definitely developed and fixed in the cells before sex differentiation and the sex instincts were born at all. It is interesting to note this for our rabid Freudians.

Fear and anger involve the adrenal gland. How comes it that two states of mind so contrasted should involve the same area? The answer lies in the bipartite construction of the adrenal. All the evidence points to its medulla as the secretor of the substance which makes for the phenomena of fear, and to its cortex as dominant in the reactions of anger.

When adrenalin is injected under the skin in sufficient quantity, it will produce paleness, trembling, erection of the hair, twitching of the limbs, quick or gasping breathing, twitching of the lips--all the classic manifestations of fear. These are the immediate effects of fear because they are the immediate effects of excess adrenalin in the blood upon the vegetative viscera and the muscles. The perception by associative memory of these effects of adrenalin, the sensations arising from the organs affected, constitute the emotion of fear. Flight follows by muscle prepared for flight, for the disturbance of the inter-muscular equilibrium tenses the flexor muscles, the muscles of flight, and relaxes the extensor muscles, the muscles of attack.

If, it would seem, the cortex secretion now pours into the blood, enough to more than overcome the effects of the medulla secretion, the inter-muscular equilibrium is disturbed in the opposite direction, for fight rather than flight, and anger results. Or if the cortical secretion pours in an overwhelming amount of its secretion from the first into the blood there will be no fear, but anger immediately. Habitually charging and fearless animals like the bison, bull, tiger, or lion have a relatively larger cortex in their adrenals. Habitually fleeing and fearful animals, like the rabbit, have a small cortex and a wide medulla in their adrenals. The reinforcing action of the thyroid is important. The adrenal medulla reinforced by the thyroid makes for terror, the adrenal cortex reinforced by the thyroid makes for fury.

Some people are not easily frightened, others are more readily frightened, and still others are of an extremely fearful nature. It depends upon the proportion of adrenal cortex to medulla secretion in them. And their reaction to fear stimuli is a pretty good measure of the ratio. These formulations apply more particularly to fear in general and anger in general. But even in the least fearsome, i.e., an individual in whom cortex dominates medulla, there may be fear--complexes, dating back to events and times when medulla overtopped cortex, especially childhood. So in the coolest people, certain persons, objects, episodes, may send a wave along an old line of nerve cells and paths which lead to the adrenal medulla, and so flood him with fear, terror or even panic before his usual cortex response occurs. Impressions during the early years of childhood, probing of the unconscious by various methods, have been shown to be the most potent in this respect. Sometimes the episode goes further back than childhood, and one must assume an inherited conditioning of the vegetative and endocrine systems. An animal leaping upon an ancestor in a forest during the night might account for the panic fear some people experience when alone in the dark, that nothing of their childhood history may account for.

In women, the adrenal medulla naturally tends to overtop the cortex, because the latter makes for masculinity. Besides, the recurring cycle in the ovary, making the corpus luteum, evolves an additional stimulant to the medulla, through its irritating influence upon the thyroid. Then the influence of the post-pituitary is anti-adrenal cortex. So that, on the whole, a number of endocrines work to render woman naturally fearful, as we say.

Courage is so closely related to fear and anger that all are always associated in any discussion. Courage is commonly thought of as the emotion that is the opposite of fear. It would follow that courage meant simply inhibition of the adrenal medulla. As a matter of fact, the mechanism of courage is more complex. One must distinguish animal courage and deliberate courage. Animal courage is literally the courage of the beast. As noted, animals with the largest amounts of adrenal cortex are the pugnacious, aggressive, charging kings of the fields and forests. The emotion experienced by them is probably anger with a sort of blood-lust, and no consideration of the consequences. The object attacked acted like the red rag waved at a bull--it had stimulated a flow of the secretion of the adrenal cortex, and the instinct of anger became sparked, as it were, by the new condition of the blood. In courage, deliberate courage, there is more than instinct. There is an act of volition, a display of will. Admitting that without the adrenal cortex such courage would be impossible, the chief credit for courage must be ascribed to the ante-pituitary. It is the proper conjunction of its secretion and that of the adrenal cortex that makes for true courage. So it is we find that acts of courage have been recorded most often of individuals of the ante-pituitary type. Photographs are obtainable of thirty-four winners of the Congressional Medal of Honor for extraordinary bravery in the War with Germany. Of these twenty-three exhibited the somatic criteria or hormonic signs of the ante-pituitary type. A prerequisite for adequate ante-pituitary function is a normal secretion of the interstitial cells of the reproductive glands. Cowardice is said to be a feature of eunuchs.

THE PITUITARY AND INSTINCT

We have seen that, more than any other gland or tissue of the body, the post-pituitary governs the maternal-sexual instincts and their sublimations, the social and creative instincts. A great deal of evidence is in our possession concerning the disturbances of emotion accompanying disturbances of this gland, and controllable by its control. It might be said to energize deeply the tender emotions, and instead of saying soft-hearted we should say much-pituitarized. For all the basic sentiments (as opposed to the intellectualized self-protective sentimentalism), tender-heartedness, sympathy and suggestibility are interlocked with its functions. Its secretion must act upon the great basal ganglia, at the base of the brain, which contain the nerve cells and fibres that are the centers of emotional control and co-ordination.

The ante-pituitary has been depicted as the gland of intellectuality (to use that term for lack of better). By intellectuality we mean the capacity of the mind to control its environment by concepts and abstract ideas. The frontal lobes of the brain are the central offices for higher thought. Their cells are the most complex, have the most numerous branches and association fibres. They store the fruits of abstract thinking, mathematics, for example. The anterior pituitary is in the closest relation and contact with them. Its secretion is tonic to them. Now the instinct that is the forerunner of intellectuality is the instinct of curiosity, with its emotion of wonder, and its expression in the various constructive and acquisitive tendencies. Studies of intellectual men, and of those with a keen instinct of curiosity and a constructive-acquisitive trend prove them to be ante-pituitary dominant in their make-up. The administration of ante-pituitary extract to some defectives increases intellectual activity and self-control. The future of intelligence may expect a great deal from the newer chemistry of the secretions of the ante-pituitary.

Two most important instincts, therefore, which in the complexity of their sublimations have created most of the institutions of society, the maternal and the intellectual, are connected directly with a proper function of the pituitary endocrines. So it happens that disturbances of these instincts, reaching far into the normal and intellectual spheres of the mind, are definitely connected with disturbances of the pituitary. As we shall note in reviewing the essentials of the pituitary-centered or pituito-centric personality, the personality governed by the fluctuations of activity within the pituitary, people with injured, diseased or mechanically limited pituitaries (because of the smallness of the bony case enclosing them) exhibit defects and perversions of conduct and intelligence directly attributable to affections of the very instincts and functions the pituitary governs. Children with small, mechanically cramped pituitaries lie and steal, are bed-wetters, have poor control over themselves, and a low learning capacity.

THE THYROID AND INSTINCT

The chemical mechanism of the instincts described: sex libido, passion and jealousy in relation to the ovaries and testes, fear and anger in relation to the adrenals, sympathy and curiosity in relation to the pituitaries, suggests that a similar explanation will hold for the dynamics of the other instincts. In the closest relation to the thyroid appear the instincts first isolated, so to speak, by McDougall as the instincts of self-display and self-effacement, accompanied by emotions of pride and shame respectively. In certain states of excessive thyroid activity there is an extra stimulation of the instinctive display of the person which may go on to boasting, mania and exhibitionism. On the other hand, in states of thyroid insufficiency, depression is produced, which may go on to melancholia, a desire to be alone, to hide, to sit apart and even a tendency to accuse the self of various uncommitted crimes and sins. In the form of cyclic insanity known as the manic-depressive psychosis, mania alternates with depression, as if the personality were dominated wholly in turn by one or the other of these two instincts of the ego. There is a good deal of evidence that behind them is a corresponding fluctuation in the amount the thyroid secretes into the blood. Among the thyroid-centered attitudes toward the self gyrate more than in any other type. Egomania and megalomania occur most often in thyroid unstable individuals.

ENERGY AND SENSITIVITY

In his classic Inquiries into Human Faculty, Francis Galton laid down some fundamental considerations concerning energy and sensitivity as mental traits. Energy he defined as the capacity for labor, and declared it to be the measure of the fullness of life or vitality. Statistical study by him of men of genius and their ancestors showed them to be endowed with a large amount of energy. It has been said to be the absolute prerequisite of genius. Now if there is a single fact that has been well established by investigations of the internal secretions, it is that the energy quantum of an individual is a function of and determined by his thyroid. The more thyroid he has, the more energetic will he be--the less thyroid the less energetic, and the lazier. The thyroid-centered individual, of the excess thyroid type, actually burns up more food and produces more heat than the ordinary organism. He burns himself up faster in general.

When the thyroid sends more secretion into the blood, more thyroxin, it accelerates all the functions and activities of the organs. Tea and coffee produce loquacity because they stimulate the thyroid. People with thyroid dominant constitutions talk fluently, rapidly, and continuously. Their energy makes them doers, actors rather than spectators. They get up early in the morning, are on the go all day without surcease or fatigue, go to bed late, and often suffer from insomnia.

Thyroid deficients, however, are definitely the opposite. They are quite conscious of the limited reserve of energy at their command. Also that they need plenty of refreshing sleep. Early to bed and late to rise remains the leading maxim of health for them. In addition they find it necessary to sleep during the day. Forty winks or more in the afternoon makes a good deal of difference to them. Taciturn, inarticulate, lazy, slow, tired, are the adjectives applied to them by their friends as well as by their enemies. All because of an insufficient or inefficient supply of the thyroid's iodine to their cells. The mobility of energy in an organism is a measure of the amount of active iodine in it. The physiologic synonyms for "energetic and lazy" are "well-iodinized" and "poorly iodinized."

Sensitivity, the ability to discriminate between grades of sensation or acuteness of perception is another thyroid quality. Just as the thyroid plus is more energetic, so is he more sensitive. He feels things more, he feels pain more readily, because he arrives more quickly at the stage when the stimulus damages his nerve apparatus. The electric conductivity of his skin is greater, sometimes a hundred times greater, than the average. Conversely the thyroid deficient type has a low discriminative faculty. Galton has recorded that idiots hardly distinguish between heat and cold and that their sense of pain is so obtuse that some of the more idiotic seem hardly to know what it is. Cretins may moan but never shed tears.

Energy and sensitivity in an individual should direct attention to the thyroid element predominating in his composition. Lack of energy and insensitivity to the degree of thyroid insufficiency in their make-up.

MEMORY, JUDGMENT, AND POISE

In between sensitivity and energy, the sensation and the reaction, comes a passage of the stimulus through the gauntlet of the stored past experience of the individual known as memory. Many hypotheses have been advanced by philosophers, psychologists and physiologists to explain the phenomenona of memory. To conceive of memory materially at all one must admit some sort of memory trace as the basis for the persistence of memory. This memory deposit facilitates the occurrence of the chemical reaction constituting the memory along the same path the next time. Forgetting then consists in a disappearance of these memory traces or deposits. Forgetting is greatest in the first hour after remembering, more than half of the memory trace being lost in that time. Comparison of the curve of forgetting, and the curve of diffusion of a colloid like gelatine from its solution, into a surrounding medium, shows them to be exceedingly similar. Forgetting may be explained by some such loss of the memory trace or deposit into the blood continually flowing by it.

The internal secretions influence the amount and duration of the memory deposits. The thyroid appears to be essential to the ***laying down*** of the memory trace. Cretins have poor memories on the retention side and so cannot learn. The memory of thyroid insufficients is wretched. In the extreme grades, the memory for recent occurrences becomes completely lost. Iodine and thyroid increase the electric conductivity of the brain, so that the memory trace must be deposited more easily in those who have an excess of thyroid. Removal of the thyroid produces a degeneration of nerve cells and their processes, and associative memory becomes difficult or impossible because conduction from cell to cell is interfered with. If sufficient thyroid is fed in excess, brain conduction may be so facilitated that epilepsy may result upon slight irritation.

On the other hand, the pituitary seems to be related to ***preservation*** of the memory deposit. In conditions of disease of the pituitary, loss of memory for past experiences is more marked. As regards recent experiences, they are better held, although in a sort of subconscious manner, recoverable when the condition improves or is cured. But the greatest difference between the thyroid and pituitary effects upon memory exists as regards material: the thyroid memory applies particularly to perception and percepts, the pituitary to conception (reading, studying, thinking) and concepts.

Judgment is another mental process that often intervenes between sensation and the energy-reaction. It involves memory and association of experiences. Behind it is an attitude as much as there is in an emotion or the arousing of an instinct. Beliefs and reasonings are complex judgments. They form the units of the intellectual process.

There is an element of speed in judgment on reasoning as in perception and memory. And as in the latter, the thyroid determines the velocity. Quick thinking, as we call it, means good thyroid action, and slow thinking deficient thyroid action. The other element in judgment, accuracy, is influenced by the ante-pituitary. During adolescence there is physical growth which consumes most of the secretion of the ante-pituitary. After adolescence, after the early twenties, when physical growth has ceased, the ante-pituitary secretion sensitizes the cells of the brain to mental growth. The reaction potential of the ante-pituitary, that is its inherent, latent ability to supply a maximum of its endocrine for the nerve cells of the frontal lobes, is the best-known chemical determinant of intellectual genius. It makes for the greatest co-ordination of experience, knowledge, information, tastes and problems into one harmonious whole. And curiously, not only does it cause a fusion of intellectual material: it creates a desire for and a love of such material.

We should expect to find extraordinarily well-developed ante-pituitary action among eminent philosophers and men of science, and we do. Adequate action of it is present throughout the range of normals who evidence sufficiently ripened judgment as they progress through life. The ability to profit by experience, and to make more and more accurate judgments as one grows older implies at least a maximum efficiency of it. This maturation is not at all universal. Even after middle age, after forty and fifty years of reasoning, some individuals retain the juvenile mind of their youth. Like the Bourbons, they have learned nothing and forgotten nothing. Their ante-pituitary insufficiency often coupled with a post-pituitary excess, and other instabilities and disequilibriums in the endocrine system, render them immature morons, compared with what might be expected of them for their years. They are the people who are old enough to know better. For the same reasons, inhibition and emotional control are poor in them.

Besides the ante-pituitary, in the evolution of judgment, and the judgment faculty, due stress must be laid upon the influence of the internal secretion of the testes or ovaries, the product of the interstitial cells. Although the probability is that the effects are indirect, through a stimulation of the ante-pituitary, the fact remains that, in a child, memory may be marvelous and judgment poor (such memory is possibly purely thyroid in its determination). With the advent of the gonads upon the scene, judgments become the centre of the play's plot undoubtedly. The intelligence of eunuchs and eunuchoids is in general low. The skull and brain of castrates, animal and human, is smaller than the average. Gall, the physiologist who popularized ideas concerning the meaning of the protuberances and depressions of the head in relation to faculty and character, early in the nineteenth century, was the first to prove this. Among historic castrates, eunuchs, not a single example of great intellect, of the creative type, is known. On the contrary, the native gifts of the mind were destroyed. Thus Abelard, who was punished with castration by his uncle for his love affair with Heloeise, never composed a verse of poetry thereafter.

IMAGINATION AS AN ENDOCRINE GIFT

That brings us to the consideration of imagination as influenced by the endocrines. The physical conditions of exercise of the imaginative faculty have not been sufficiently investigated. Alcohol has long been known to act as an evocant of strange images. The hallucinations of delirium tremens are the results obtained in extreme intoxication. A strangely imaged flow of consciousness, the imaginative state, may also be evoked by morphine and cannabis indica. There is no doubt that the brain cells may be made to combine in the fresh, novel, and unfamiliar associations that are recognized as unreal.

Francis Galton, pioneer student of the conditionings of human faculty, left an interesting study of the visualising capacity, so far as it could be attacked by the statistical method. Two of his conclusions are worth repeating for our purposes. One is that the power to imagine is poor in philosophers and men of science. The other that it is higher in the female sex than in the male. We have seen that the philosophic, scientific, intellectual mind, the capacity to abstract, and think in terms of abstractions, is definitely dependent upon proper secretion by the ante-pituitary. In woman, the post-pituitary is generally predominant over the ante-pituitary. Though we are in need of a series of studies of the endocrine traits and composition of men endowed with high imaginative qualities, and so are at a loss, we have indications of an endocrine control of the state of consciousness we speak of as the imaginative.

Most of the evidence accumulated in the examination and treatment of morbid conditions characterized by a restless, incoordinate activity of the brain cells points to excess of the post-pituitary secretion as the cause, or as one of the most important causes. The thyroid and the adrenal medulla also exert their influence. But the strongest appears to be the post-pituitary. Phobias, fears which obsess the mind, anxiety neuroses, suspicions, hallucinations, delusions, nervousness, all expressions of what we may sum up technically as the imaginative state of mind, occur and occur frequently, associated with other symptoms of posterior pituitary overactivity. Persons in whose make-up it rules are more liable to imagine disturbances of their mentality, or exhibit a well-developed imaginative streak. Normal states of overactivity of the post-pituitary such as occur in some women during the menstrual period and pregnancy, and in some men as part of the endocrine cycle of their everyday lives, are accompanied by increase in the susceptibility and vigor of the imagination. Whether the feeding of excess post-pituitary would lead to a stimulation of the tendency or ability to imagine is still to be decided. But it is known that quieting the post-pituitary by various means will cause a depression of the faculty, and eliminate its pathologic manifestations.

Psychologists distinguish between the constructive imagination that expresses itself in an ordered activity and the unbalanced fancies of the fearful neurotic for example. The post-pituitary confers the lability of the underlying state of brain in all of these imaginative tincturings of consciousness. The constructive imagination, one of the few truly precious gifts of a personality, is probably the expression of a certain balanced activity of the ante-pituitary and the post-pituitary.

MOODS AND THE ORGANIC OUTLOOK

The lability the post-pituitary confers upon the combinations of perceptions and conceptions, grouped as the imagined, extends to the ruling mood that may be spoken of as the organic outlook. Post-pituitary in excess, without compensation or balancing by one or some of the other endocrines, is associated with an instability of mood and the organic outlook. Concomitant is a defective self-control. Typically, one sees the effects in the mental abnormalities of women during the premenstrual period. A number of them have their pituitary balance upset then, with an overtopping of the ante-pituitary by the post-pituitary. Irritability, a sub-hysteria, or an actual hysteria may emerge in the usually most placid characters. A quiet wife and mother may go for her husband, curse and mortify him, even strike and beat him. She may slap her children at that time and no other. It is well known that most of their crimes are committed by women during the menstrual period. So are the suicides. Deterioration of mentality and character so often observed during the menopause, with its apathies or excitements, melancholia or mania, the fits of weeping or gaiety, the loss of grip upon reality, the complete change in mood and temperament that reflect the transformation of the organic outlook, demonstrate clearly the overwhelming influence of the endocrines upon the attitudes of the self toward the self.

It is possible to speak of thyroid moods, adrenal moods, ante-pituitary or post-pituitary moods, gonadal moods. Each of these is the echo in the mind of cells stimulated or depressed, by concentration or dilution in the blood of particular internal secretions. Restlessness and excitement can be produced experimentally by feeding thyroid. Vague anxiety, depressive fancies and fears, imaginative overactivity can be removed by inhibiting the post-pituitary. Hypersecretion of the ovary will cause a sexual susceptibility and a mood of genital obsession, capable of the most remarkable sublimations and perversions.

CHAPTER IX
THE BACKGROUNDS OF PERSONALITY

The question of moods and sublimations once raised introduces the problem of the relation of neuroses, nervous disorders without an organic disease basis, and mental abnormalities, to the endocrine system. Obviously, in view of all the influences exerted by the ductless glands upon every organ and function of the body and mind, and their intermediary, the vegetative nervous system, a relation must exist. Observations accumulated, some of which have been referred to in the preceding chapters, prove the complete, though complex, reality of such a deduction.

The history of attitudes toward nerve and mental disorders is a remarkable illustration of the vicissitudes of ignorance playing with words. The Greeks, swayed and dazzled as they were by the magic of words which they discovered, yet never permitted themselves to be fooled by them. As an explanation for the phenomena of hysteria in women, that benign mental disorder par excellence, they had the theory of a wandering about of the womb in the organism as a cause. That provided an image of something material happening as an explanation. With the triumphs of anatomy after the Renaissance, that naive view had to be discarded. In its place the humoral theory held sway, with its good humors and its bad humors, and their bilious, lymphatic, nervous and sanguine admixtures. But that, too, went the way of all flesh. During the first half of the nineteenth century, a popular phrase, "nerves," paraphrased by practitioners of medicine as neuroses, then came into vogue as the efficient cause of these troubles. "Nerves" indeed today have filtered everywhere into the common consciousness.

Because of the irritant effects of light, food and social conditions, America has come to swarm with neurotics of every type, especially the sexual. A rich field was created for cults of treatment, which spring up like weeds periodically all over the country. We have seen how the American, Beard, was inspired by the idea that "nerves" represented a loss of tone, a flabbiness, weakness and softness of the nerves, to coin the word neurasthenia. Nerve exhaustion he believed was the cause of the nerve weakness. Weir Mitchell, another American, introduced the rest cure combined with overfeeding as a treatment for it.

An analytical French neurologist, Charcot, was not to be satisfied by words of Latin-Greek derivation. Insisting upon the significance of the individual mental workings of each case, he and his pupil Janet began to unravel a tangle which has led to the present revolution in psychology. For Freud, Jung and Adler took up the story where Janet left off.

Janet elaborated the ideas of a subconscious and an unconscious, a dissociation of the components of the mind, and a splitting of the personality. Lumping the phenomena of amnesia, somnambulism, hypnotism, anesthesia, obsession and hysteria into the grand group of mental dissociations and disintegrations, he achieved a unification never considered possible before him. Suggestion as a mode of cure was also emphasized and elaborated by him to an undreamed-of degree.

Freud, in 1895, studying a case of hysteria with Breuer, had attempted cure by the method of free association, attempting to get the hysteric to pour out her mental life. Not succeeding, and his interest aroused by her continual references to her dreams, he discovered that by means of those dreams he could tap the subconscious and unconscious in regions hitherto inaccessible. For in the dreams, ideas, persons, and experiences appeared that never came upon the stage of the conscious. From that finding he developed the concept of repression, i.e., the relegation of a painful experience into the unconscious, and kept imprisoned there by the censor. Also how there it became the complex, which, like a stage manager, never appeared before the footlights of the conscious, but determined its content just the same by inhibition or stimulation of any character or scene to be enacted upon it.

A complete critique of Freudianism cannot be attempted here. But in relation to the endocrine system as controllers of nerve function in health and disease, a valid criticism can be made. Firstly, the Freudian jargon, its technicalities and explanations, are metaphors. Some may regard them as justifiable descriptions of mental processes. But it certainly can be urged against them that they provide us with no idea concerning what is happening in the cells of the body and brain as explanation for the event, normal or abnormal, supposedly explained. Words like sublimation or transference are figures of speech and nothing else. Secondly, they ignore totally the powers of the vegetative apparatus, the viscera, muscles and secreting glands together, as originators and determiners of the wish and its adventures.

How utterly different, from the point of view of the physiologist, the two explanations are as pictures, can be seen from a single example. The idea of repression, to the Freudian, means the pushing down into the subconscious of some experience. Pushing down is a process controlled by the laws of physics: it involves the concepts of matter and force. Hence, the expression, as a description of a psychic episode, is a metaphor pure and simple. From the standpoint of the process of repression as pictured by the student of the vegetative apparatus, the term signifies a real bottling up of energy. For the repression means actual compression of muscle, the muscle contained in the viscera. And the repression means a real interference with the release of energy, which remains bound up, tugging for room for expression as much as a spring tightly coiled in a box. In the production of that tension an endocrine has often been decisive. The endocrine nature of the individual may decide whether a subconscious, i.e., visceral or vegetative tension, is to come into being, live or die, in the face of a given situation. If thereby, a permanent disturbance of the equilibrium between the components is brought about, a neurosis, expression of an unsatisfied vegetative tension, follows.

It has been hailed as a brand new discovery by those following the latest in psychology that the subconscious and the unconscious constitute a more essential component of the personality than the conscious. As a matter of fact, common practice has recognized the fact, if not the mechanism and its significance, for ages. It is not what people say or do--it is how they say it: that is how the true reactions of personality are recognized instinctively even by animals. Tone and gesture (when not acted or posed) are accepted as symbols and symptoms of states of the inmost sancta sanctorum that words and wit never give entrance to, nay disguise and block. Tone and gesture as revelations of the Inner-Me, the True-Me or Intra-Me if you will, are so potent because they are direct expressions of the vegetative apparatus. The curl of a lip, the flicker of an eye-lash, the twitch of a shoulder are the overflow of energy cramped in the increased intravisceral pressure, determined by increased outflow of endocrine secretion. Wittingly or unwittingly we interpret the little signs as messages from the deepest self, which they truly are.

NERVOUS BREAKDOWNS AND SHELL SHOCK

In civil life, the complex of symptoms Beard jumbled together as neurasthenia, when associated with a loss of self-control, so that the sufferer is incapacitated for the duties of everyday life, has become the popular "nervous breakdown." A sanitarium appears to be one of the necessary components of the condition. It is the last act, the climax of "nerves."

During the War of 1914-1918, thousands of cases of functional disorders of the nervous came to be grouped under "Shell Shock." The psychic phenomena in the wake of concussion of the brain due to explosives suggested the term, and its application to affections of self-control, or dissociations of the personality, with paralysis, blindness, speechlessness, loss of hearing and so on. The War neurosis (including those arising in home service) is still a topical subject because thousands of mentally disabled soldiers are alive.

In view of what has been said concerning the endocrine mechanism of the instincts and the vegetative apparatus, it could be predicted that a number of these nerve casualties of peace and war would be caused by an upset of the equilibrium between the glands of internal secretion. A study of war neuroses by the great Italian student of the endocrines, Pende, confirms this assumption. As emphasized, the internal secretions are like tuning keys, and tighten or loosen the strings of the organism-instrument, the nerves. War for the soldier, or the civilian combatant as well, sets the strings vibrating, and with them the glands controlled by them. Excessive stimulation or depression of an endocrine will disturb the whole chain of hormones, and the vegetative system, and their echoes in the psyche. The nervous disorders of war that have been lumped as shell shock or war shock may be looked upon as uncompensated; airings of the endocrine vegetative mechanism, as dislocations of parts and processes that are reflected outwardly as ailment or disease.

AN ENDOCRINE NEUROSIS

An exquisite example of an endocrine neurosis, that is a disorder of nerves and brain dependent upon an upset of the equilibrium between the internal secretions due to a trying experience, was furnished recently by the reactions of three naval officers lost in the snow wilds of Canada through a balloon adventure. The cases aroused a good deal of interest at the time, and the details were reported by the newspapers as if they were the episodes of a serial mystery story.

The three officers started out late one fine evening from Rockaway Air Station in a balloon for a practice trip. Atmospheric conditions suddenly changed, they became lost in the clouds, and finally landed somewhere in the Canadian wilderness. The commander of the balloon crew, Lieut. A., 23 years old, was the youngest of the three; the oldest, Lieut. B., being 45, and the third man in the thirties, Lieut. C.

According to the testimony given at the Court of Inquiry held afterwards, two hours after they abandoned the balloon and started struggling through the snow, B. became tired and complained of his fatigue. B.'s fatigue increased, and two days later became so great that the party had to stop for an hour and build a fire in order to permit him to rest. However, an hour proved too little: and in another half hour he was falling and fainting.

Letters written by C. to his wife and gotten hold of by reporters declared that B. at this juncture passed into a semi-sane state, in which he accused himself of a number of sins, and volunteered to commit suicide, so that the others would not be burdened by his weakness. Also, that they might use his body to fortify themselves. A. discussed with C. the advisability of taking B.'s knife away from him. Living on their carrier pigeons, they continued on, moved by a desperate hope of finding someone. B. had several fainting spells after drinking water traced by moose tracks.

Luck favored them, and they encountered an Indian who guided them to a place called Moose Factory. Here they wrote the letters home which reached their wives and the daily press before they themselves returned to civilization. A great hue and cry was raised by the newspapers about their plight. Newspaper correspondents vied with each other for the honor of being the first to meet them and get their story.

They arrived at a collection of houses named Mattice. A. and C. proceeded ahead and found instructions for them not to talk. C. went back to B., who was in a shack with the correspondents full of the story of the letters. B. became enraged and struck C. who retained his self-control.

Differences were patched up, and the three returned together to New York. There the medical examination of the three showed that the four days in the wilderness had left its deepest effects upon the physique and mind of B. In a few days he developed an attack of tonsillitis, with fever, and a mental disturbance described by the medical officer as exhaustion psychosis. He believed this condition to be the result of severe exhaustion, prolonged anxiety, worry, and extreme exposure. Extreme restlessness and irritability, confusion of thought and an undefined perplexity, all the prominent symptoms of exhaustion psychosis, making him hyperactive and inclined to acts of violence, were in evidence.

The physique, character and reactions of Lieut. B. are what interest us in the case. The pictures of him published, and the structure of his skull, face and teeth, his hair and other physical traits point to his being an adrenal-centered type, of the unstable variety, so far as his internal secretion make-up is concerned. As we shall see in the next chapter on the different kinds of endocrine personalities, the unstable adrenocentric (convenient name for the class) is characterized by rapid exhaustibility because under conditions of stress and strain, the reserve of the gland is consumed. The adrenal glands, we noted in a preceding chapter, are concerned with the maintenance of muscle and nerve tone in emergencies. They are the glands which, during crises especially, control the production and supply of energy to the various organs and tissues called upon to function to the utmost in emergencies. When the adrenals fail, as they do readily in these labile adrenocentrics, it is as if the adrenals were cut out of the body. And it has been repeatedly shown that extirpation of the adrenals is immediately followed by degeneration and breakdown of the brain cells.

These facts explain the reactions of Lieut. B. The acute call upon his adrenals made by his dangerous situation probably soon exhausted them of their content of reserve secretions. Overwhelming fatigue with loss of muscle tone followed. The changes in the brain caused him to talk as he did in the wilderness. Returned to safety, the news that his reputation was under fire because of C.'s letter brought out another adrenal characteristic: the excessive instinct of pugnacity, easily stimulated, with its emotion of anger and the tendency to violence. What is spoken of as a quick temper is an adrenocentric trait. Returned to New York, an infection, tonsillitis, attacked him. Infections in adrenocentrics use up the content of the adrenals as rapidly as physical exhaustion or emotion. So the tonsillitis, which in another type of individual would have been combatted continuously by the adrenals and so passed by as a mere sore throat, presented him with a high temperature, and the brain disturbance described by the medical officer as exhaustion-psychosis, with again a tendency to violence. In short, the history of his adventure is the history of his adrenals under stress and strain. It illustrates the mechanism of a typical endocrine neurosis.

THE UNCONSCIOUS AND THE VISCERA

In the chapter on the glands of internal secretion as an interlocking directorate, certain generalities were stated as the laws of the government of the organism's life by them in association with the vegetative apparatus. It was put forward as a fundamental revision of the theory, hitherto accepted, of the limitation of mind to the brain cells. We think and feel not alone with the brain, but with our muscles, our viscera, our vegetative nerves, and last but not least our endocrine organs. In short, we think and feel with each and every part of ourselves.

Among these pristine factors determining the content of consciousness, the endocrines are most important, because they alone to start with, of all the other factors, are different in each and every individual. They are what render him unique at birth, even though he looks the counterpart of millions of other babies born at the same time. They constitute his inner destiny. As he grows, the external factors, social experiences, climate, accidents, and disease modify and condition the reactions and complexity of the endocrine system. As these modifications and associations are of the greatest import for the final elaboration of the personality, composing as they do the elements of the unconscious which confers the unique stamp of normal, abnormal, supernormal, or subnormal, it is worth while now to review the most general of the determining laws. Man is an energy phenomenon, both conscious and unconscious, with the energy emanating from the endocrine-vegetative mechanisms. So it becomes possible for us, by their aid, to analyze the conscious, the subconscious and the unconscious with the terms long current in the analyses of physics.

1. Man is an energy machine which, though it is constantly losing energy as a whole; consists of parts constantly accumulating energy (as a result of inherent chemical reactions accelerated by the absorption of food). This process of local accumulation of energy associated with general loss of energy may be observed even in the ameba, in the form of stored reserve food material. Evolution created a system of organs, the viscera, as specialists in energy conservation, utilization or trans-

formation.

For intercommunication and interaction between the viscera two systems were elaborated: a younger system of direct contacts, the nerves, and nerve cells, through which influences could be conducted for the stimulation, acceleration, retardation or inhibition of an energy process in them; and the older, the endocrine gland association, for the production of chemical substances to act as messengers to be sent from one viscus to another, and also to the nerves, through the blood or lymph which bathe all the cells. They could affect only one or certain organs, because by selection only the chosen organ or organs knew the code, as it were. The chemical system is much the older system, and preceded the nerve system by aeons of time. The whole system, viscera, visceral nerves and the endocrines gradually united into a complete autonomous organism within the organism, and as such functions as the vegetative apparatus.

EVOLUTION OF THE ENDOCRINES

2. In the course of evolution, variations occurred in all three components of the apparatus, the viscera, the nerves, and the endocrines. Now variations in the viscera and the nerves are essentially grossly physical and quantitative. That is, there may be a bigger stomach or a smaller stomach, larger nerve fibres or smaller. And as Life always has worked with a large margin of safety, and always played for safety first as regards quantity, these variations have not become of much significance for the history and destiny of the animal.

But variations among the endocrines made a tremendous difference. To have very much thyroid and very little pituitary, much adrenal and not enough parathyroid meant a great deal to the Organism as a whole, as well as to the vegetative apparatus. For states of tension and relaxation, activity and inactivity in the nerves and viscera would be determined by these variations in the ratio between the variants. The vegetative apparatus in its virginity, say in the new-born infant, may be said to have its development primarily determined by the reaction potentials of the endocrine part of it, that is the latent power of each gland to secrete at a minimum or a maximum, and the balance between them.

EDUCATION OF THE VEGETATIVE SYSTEM

3. Training or education involves, beside other effects, a training of the endocrines, and hence of the entire vegetative apparatus, to respond in a particular way

to a particular stimulus. Experience is like the introduction of new push-buttons, levers, and wheels into the mechanism. All learning which calls out or arrests the functioning of an instinct, must, from what we have learned of the chemical dynamics of instincts as reactions between hormones, nerves and viscera, affect the vegetative system. When there is a conflict between two or more instincts, between pressures of energy flowing in different directions, there may be compromise and normality, or a grinding of the gears and abnormality.

Where does the brain come in, in all this? As the servant of the vegetative apparatus. To call it the master tissue is manifestly absurd, when it can only be the diplomatic constitutional monarch of the system. It can, in fact, act only as the great central station for associative memory, as only one of the factors implicated in education.

The most powerful educative agents of the vegetative apparatus of a human being are the other humans around him. And they comprise the most powerful of the external effectors of education, for better, for worse. The training and education of the endocrine-vegetative system is the basis of all social rules (Habit, Custom, Convention, Law, Conscience). An unresolved discord, a continued conflict among the parts of the vegetative system, in spite of such education, is the foundation of the unhappiness of the acute or chronic misfits and maladjusted, the neurotic and the psychotic.

THE PHYSICAL BASIS OF THE UNCONSCIOUS

4. Another vastly important law that governs the content of the conscious and the unconscious, and resultant behaviour is the fact that the nerves and nerve cells of the vegetative apparatus, the nerves leading to the viscera and the endocrine glands, like the solar plexus, are affected by stimuli of lower value than those which arouse the brain cells. In the metaphorical language of the old psychology, the threshold value, that is the strength or loudness of stimulus sufficient to make itself felt or heard, is less for the vegetative apparatus than for the brain. So we begin to glimpse why an emotion seems to be experienced before the visceral changes that really preceded it, but pressed their way into consciousness later. This gives us a clue to the unconscious as the more sensitive and deeper part of the mind.

More than that, it supplies us with a physical basis for the unconscious which will explain much of the observed laws of its workings. It provides a reason for the apparent swiftness, spontaneity, and unreasonableness of what is called intuition. And it may show us a source for a good deal of the material of dreams and dream states.

We have said that we think and we remember, not alone with the brain, but with the muscles, the viscera and the endocrines. So do we forget not alone with the brain, but with the muscles, the viscera, the endocrines and their nerves. The utmost importance of muscle attitudes in remembering has been established in the experimental laboratory.

It is one of the great services Freud rendered to psychology (and one, by the way, largely responsible for the acceptance of his doctrines by the disinterested intelligence) that he showed that a species of forgetting is nothing casual, but active and purposeful, a manifestation of the life of the unconscious. However, though his description of the process was correct, he left it to occur in a vacuum. As a matter of fact this forgetting consists in the inhibition of associative memory by a process in the vegetative apparatus, so as to maintain the equilibrium within itself which is reflected in consciousness as comfort.

The unconscious, in short, consists of the buried associations among the parts of the vegetative apparatus and the brain cells. We seem to be much nearer to grasping the nature of the unconscious, when we look upon it as a historical continuum, a compound or emulsion of different and various states of intravisceral pressure and tone, in the vegetative apparatus, dependent upon the balance between the endocrines, as well as upon past experiences of the viscera in the way of stimulation or depression. We forget that which is held down, literally, in the vegetative apparatus. This explanation of forgetting tells, too, why the forgotten (stored in the sub-brain, the endocrine-vegetative system) continually projects itself into and interferes with the regular flow of consciousness, e.g., in slips of the tongue, mistakes of spelling, and so on: because the energy bottled in the vegetative system tends to erupt into the consciousness into which it would ordinarily flow.

In the evolution of the mind, there have been elaborated devices to protect it against the vegetative apparatus. Consciousness, or awareness, must be accepted as a fundamental, primal fact, like protoplasm. Consciousness and protoplasm may be the complementary sides of the same coin. Whatever the truth, the fact stands out that the oldest, deepest, most potent consciousness is that of the traditionally despised lowest organs, the vegetative organs, the heart and lungs, stomach and intestines, the kidneys and the liver, and so on, their nerves, e.g., the solar plexus, and the glands of internal secretion. They invented and elaborated muscle, bone and brain to carry out their will. Evolution has been in the direction of a greater perfection of the methods of carrying out their will. Their consciousness, working upon the growing and multiplying brain cells, has created what we call self-conscious mind.

Mind, reacting upon its creator, has, in a sense, come to dominate them, because it has become the meeting ground of all the energy-influences seething and bubbling in the organism, and so developed into the organ of handling them as a whole, their Integrating-Executive. But just the same and all the time, the underlying consciousness of the viscera and their accessories stand as the powers behind the throne, but as what we have now learned to speak of, in relation to the Mind, as the Unconscious.

PSYCHOPATHOLOGY OF EVERYDAY LIFE

To sum up these relations of the viscera, the endocrines, the unconscious and the mind, it may be stated as a far-reaching generality for the understanding of human life: that character and conduct are expressions of the streams of energy arising in the vegetative apparatus, primarily endocrine determined at birth, and secondarily experience determined after the organism has learned to react as a whole, as consciousness. The result of such a reaction as a whole tends to balance the disturbance of energy, so as to maintain or restore the equilibrium, or sense of harmony and comfort, when consciousness again disappears. This law is an attempt at synthesis of the labors of the psychanalysts, the behaviourists, and the students of the internal secretions (Freud, Jung, Adler, Sherrington, Watson, Von Bechterew, Kempf, Crile, Cannon, Cushing, Fraenkel are the great names of the movement). Most of the details, and all of the quantitative applications of the law still remain to be worked out. But a statement like the following of Cushing, the eminent surgeon-student of the endocrines, that "it is quite probable that the psychopathology of everyday life hinges largely upon the effect of ductless gland discharges upon the nervous system," shows which way the wind is blowing.

In the face of these conceptions the position of the psychanalyst as a practical therapeutist becomes clearer, and the causes of his failure when he fails. In the first place, he deals with psychic results as processes, and ignores the physiology of their production. Since a true cure of the neurosis, what he is after, is impossible without a removal of the cause, a disturbance in the vegetative apparatus, he cannot succeed where an automatic adjustment among the viscera does not follow his probings and ferretings of the unconscious. In the second place, he disregards the existence of a soil for the planting of the malign complexes in the individual in whom they grow and flourish. That soil is composed in part of the endocrine relations within the vegetative apparatus. And as we can often attack that soil more effectively and radically from the endocrine end than from the experience end (e.g., repressed episodes) we may transform the soil and make it barren rock for morbid complexes, at any rate. The concept of the endocrine-vegetative apparatus as the determinant of normal and abnormal behaviour, emotional reactions and disturbances of power should in time cause even the most fanatic of the psychanalysts to recognize the functional basis of the mental acrostics they are so fond of dissecting.

NATURAL ABILITY

Another achievement of the psychanalysts is the recognition of the influence of organic and functional inferiorities of the individual upon the history of his personality. Gross organ inferiorities are those which are definite handicaps in the struggle for success in society, such as heart disease. Such handicaps, however, are limited to relatively few of a population. The raison d'etre of the greater number of minor mental inefficiencies the psychanalyst puts down to handicaps in the unconscious. Again he mistakes figurative imagery for explanations. The conception of endocrine diversity in the make-up supplies us with the rationale of the vast majority of organic and functional defects and inferiorities, in short, subnormalities of any group, large or small.

Moreover, how would the psychanalyst explain the occurrence and influence of organic and functional *superiorities* and their tremendous influence upon the individual and society? We live in a generation which has acquired a flair for the pathologic. Undoubtedly it is a soul-sick generation, and its interest in sickness of the mind is only natural. Just the same, whatever advances, improvements, progress, have been made (and certainly a number of the changes in his environment, external and internal, must be admitted to be changes for the better) have been made, not by natural disability, but by natural ability. What is the physiology of natural ability?

The finest study of natural ability that has as yet been composed is Francis Galton's on Hereditary Genius. It also remains the best study of the natural conditions of success. He showed that of the type of man he classed as "illustrious" there occurred about one in a million, and of the type "eminent" about two hundred and fifty in a million. Of the qualities which determine natural ability of this kind, he selected inherent capacity, zeal, and perseverance as the three prerequisites. And he states that "If a man is gifted with vast intellectual ability, eagerness to work, and power of working, I cannot comprehend how such a man should be suppressed." "Such men (those who have gained great reputations) biographies show to be haunted and driven by an incessant, instinctive craving for intellectual work." "They ... work ... to satisfy a natural craving for brain work." "It is very unlikely that any conjunction of circumstances should supply a stimulus to brain work commensurate with what these men carry in their own constitutions."

What is this inherent craving for brain work? What is this zeal? And what is power of endurance and perseverance, the quality of stamina? How are they to be interpreted in terms of the internal secretions?

In view of what has been said of the ante-pituitary as the gland of intellectuality, studies of intellectually gifted people having shown well functioning large pituitaries, and of mental defectives in a certain number of cases a small limited pituitary, it is justifiable to regard the factor of inherent capacity as a function of the ante-pituitary. The factor of zeal or enthusiasm points to the thyroid. Markedly enthusiastic types are thyroid dominant types. Vigor as a third factor, the ability to stand stress and strain of continued effort is dependent upon good adrenal and interstitial cell function. So we may say that craving and capacity for brain work plus ardor plus perseverance in its pursuit, the triplicate of natural ability, are the reflections in conduct and character of balanced and sufficient ante-pituitary, thyroid, and adrenal-interstitial contributions in the chemical formula of the personality. In the chapter on historic personages analyzed from the endocrine viewpoint, we shall see that some of the most eminent and illustrious people of history have been pituitary-centered.

MENTAL DEFICIENCY

Natural ability grows in an endocrine soil of a particular kind, perhaps affected by the internal secretions much as natural soil is by fertilizers like phosphates or nitrates. Increased production follows increased fertilization. Natural disability must vary similarly with a perversion or improper mixture, deficiency or absence of the hormones that combine in natural ability.

It is assumed as a matter of course that the brain itself is there, which, to carry out our analogy, means that the crude soil or earth is there. Sufficient quantity and adequate quality of nerve tissue must be regarded as prerequisite. If the brain has been damaged in any way during development or birth, if it has been smashed up in any way, or if it has failed to evolve the minimum number of healthy nerve cells, the endocrine influence becomes negligible. It is like attempting to insert a key into a door which has no lock.

It is among the specimens of normality of the brain cells that we may look for our examples of endocrine mental deficiency. Included are all sorts of examples of feeble-mindedness varying from the moron to the imbecile and idiot, arrested brain life. The cretin is the classic type of mental deficiency due to endocrine insufficiency, curable or improvable by the proper handling.

Insanity, degeneration of the normal brain life, may be caused by an upset of the endocrine balance. Among the commonest manifestations of insanity are excitements and depressions, apathies and manias, hallucinations, delusions and obsessions, all of which are reproducible under known conditions of internal secretion excess or failure. Alternating states of mania and depression are caused in some instances by extreme hyperthyroidism. The critical periods of life, when a profound revolution is overturning the endocrine equilibrium, puberty, pregnancy, and the menopause, are the periods of most frequent occurrence of insanity, when mental instability reveals endocrine instability (Dementia praecox, pregnancy psychosis, menopause neurosis). Actual insanity need not be the only manifestation. By far the greater number of mental disturbances due to aberrations of the internal secretions never see an asylum or a doctor. They live more or less close to the borderline of insanity as persons who have spells, eccentricities and peculiarities, hysteria, tics or just "nervousness."

About two-thirds of mental deficiency is definitely inherited, about one-third acquired. It is the opinion of a number of psychologists that it is inherited as what the Mendelians call a recessive, that is as a trait which will be overshadowed, if there is admixture of normal mentality, but will crop up by breeding with another mental defective. What we know of the endocrine factors in heredity leads us to suppose that it is the mating of one marked endocrine insufficiency with another that is often responsible for the inherited tendency to feeble-mindedness and insanity. The effect of the hormone system upon the vegetative apparatus may create the more obscure insanities and quasi-insanities. The direct action of the internal secretions upon the brain cells, producing a sort of hair trigger situation within them, may cause the explosive discharges from them which appear as overpowering impulses or uncontrollable conduct. The waves of feeling which precede them are unquestionably endocrine determined. The wave of fear a cat experiences upon seeing a dog is accompanied and indeed preceded by an increase of the amount of adrenalin in the blood. The picture of fright, as observed in a so-called normal person, staring eyes, trembling hands, dry lips and mouth, corresponds to the portrait of the appearance in hyperthyroidism. In persons afflicted with uncontrollable impulses, the inhibiting hormones may not be present in sufficient quantity.

Feeble-mindedness, ranging from stupidity to imbecility, may also be a direct effect of insufficient endocrine supply to the brain cells. When there is not enough of the thyroid secretion in the blood, the tissue between the cells in the brain become clogged and thickened, so that a gross barrier to the passage of the nerve impulses is created. We have here an illustration of internal secretion lack actually producing gross changes in the brain. But without a doubt, most endocrine influences upon the brain, at work every minute and second of its life, are the subtle ones of molecular chemistry and atomic energetics. We know that such mental qualities as irritability and stupidity, fatigability, and the power to recover quickly or slowly from fatigue, sexual potency and impotence, apathy and enthusiasm are endocrine qualities. We know also that the thyroid dominant tends to be irritable and excitable, the pituitary deficient to be placid and gentle, the adrenal dominant to be assertive and pugnacious, the thymus-centered to be childish and easy-go-lucky and the gonad deficient to be secretive and shy. This brings us to the relation of the internal secretions to the type of personality as a whole.

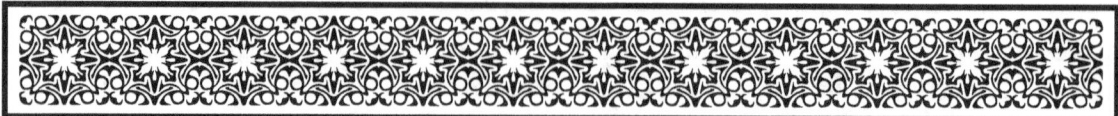

CHAPTER X
THE TYPES OF PERSONALITY

THE ENDOCRINE PERSONALITY

If a single gland can dominate the life history of an individual it becomes possible to speak of *endocrine types*, the result of the *endocrine analysis* of the individual. Studying endocrine traits of physique, life reactions, disease tendencies, hereditary history and blood chemistry, one may gain an insight into the composition or constitution of an individual. The endocrine type of an individual is a summary of these, his behaviour in the past, and is also a prediction of his reactions in the future, much as a chemical formula outlines what we believe to be the skeleton of a compound substance as deducible from its properties under varying conditions. Only, admittedly, as yet the endocrine label is but roughly qualitative and most crudely quantitative, whereas the chemical formula is the essence of the exact.

However, the fact remains that though we are only upon the first rungs of the ladder, we are upon the ladder. The horizon undoubtedly broadens. We possess a new way of looking upon humanity, a fresh transforming light upon those strange phenomena, ourselves. Of the ugly achievements of that dreadful century, the nineteenth, the most illuminating was the discovery of itself as the *ape-parvenu.* Yes, we are all animals now, it said to itself, and set its teeth in the cut-throat game of survival. But there was no understanding in that evil motto of a disillusioned heart. The ape-parvenu, desperately lonely and secretive, has still to understand himself.

Let us be clear if we can. There is perhaps a certain presumption in the phrase, the endocrine type. It is ambitious, and perhaps will not fulfill its promise. But it is useful because it points a parallel and an ideal. As Wilhelm Ostwald never tired of repeating, H_2O is a complete shorthand record for the bundle of qualities commonly known as water. It is an example of that highest task of mind, synthesis. It is the highest synthesis of the studies of the internal secretions that certain combinations of them, permutations and blendings of them, are responsible for those unique wonders of the universe, personalities.

The riddle of personality! Are we at last upon the track of its uncovering? That elusive mystery, which philosophers have wrapped in the thousand veils of Greek and Latin words, and psychologists, even unto the third and fourth generation of Freudians, have floundered about in, moles before a dazzling sun, is it to be unwound for our inspection? Think of the human soul. What an invisible, intangible chameleon is its true reality! Watch it, and you see something that seems to uncurl and expand like a feather with exultation and delight and joy, to contract and stiffen into a billiard ball with fear and pride, shrewd caution and vigilant malevolence, to rear back and spark fire like lightning with anger and temper, and to crawl and slither with abjection and smirking slyness, when it needs to. This multiplex Thing-Behind-Life, are we really about to dissect it into its elements?

Personality embraces much more than merely the psychic attributes. It is not the least important of the lessons of endocrine analysis that there is no soul, and no body, either. Rather a soul-body, or body-soul, or the patterns of the living flame. The closer tracking of the internal secretions leads us into the secrets of the living flame, why it lives, and how it lives, the strange diversities of its colorings and music and the odd variations in its energy, vitality and longevity. Why it flickers, why it flares and glares, spurts, flutters, burns hard or soft, orange-blue or yellow.

The medieval scholiasts, who fought as fiercely about names as nations about territories, divided men into the sanguine, the bilious, the lymphatic and the nervous. It was a pretty crude classification of different constitutions. The endocrine criteria, more exact and concrete, divide them into the adrenal centered, the thyroid centered, the thymus centered, the pituitary centered, the gonad centered, and their combinations.

THE ADRENAL PERSONALITIES

An adrenal personality is one dominated by the ups and downs of his adrenal gland. In the large, the curve of his life is the curve of secretion by this gland, both of its Cortex and medulla. Such an adrenal personality is entirely normal, within the definition of the normal as something not threatening the duration of life, nor comfortable adaptation to it. So are the other glandular types. No sharp line can be drawn between the normal and the abnormal in any case, the borderland is wide, the transitions many.

The skin is one of the chief clues to the adrenal personality. The relation between the adrenal and the skin dates way back in the evolutionary scale, for adrenalin has been isolated directly from pigment deposits in the epidermis of frogs. Skin pigment bears a direct relation to the reaction of the organism to light, especially the ultraviolet rays, to the radiation of heat, and hence to the fundamental productions and consumptions of energy by the cells. So the gland of energy for emergencies writes its signature always all over the skin.

In an adrenal personality, the epidermis is always slightly, somewhat, or deeply pigmented. The pigmentation is due to a dark brown deposit lightly or thickly scattered over the skin. With the general diffuse pigmentation or darkening there are often the black spots, the pigmented birth marks, or the lighter ones of freckles. The latter signify some permanent or transitory adrenal inadequacy in the past, antenatal or post-natal, of the individual, and presage the same in his future. These spots have been frequently observed to appear after an attack of diphtheria or influenza. There seems to be more tuberculosis among those who have them than those who do not. We therefore say that diphtheria, influenza and tuberculosis stand out as adrenal-attacking diseases, which have a greater power to kill, cripple or hurt those with defective adrenal constitutions than others.

The hair of the adrenal type is characteristic: ubiquitous, thick, coarse and dry. It is prominent over the chest, abdomen and back, and has a tendency to kink. Often its color is not the expected: an Italian's will be yellow, a Norwegian's jet black. It has been stated that most red-haired persons are adrenal types. Such persons also have well-marked canine teeth which is another adrenal trait. They also have a low hair line.

When the adrenal type has a properly co-operating pituitary and thyroid, he possesses a striking vigor, energy and persistence. With a fortunate combination, he develops into a progressive winning fighter, arriving at the top in the long run every time.

Brain work is pretty well lubricated in the well-compensated adrenal type. Brain fag is closely associated with, if not dependent upon, adrenal fag, particularly of the cortex. Brain tissue and adrenal cortex tissue are near relatives, and a normal human brain never develops without a normal adrenal cortex. The adrenal type with an hypertrophied adrenal cortex is always efficient.

Among women, the adrenal type is always masculinoid. If physically feminine--due to adequate feminine reactions on the part of the other endocrines--she will at least show the qualities of a psychic virilism. A generation ago, such a woman had to repress her inherent trends and instincts in the face of public opinion and law, and so suffered from a feeling of inferiority. Nowadays, these women are striding forward and will attain a good many of the masculine heights, commanding responsible executive positions and high salaries. An adrenal type will probably be the first woman president of the United States.

However, that presupposes a normal range of action of the other endocrines. Let there be some quirk or weakness elsewhere in the chain of hormones, and instead of the successful woman, behold the spinsters, the maiden aunts, the prudes and cranks who never satisfactorily adapt themselves in society. To them must be given a good deal of credit for the suffrage revolution. These unadapted adrenals, as we may call them, once sowed the seeds, expending their masculinism in the struggles of the pioneers' martyrdoms, preparing the harvest their sisters, the more adequate adrenal types, will now reap. The unadapted adrenals of today will have to look for new worlds to conquer.

So much for the compensated adrenal types. They are the good workers, the efficients, the kinetic successes of the driven world. They make, at a certain level, good slave drivers because they feel within themselves a driving force. But suppose the adrenal type becomes uncompensated, or perhaps is inadequate to the demands of life to start with. Then the story becomes different. The perfect efficient super-man of business or profession begins to lag. Though he is himself in the morning, he begins to lag in the afternoon. That is when he tires. In the evening he is all in. More sleep, recreational trips, vacations slip into the rank of necessities, whereas previously they had been laughed at as luxuries. More minute or large moles emerge in the skin, especially if the individual is of a fair type. If a strenuous effort is not made to give the adrenals an opportunity to recuperate, or if adjustment on the part of the other glands does not occur, this stage of intermittent and remittent adrenal inadequacy gives way in turn to the state of permanent adrenal insufficiency.

The adrenal insufficient is important because he is to be seen everywhere. Built along the same lines as the adrenal adequate and apt to be taken for him, he differs and contrasts vividly below the surface. One may sum him up by saying that he is one variety of neurasthenic, perhaps the most frequent variety. Cold hands and feet plague him, cold feet psychically as well as physically, for a chronic and obsessive indecision is one of his most prominent complaints. A fatigability, that goes with a low blood pressure, lowered body temperature and a disturbed ability to utilize sugar for fuel purposes, is another of his chief complaints. The skin often presents an instability of the blood vessels, so that they now react to stroking with a blanched instead of a reddened effect. Irritability, a liability to go off the handle at the slightest provocation, and a consequent complete exhaustion that, after an outburst, sends him to bed, is conspicuous. Dismissed sometimes contemptuously as weaklings, they are accused of laziness, craziness, and haziness. In their psychic attempts to compensate, they land into all kinds of hot water, from which friends, relatives or luck extricate them sometimes. The other times they go to the wall.

The congenital adrenal deficient is a special problem. If the history of such an individual is followed from birth, one gets a pretty typical story. The genealogy is nervous. Nervous is a word of many meanings. But when parents confess themselves nervous, it generally means a mental and emotional instability of some sort. Sometimes the idea is camouflaged as high strung. In the feeding narrative of the child, one finds not occasional incidents or episodes, but continued trouble, difficulties, adventures. Even after the first year or two, the nutritional chronicle is not satisfactory. Lack of appetite, lack of energy, lack of response to stimuli are its keynotes and the motifs of the later years of childhood.

Growth is a strain. It becomes a task to make these children grow and gain. Chronically below the average weight and height, herculean efforts are made by the conscientious parents, but with small success.

With the entry of school life and competition, the curtain rises upon the real tragedy, a tragedy in which the avenging Fates are the usual ignorance, stupidity and misunderstanding. If the teachers alone are duty-obsessed, or perhaps sadistic, the child endures the agonies of repeated admonitions, demotions, and punishments. However, a certain thick-skinned indifference may develop to protect the sufferer.

If the parents are in addition ambitious, or proud, or competitive, then woe betide the victim. With their nervous dispositions, it is the school and the tutor who are to be blamed, if not the child. From school to school, from system to system, from novelty to fad, from doctor to doctor, from fakir to charlatan, from pillar to post, they wander in search of an education. Educational cults by the dozen have sprouted and grown fat around these unfortunates.

The chief defect of the congenital adrenal inadequate is an insufficiently developed adrenal cortex. That means an insufficiently developed brain and nervous system. For we have seen how closely all these are related in development. Now education can never be the education of a vacuum. And we have to deal here with a relative vacuum. When there are no potentialities, there can be no education. Where the potentialities are limited, education must be limited. The congenital adrenal inadequate is defined in physical and mental energy. Hence educators cannot drive him. Up to a certain point he can be led, but no farther. He should not be expected to go to a college, and waste the opportunity of some one financially unlucky, but whose endocrine system is more generously endowed.

Not that the outlook is absolutely hopeless. Puberty, with its tremendous changes in the glands of internal secretion, when one can almost hear the clicks and the whirring of the wheels in the internal machinery, may transform. The unfathomed possibilities of gland therapy are still to be probed. But the general rule remains.

THE REACTIONS TO MODERNISM

The adrenal personalities in all their variations must be safeguarded and carefully looked after in the strained complexities of modern post-bellum civilization. In a sense, the adrenal type is the Atlas of the twentieth century world, and small wonder that he and his descendants stagger beneath the burden. The adrenals are organs for the mobilization of energy, physical and mental, for emergencies. They are the glands which meet shocks and neutralize the effects of shock. In the solitary animal, the everyday producers of shock are pain, fright and wounds. The adrenal mechanisms oversecrete to encounter the enemy, and then there is a period of rest and recuperation. Man, however, with the growth of his imagination and the increase in number and density of his surrounding herd, has become the subject of continuous stimulation. In the past, this was balanced by the almost universal dominance of some religious belief, as an effective opiate. Concepts like Fate, Predestination, an all-guiding and all-wise Providence, relieved and shielded the adrenals, and acted as valuable adjuvants for the preservation of normality.

The nineteenth century witnessed the birth and expansion of a great number of new stimulant reagents, the discoveries of physics and chemistry, which, with the climax of the World War of 1914-1918, have made for a more or less complete deliquescence of accepted religion. For the great majority there was no faith to take its place. War, pre-war, and post-war shocks have continued with their incessant pounding upon the reserves of energy. Under these conditions the adrenal personalities are bound to suffer. The other endocrine types suffer, too, but quite differently.

Today, anti-adrenal, anti-religious ideas are epidemic. Of these, first prize belongs to a cult of egotism fathered by the Napoleonic Idea, consciously assertive and self-conscious in Max Stirner's "The Ego and His Own," which engendered a swarm of imitators and plagiarists. Human beings are all incorrigible egoists more or less, furtive or frank. But social and religious codes curbed the most narcissistic of kings and conquerors. Before Napoleon, all of them vowed allegiance and expressed submission to some sort of deity, confessed some fear of the Lord in their hearts. But the ideas of Napoleon flouted all that. The unscrupulous predatory who put effectual scheming for the self plainly above every other consideration and rode rough shod over all his fellows appealed powerfully to the latent animality of the adrenal types. Then came the dawning awareness of capital and labor of themselves as classes fiercely opposed forever in the policy of cut-throat versus cut-throat. The labor organizations and the commercial companies and corporations pitted themselves against each other consciously. Doctrines like "Property is but Robbery," "Everyone for himself and the devil take the hindmost," the "Iron Law of Wages" and the "Facts is Facts" of the Gradgrinds were the phrases of the nineteenth century that assisted. Finally came the Darwinian revelation of man as the ape-parvenu, which completed the disintegration of the old restraints.

Man seemed to see himself now for the first time stark and naked. But Man consists of many varieties, and all reacted differently to the image in the clouded mirror. There was universal attempt at suppression. But slowly the anti-adrenal forces infiltrated every activity and every soul. Like a hidden focus of infection in the body, it germinated and poisoned. A slow fever crept into life. A febrile quality tinged the acquisition of wealth, the concentration upon sex, and the desperate pursuit of the novel stimulus.

Then, like the hand that appeared at Belshazzar's Feast, came the War, only it was a hand that stayed with a long flashing lightning sword in its grip, sweeping pitilessly among the erstwhile dancing multitudes to mutilate and destroy. A good many people, with that sturdy animality George Santayana speaks somewhere of as a trait of mankind, set out to enjoy the War. It was a new sort of good time upon an incredibly large scale. It was an undreamed-of opportunity. The mechanisms of suppression of the mind render it incapable of appreciating horror until encountered. And so thousands with dangerously unstable adrenals were plunged into the most trying conditions possible. Hundreds of them, already shaken, on the borderland of instability, reacted with the phenomena of breakdown of control, lumped with a host of other phenomena, under the general rubric of "shell shock."

That alone was not all. If hundreds collapsed, thousands approached the verge of collapse. They survived and were discharged from the armies as normal. They reappear in civil life as cases of "nerves." Ordinarily that would mean that they would be classed as failures. But such have been the psychologic reactions to the war that all kinds of compensations in the way of dangerous mental states have become frequent in these inadequate adrenal types. A trend to violence and a resentful emotionalism are combined with desperate attempts to spur the jaded adrenals with artificial excitements. Consequent melancholia and depression, the "blues," are inevitable. A survey of drug addicts would probably show a definite percentage of this type. The same applies to certain petty criminals and law breakers.

The adrenal element in the personality must be considered in every disturbance, morbid, personal, or social involving brunette types, Huxley's dark white, Mediterranean-Iberians, red-haired persons, and even pigment-spotted fair people. Historians have traced the earliest civilization to the doings of a brunette people, the Sumerians, the first to build cities in the Euphrates-Tigris region more than five thousand years before Christ was born. An adrenalized people one would, expect to be the first to take advantage of possibilities because of their energy capacity. The earliest Sumerian stone carvings of warriors exhibit an undersized skeleton compared with the large head, broad face, a low hair line and prominent nose that would fit into the ensemble of the adrenal type. Certain other historical aspects of the adrenal personality have yet to be worked out.

THE PITUITARY PERSONALITIES

The presence of two antagonistic elements in the one gland complicates any attempt at even the most abstract analysis of a personality dominated by that gland. The pituitary, composed of an anterior lobe and posterior lobe, supplies two fairly uncomplicated corresponding types, best described as the masculine pituitary type, and the feminine pituitary type. The masculine pituitary type is one determined by the rule of the anterior pituitary, representing superlative brain tone and action, good all-around growth and harmonious general function, the ideal masculine organism. The feminine pituitary type has an excess of post-pituitary, with susceptibility to the tender emotions, sentimentalism, and emotionalism, feminine structural lines. Ante-pituitary dominance in a male reinforces the general masculinity while the post-pituitary depresses it. The post-pituitary in a woman augments her natural trend, ante-pituitary tending to counteract it. In other words, post-pituitary and ovary are conjunctive, ante-pituitary and ovary are disjunctive, post-pituitary and testis are opponents, ante-pituitary and testis are allies.

One mechanical circumstance involved in the pituitary personalities may be the determinant of the entire life history. That is the emphasized fact that the pituitary is encased in a small bony box, at the base of the skull. The size of this bony box, and its capacity to yield to the various pressures of a pituitary enlarging to meet the demands of the organism, will often spell happiness or misery, success or failure, genius or idiocy for the man or woman. Certain possibilities are conceivable. All of them occur, for the developments of X-ray technique have rendered available almost a direct view of the sella turcica.

In the first place, the bony box may be definitely too small to start in with. That means a small and so potentially inadequate pituitary, both anterior and posterior, potentially inadequate in that it will become impossible for it to grow and produce extra secretion upon demand. Handicapped thus, the unfortunate so born is doomed to inferiority and very little can be done for him. He will not develop satisfactorily. He possesses small genital organs which will not evolve properly in adolescence, or if they will not stand still, tend to revert to the opposite sex type. Then he tends to be dwarfed, fatigable, adipose. Among these types are included subjects of obsessions and compulsions who are dull and apathetic, cannot learn or maintain inhibitions, and so, without initiative, evolve into moral and intellectual degenerates, liable to epilepsy and the most remarkable sex aberrations. All because a cranny of the skull, about the size of a thimble, is not large enough for their dominating gland.

If the bone of the cavity of the pituitary is softer and yielding, so that some enlargement of the gland is possible, especially of the anterior, there appear rapid growth with a tendency to high blood pressure, great mental activity associated with frequent and severe headaches (often of the migraine type), a combination of initiative and irritability and a marked sexuality. X-ray examination of the sella turcica shows what is called erosion of the bone as it yields to the pressure of the growing gland.

The ideal sella turcica for the ideal pituitary type is a large room in which the gland may grow and reach its maximum size and so its maximum function, without needing to exert pressure or destroy and erode bone in front of it, to the side of it or behind it. The distinctive masculine and feminine types, classed as the normal, belong to this group. Sometimes, the bone in front of the pituitary will yield, while the one in the rear will not, and sometimes the conditions are reversed. Thus we may have ante-pituitary sufficiency with post-pituitary insufficiency, or ante-pituitary insufficiency with post-pituitary sufficiency, complexes which contribute to create the grosser functional hermaphrodite types of mixed sex.

In the average feminine pituitary type of personality, post-pituitary dominates. In a woman and to a lesser degree in a man, the general build is slight and rather delicate. The skin is soft, moist, and hairless, the face is the doll or Dresden China sort, with a roseate or creamy complexion, flushing easily, eyes large and prominent. The mouth shows a high arched palate and crowded teeth rather long. The voice is high-pitched. One recognizes the traditional womanly woman, petite and chic, who always marries the hero in stories. She is usually fond of children, easily moved, has a good libido, and the traditional feminine traits. When unstable, the post-pituitary type is restless and hyperactive, craves excitement, and continual change of interest and scene, a new pleasure every moment. A good many of the women of today, who fifty years ago would have been nice sedate girls because of their excellent post-pituitary constitution, have been irritated by the atmosphere of post-1914 into the excess post-pituitary state, the adventurous never-satiated avid pleasure hunter, in whom the craving for stimulation will stop at nothing. F. Scott Fitzgerald portrayed an exquisite specimen of the kind in his short story "The Jellybean," with a quasi-heroine of a good Southern family, built to be a high standard wife and mother, who drinks, swears, gambles, and finally marries on a dare. Modern post-pituitary woman is excitement mad and thrill chasing. The worst of it is that the resultant personal tragedies cannot be dismissed as transient inevitables. The heredity of the internal secretions determines that the offspring of these women are bound to be pituitary unstable, the least desirable of endocrine instabilities because of the concomitant mental effects. Even from the purely selfish point of view, the standpoint of enlightened selfishness, the post-pituitary type must beware of excesses. For disturbances of menstruation, psychic fears, anxieties, states of suspicion and obsession, various pains are among the penalties.

A period of post-pituitary excess as an effect of disease, pregnancy, or the rapid life, may be followed by post-pituitary deficiency as a result of exhaustion of the gland. The girl or woman then becomes fat and suffers from headaches (the fair, fat and forty type) yet retains a certain capacity for enjoyment which enables her to continue gay, happy and gentle, kind, interested. So she contrasts with the thyroid deficient who gets fat, but also dull, stupid, even morose.

The masculine pituitary personality, the man with a dominant anterior pituitary gland in a roomy sella turcica with plenty of space to grow in, is the ideal virile type. They are generally tall (unless the growth of the long bones was checked too early by a social precocity of the testes) with a well-developed strong frame, large firm muscles, and proportionately sized hands and feet. The head is of the marked dolichocephalic type, flattened at the sides, face is oval more or less, with thick eyebrows, eyes rather prominent, nose broadish and long, lower jaw prominent and firm. Prominent bony points like the cheek bones, the elbows and the knees, the knuckle joints of the hands and feet. The teeth are large, especially the upper middle incisors, and they are usually spaced. The arms and legs are hairy. High grade brains, the ability to learn, and the ability to control, self-mastery in the sense of domination of the lower instincts and the automatic reactions of the vegetative nervous system, the rule by the individual of himself and his environment are at their maximum in him. The ante-pituitary personality is educable for intelligence, and even intellect, provided the proper educational stimulus is supplied. Men of brains, practical and theoretical, philosophers, thinkers, creators of new thoughts and new goods, belong to this group. The distinction between men of theoretical genius, whose minds which could embrace a universe, and yet fail to manage successfully their own personal everyday lives, and the men of practical genius, who can achieve and execute, the great engineers, and industrial men lies in the balance between the ante-pituitary and the adrenal cortex primarily. Men like Abraham Lincoln and George Bernard Shaw belong to this ante-pituitary group.

The feminine pituitary personality, in whom there is predominance of the post-pituitary over the ante-pituitary, occurs in men. The type is short, rounded and stout. They have heads that seem too large for their bodies, the general hair distribution on the trunk and extremities is poor, although that of the scalp and face is plentiful, and they acquire an abdominal paunch early. They exhibit the feminine tendency to periodicity of function, their moods, activities, efficiency are cyclic, reminding one of the menstrual variations of the female. This rhythmicity saturates their personalities, so that poetry and music almost morbidly appeal to them. A number of the great poets and musicians are to be classified as of the feminine pituitary species. Last, but not least, they are the hen-pecked lovers and husbands. Sex difficulties are frequent in their history.

The determination of endocrine type and tendencies, the prediction of the future personality, during childhood is one of the developments confidently to be looked for, as our knowledge of the internal secretions will grow. The possibilities of control loom as one of the most magnificent promises of science. Yet the high expectations for tomorrow should not depress our respect for the achievements of today. In the case of the pituitary, for instance, a hint as to the method of approach is furnished by the tabulation of the traits of pituitary dominance and pituitary inferiority in children.

Pituitary sufficient and dominant:
  Large, spare, bony frame
  Eyes wide apart
  Broad face
  Teeth, broad, large, unspaced
  Square, protruding chin and jaws

Large feet and hands
Early hair growth on body
Thick skin, large sex organs
Aggressive, precocious, calculating, self-contained

Pituitary inferior:
Small, sometimes delicate skeleton
Rather adipose, weak muscles
Upper jaw prognathous
Dry, flabby skin
Small hands and feet
Abnormal desire for sweets
Subnormal temperature, blood pressure and pulse
Poor control of lower vegetative functions
Mentally sluggish, dull, apathetic, backward
Loses self-control quickly, cries easily, discouraged promptly,
   psychic stamina insufficient

The pituitary personality in childhood produced by limitation of the size of the gland, because its bony box is completely or partially closed, presents typical hallmarks. He supplies the second and third offenders in the juvenile courts, the delinquents and pathological liars of childhood, the incorrigibles, the precocious hoboes, mental and moral deficients and defectives, the prey of the sentimental complexes of elderly virgins and helpful futility all around. Not utilitarianism or futilitarianism is needed, but pituitarianism. The feeding of pituitary gland in large enough quantities to these unfortunates may do more than ten charity organizations, with the most patrician board of directors complete.

THE THYROID PERSONALITIES

The accessibility of the thyroid gland in the neck, the ease of surgical approach, the definite effects following its removal, and then the miraculous marvels of the feeding of thyroid have rendered it the centre of attack by the largest army of endocrine investigators. As a result we know more about the thyroid in childhood, adolescence, adult life and old age than about the other glands.

In childhood, the subthyroid or thyroid deficient, the cretinoid type, the type resembling the cretin, is fairly common. The peasant's face, with the broad nose and the tough skin, coarse straight hair, the undergrowth, physical and mental, a persistent babyishness and a retardation of self-control development, make up the picture. He needs an excess of sleep, sleeps heavily, needs sleep during the day, when awakened in the morning still feels tired, and rather dull and restless, dresses slowly, has to be coaxed or forced to dress, gets to school late nearly every morning, does badly at the school, reaction time, learning time and remembering time being prolonged as compared with the average, and is lazy at home lessons. He perspires little, even after exertion, yet fatigues easily, is subject to frequent colds, adenoids, tonsillitis, and acquires every disease of childhood that happens along.

Adolescence, the coming of menstruation, the first blooming of youth is delayed in the subthyroid. The secondary sex traits as they develop tend to be incomplete and to mimic those of the opposite sex. Yet in adolescence too there may be a sudden change and reversal of the whole process, a jump from the subthyroid to the hyperthyroid state. So a girl who has been dull and lackadaisical, with no complexion and every prospect of evolution into a wall flower, may be transformed into a bright-eyed woman, generally nervous and restless, high colored, and possessed of a craving for continual activity and excitement. Skin, hair and teeth become of the thyroid dominant type. The heart palpitates under the slightest stimulus, she perspires almost annoyingly, heat and emotion are prostrating. If such a transfiguration does not occur, the effect of the reconstructions of puberty is to create a person with about the following characteristics.

1. Height below the average
2. Tendency to obesity (toward middle age)
3. Complexion sallow
4. Hair dry--hair line high
5. Eyebrows scanty, either as a whole or in outer half
6. Eyeballs deep-set, lack lustre, in narrowed slits
7. Teeth irregular, become carious early
8. Extremities cold and bluish
9. Circulation poor. Subject to chilblains

Intellectually, these people vary enormously, depending upon which of the other glands will enlarge to compensate for the deficiency of the thyroid. If the growth of the skull has left a roomy sella turcica for the pituitary to grow in, the intellect may be normal or even superior, though energy is below par. If this is not possible and the adrenals have to predominate, a lower, more animal and less self-controlled type of mentality is produced.

In direct contrast to the subthyroid types is he who originally was hyperthyroid. During childhood he is quite healthy, thin, but striking robust, active, energetic, generally fair-complexioned with nose straight and high bridged, eyes rather "poppy," teeth excellent, regular, firm, white with a pearly translucent enamel. These children are always on the go, never get tired, require little sleep. Seldom will one of the classical children's diseases strike them, measles perhaps, but no other. Adolescence for them, however, is more apt to be stormy and episodic, adjustment to the new world of people and things is much more difficult, wanderlust is acute. All an expression of cells keyed up, charged with energy that must flow somewhere or explode.

The ruddy live-wire, recognized everywhere as bubbling with vitality, the life of any group, the magnetic personality may, however, be shocked by some seismic event like the death of a father or mother, or the ruin of some cherished ambition. A break in the balance of the other glands follows quickly and disablement and invalidism, which may cure itself after some years, remain stationary, or descend to the worst forms of thyroid deficiency.

During maturity, the type are characterized usually by a lean body, or tendency rapidly to become thin under stress. They have clean cut features and thick hair, often wavy or curly, thick long eyebrows, large, frank, brilliant, keen eyes, regular and well developed teeth and mouth. Sexually they are well differentiated and susceptible. Noticeable emotivity, a rapidity of perception and volition, impulsiveness, and a tendency to explosive crises of expression are the distinctive psychic traits. A restless, inexhaustible energy makes them perpetual doers and workers, who get up early in the morning, flit about all day, retire late, and frequently suffer from insomnia, planning in bed what they are to do next day.

Certain types of thyroid excess associated with the thymus dominant next to be described are peculiarly susceptible to emotional instability. They are subject to brain storms, outbreaks of furious rage, sometimes associated with a state of semi-consciousness. To emphasize the analogy to epilepsy, their attacks have been called psycholepsy. Among the Italians especially they were watched and reported during the War, when the explosive fits were seen to take the form of irresponsible acts of insubordination or violence.

THE THYMO-CENTRIC PERSONALITIES

During the first period of childhood, up to five, six or seven, or more accurately, up to the point at which the permanent teeth begin to appear, every child may be said to be a thymus-dominated organism, because the thymus, holding the other endocrines in check, controls its life. That is why up to the third and fourth years at any rate, most children seem alike. Closer observation, however, reveals points of differentiation and signs of the coming potencies of the other hormones. During the second period, up to puberty, these marks of the deeper underlying forces of the personality make themselves more and more felt. The thymus, like a brake that is becoming worn out, continues to function in a progressively weaker fashion. Until with the arrival of the gonadal (ovaries' or testes') internal secretion, its influence is wiped out.

There is a definite degree of thymus activity during everyone's childhood, unless by its premature involution, precocity displaces juvenility. Yet even during childhood, there are certain individuals with excessive thymus action, foreshadowing a continued thymus predominance throughout life. The "angel child" is the type: regularly proportioned and perfectly made, like a fine piece of sculpture, with delicately chiselled features, transparent skin changing color easily, long silky hair, with an exceptional grace of movement and an alertness of mind. They seem the embodiment of beauty, but somehow unfit for the coarse conflicts of life. In English literature several characters are recognizable as portraits of the type, notably Paul Dombey, whose nurse recognized that he was not for this world. They may look the picture of health, but they are more liable than any other children to be eliminated by tuberculosis, meningitis or even one of the common diseases of childhood.

It is after puberty, when the thymus should shrink and pass out of the endocrine concert as a power, that the more complex reactions of personality emerge when the thymus persists and refuses to or cannot retire. The persistent thymus always then throws its shadow over the entire personality. To what extent that shadow spreads depends upon the strength of the other glands of internal secretion, their ability to compensate or to stay inhibited. Whether or not the pituitary will be able to enlarge in its bony cradle seems to be the most important factor determining these variations. If there is space for it to grow, at any rate normally, the individual may pass for normal, although he will have difficulties throughout life he may never understand, particularly in sexual directions. If the pituitary is limited. partially or completely, the thymus predominance is more prominent and fixed, and the abnormalities become obvious, both of person and conduct.

The anatomic architecture of the latter thymo-centric personality is fairly typical. The reversion in type of the reproductive organs, the slender waist, the gracefully formed body, the rounded limbs, the long chest and the feminine pelvis strike one at the first glance. The texture of the skin is smooth as a baby's, and sometimes velvety to the touch. Its color may be an opaque white, or faintly creamy, or there may be an effect of a filmy sheen over a florid complexion. Little or no hair on the face contributes to the general feminine aspect in the more extreme types. They are often double jointed somewhere, flat footed, knock-kneed.

In women, the external manifestations of a thymo-centric personality may be limited to thinness and delicacy of the skin, narrow waist, rather poorly developed breasts, arched thighs and scanty hair, with scanty and delayed menstruation. Or there may be obesity, with juvenility, if there is a repression of the pituitary secretion for one reason or other.

In their reactions to the problems, physical and psychic, of everyday life, the thymo-centrics are distinctly at a disadvantage. In the first place, muscular strain, stress or shock is dangerous to them because they have a small heart, and remarkably fragile blood vessels, which renders their circulation incapable of responding to an emergency, or at least definitely handicapped. In infancy, they may die suddenly because of this, either for no ascertainable cause at all, or because of some slight excitement like that attending some slight operation, a fall, or a mild illness. During the run-about epoch they are unable to cope with the necessities of an active child's existence in playing with other children. Puberty and adolescence are specially perilous to them for they may endeavour to compensate for an inner feeling of physical inferiority by going in strenuously for athletics and sports, and so risking a sudden hemorrhage in the brain, producible by the tearing of a blood vessel, as if constructed of defective rubber. Reports published in the newspapers from time to time of children or young men instantly killed by a tap on the jaw in a boxing contest, or some other trivial injuries are doubtless samples of such reactions in thymo-centric people.

As an illustration of the conduct aberrations of the thymo-centric personality during adult life, the following extracts from a newspaper report of a suicide are worth quoting.

"An autopsy made yesterday by Dr. Benjamin Schwartz, first assistant to Dr. Charles Norris, Chief Medical Examiner, removed any mystery that surrounded the death on Saturday night by pistol bullets of Dr. Jose A. Arenas and the wounding of 'Miss Ruth Jackson' and Ignatio Marti.

"Dr. Schwartz said that his post-mortem examination had convinced him beyond doubt that the dead physician-dentist had killed himself after he had tried to take the life of the young woman with whom he had lived and of the youth who was his successful rival.

"'Besides that,' Dr. Schwartz said, 'my report to the police will include a statement from the young woman to me that she always had understood that Dr. Arenas had killed some one in Havana, Cuba, before he came to New York.

"The autopsy left no doubt that Dr. Arenas was a case of status lymphaticus (thymus-centered personality). I made a most complete report because of the scientific value of the autopsy.

"'This confirmed my first deductions after seeing the body on Saturday night in the doctor's furnished room with alcove bedroom adjoining. You will remember that as soon as I had seen him I revealed that he was wearing corsets.

"'These cases of status lymphaticus are intensely interesting. In them the blood vessels are very small, and the lymphatic clement is greatly in excess. They die suddenly, from ruptures of blood vessels. Many of them are degenerate. Most of them are criminals. All of them are liable to commit crimes of passion. Among them are found a large percentage of drug addicts.

"'Miss Jackson, in the hospital, confirmed my scientific theory that the dead man was not normal. She was perfectly frank in her statement. She said she had left her husband, Elmer Schultz, an automobile salesman in Toledo, several months ago and had come to New York. She said she had lived with the doctor for some time.

"'About ten days ago she left him to live with Marti, a healthy, normal lad. Before she went from the doctor's room she destroyed those colored collars that were found beside the body. She cut them with scissors. But that was after, so she states, the doctor had destroyed stockings of hers by cutting them.

"'She told me in the hospital today, and with every appearance of truth, that she had met Arenas in the subway at the station on Seventy-second Street and Broadway on Friday night and that she had asked him when she could come and get her clothes. He said, according to her story:

"'Come to the house tomorrow afternoon--but come with Marti.'

"'She said that she and Marti went there according to this invitation: that first the doctor showed her the cut collars and told her that she would get her clothes back in perfect condition, and that the next thing she knew she had been shot. She couldn't remember much after that.

"'I believe that both she and Marti have told a perfectly straightforward story and the autopsy is proof of it.

"'There were six bullets in the doctor's pistol to be accounted for. One, in an undischarged cartridge, still was in the weapon. That leaves five. One struck "Miss Jackson" in the right chest squarely in front, and penetrated the flesh about one inch. If there had been any power at all behind the missile it would have gone right through, pierced a lung, caused a hemorrhage, and the chances are that "Miss Jackson" would have died. That leaves four bullets.

"'One more struck Marti in the left upper chest. It passed through the pocket there, and the skirt, grazed the skin, and then bounced over to the right hand side in front. It was a most amazing case of a bounding bullet. I was particularly careful about examining its course because at first I was suspicious of the stories that were told by Marti and "Miss Jackson." Now I know they are true.

"'But anyone might have been puzzled by the queer antics of the missiles from the pistol of South American manufacture that the doctor used. If it had had any penetrating power--or rather if the bullets that it sent out, had any real kick behind them--the chances are that both "Miss Jackson" and Marti would be dead now.

"'Two bullets, it will be remembered, entered the doctor's left chest, quite close together. Well, one nicked the heart and lodged between the lung and the heart. It didn't cause any more damage than a mosquito bite.

"'The second bullet went through the soft flesh of the chest, but it struck a rib and bounded back out again. That bullet was picked up beside the body.

"'After these vain attempts to send a bullet through his body to a fatal spot, the doctor apparently shifted the weapon to his right temple and pulled the trigger for the fifth time. Then the fifth bullet, driven likewise by a very weak charge of powder, pierced the skull at a point where it was thin and tore into his brain. Its lack of power, however, is shown by the fact that I found it this morning in the brain tissue.

"'In all my experience I have never seen anything so queer. It sounds almost like a dream--a man trying to kill with a pistol that shoots bullets that either stop after striking soft flesh or bound out of the body into which they are fired. But it is true; I have had all of the bullets in my hand.

"'They are all accounted for. They are all of the same sort. There is no reason to doubt that they are all from the same weapon, an instrument without manufacturer's name, and of a design that the police say is unfamiliar to them.

"'The dead doctor was a distinct type, and his tragic end was one that should not surprise anyone who has any knowledge of such cases. The courtroom was thronged with friends of the dead physician-dentist, who not only is reported to be of a wealthy family of Bogota, Colombia, but generally is credited with many charitable works in the uptown Spanish colony here.'"

The distinct type to which the first assistant to the chief medical examiner of the city referred is the thymo-centric personality (status lymphaticus is another technical name for it), we have been considering. The persistence of the thymus after adolescence makes for an arrest of masculinization or feminization, the end-point arrived at by the processes of puberty. That is, a partial castration takes place. Now, as the experiments of Steinach upon the transplantation of ovaries into males deprived of their testes and of testes into females deprived of their ovaries have demonstrated, the removal of the interstitial cells of one sex assists enormously in arousing the opposite sex traits that have been latent, homosexuality. In a thymo-centric, tendencies to homosexuality and masochism appear. And so all the remarkable after-effects of those processes that the Freudians have so lovingly traced: the father complex in men, the inferiority complex, and the feminoid complex in general.

The feminoid complex introduces again the character of the functional hermaphrodite, the mixed male-female. The sex index will certainly come in time as a measurement of sexuality. But until then some more available classification of sex tendency is necessary. Including sex intergrades, one may divide sex types into six classes: male, **male**-female, male-***female***, female, ***female***-male, and female-**male**. The sex intergrades, the four hyphenated classes, nearly all have some degree of persistent thymus. If its influence is partial, the emphasis is before the hyphen, upon the ostensible. If its influence is unchecked, the emphasis is after the hyphen upon the apparently latent sex. The sex difficulties produced in these people by the conflict between their conscious sex and their subconscious sex, the sex duel in the same mind, Siamese twins pulling in diametrically opposite directions, are comprehensible only from the viewpoint of the internal secretions.

Homosexuality, in one form or another, frank or concealed, haunts the thymocentric and spoils his life. The persistent thymus, like a vindictive Electra, stalks the footsteps of its victim, its possessor. He wishes to live, according to society's remorselessly rigid expectations, for virility and happiness. But his thymus condition forces him also to live for femininity and misery. That homosexuality is not purely a psychic matter, of complexes and introversion, as the newest psychology would have us believe, has been proved by observations of its development in animals with internal secretion disturbances, acquired or experimental. Thus it has been recorded that a male dog showed a large goitrous swelling of the thyroid in the neck, with a rapid heart, staring eyes, the loss of flesh and fat and the nervousness of a hyperthyroid condition. Therewith he became an absolute homosexual. Observations on the primates along the same lines have been made. In goitrous hyperthyroids thymus persistence is common.

What complicates his sex difficulties, and makes social adjustment almost impossible or completely impossible, is that his pituitary frequently cannot react to assist him. Often, as emphasized, it is bound in by bone on all sides and neither ante-pituitary nor post-pituitary can adequately secrete for his needs. So social instinct and the capacity for inhibition, the ability to control himself conceptually and somatically, are poor. As a child it is difficult to train him along the lines of the elementary habits and customs. He is into late childhood a bed-wetter, and steals and lies quasi-unconsciously.

His mother realizes soon that he cannot be made to acquire a sense of responsibility either for himself or for others. She becomes afraid to let him go into the street because of his inability to take care of himself, to acquire the right attitude toward street cars, autos, strangers, in short, danger. She dreads to take him to places because no sooner would they be out of them, than she would discover that he had taken something that did not belong to him, quite as a matter of course. He will fabricate stories with no motive, fabricate them out of whole cloth for the pure fun of it. In a word, moral irresponsibility is the keynote of the volitional traits of the thymo-centric personality from childhood up.

With so much against them, physical inferiorities, mental defects, moral lacks of every sort, it is little wonder that the thymo-centrics die young. Infections hit them badly. The cases of flu that went off in twenty-four hours belonged to the type. Fulminant meningitis, pneumonia, diphtheria, scarlet fever, the varieties that are supposed to kill in twenty-four to forty-eight hours because of the terrible virulence of the attacking microbe, are probably so malignant only because the organism attacked is a thymus subject.

In the alcohol and drug habitue wards of hospitals as well as in medicolegal cases of degenerates, gunmen and other criminals, the characteristic conformation and diagnostic stigmata of the thymo-centric are often encountered. Life treats them badly. Misunderstood and misjudged, they are the hopeless misfits of society. If the pituitary and the thyroid can enlarge to compensate for their defects, they may become the queer brilliants, the eccentric geniuses of the arts and sciences. Should they not, mental deficiency and delinquency are their portion. Epilepsy, then, is sometimes their mode of escape from the terrors of an utterly foreign world. Should they survive all other hazards, suicide may still be their most frequent fate. A study of 122 cases of suicide by one observer showed that the status lymphaticus was practically constant and often pronounced.

Certain of them, after a stormy life in the twenties, become adapted to their surroundings in the thirties because the pituitary gradually emerges and becomes dominant in their personalities. They are then recessive thymocentrics. An increase in size, a broadening, together with a greater mental tranquillity and stability, accompany the adaptation. Historically, the thymocentrics who combined brilliancy and instability played a great part as some of the famous adventurers and restless experimentalists.

THE SEX GLAND CENTERED OR GONADO-CENTRIC PERSONALITIES
(The Eunuchoid Personality)

Among the individuals whose personality is dominated by their sex glands the physiognomy, physique and life reactions are so distinctive that no better examples exist of our main thesis: that the whole life of man is controlled primarily by his internal secretions. These gonado-centric types are not all necessarily sex gland deficient, as the term eunuchoid implies. They may be rather gonad unstable with a corresponding instability of the entire endocrine system.

About the face of the eunuchoid the striking feature is the incomplete, irregular, or absent hair development. Below thirty it is chubby and ruddy, and rather childish in its texture; after thirty, there is an effect of premature senility: the skin is yellowish, leathery, and wrinkled as the faces of old women are wrinkled: the upper lip is traversed by vertical wrinkles, and wrinkles come around corners of the mouth. The expression is juvenile, effeminate or plaintive.

Invariably the voice is higher pitched than the usual masculine tones. It may be gentle and subdued, like a genteel female's, or strident and rasping. Occasionally it is a pleasant high tenor. The Adam's apple, poetic popular name for the thyroid cartilage, is never prominent, because it is not ossified, as it should be in the normal male.

Tall and slender, or generally undersized, the muscles are soft and flabby as a woman's. The hands and feet are small and gracile typically. Viewed in profile, the lines of the body are feminine. The breasts may reach almost the size of the female's and there may be a well-marked area of pigmentation around the nipple. The hair growth under the shoulders and on the lower abdomen tends to be scanty and to approximate the opposite sex in quality and distribution, as do the reproductive organs themselves.

These traits of physiognomy and physique indicate functional hermaphroditism in the underlying feminoid constitution. The feminoid constitution appears again in the supposedly masculine. The feminoid constitution should not be confused with the infantiloid constitution. The former, the gonado-centric personality, is a digression of growth, a deviated evolution of the individual because of the conflicting forces, some masculine and some feminine, in his make-up. The infantiloid constitution is one of arrested development, and may center around the arrested function in childhood or adolescence of any one or a number of endocrine glands. Yet the two may resemble one another pretty closely, at times. A cretin imitates the extreme grade of infantiloid constitution. The infantiloid is a sort of enlarged and lengthened child. The feminoid is ostensibly a man, with a good deal of woman in him. The infantiloid is a quite general type, but of course when typical is a freak, recognized and treated as such. How far the eunuchoid may deviate from the normal is suggested by the following description of one.

"Face rounded, moon-like, chubby, devoid of hair. Eyes puffed. Lips protruding and fleshy. Cheeks round and thick. Nose little developed. Skin thick and of clear color. Disproportion between the size of head and body. Hair of scalp fine. Brows and lashes scarce, trunk elongated and cylindrical. Limbs thick and plump, tapering from the root to the extremities. Good fat layers over the entire body. Reproductive organs those of a little boy. Infantile mental state: light-heartedness, naivete, timidity, easily evoked tears and laughter, promptly aroused but fugitive wrath: excessive tenderness, but unreasonable dislikes."

An almost wholly mental infantiloid state or one purely physical may occur. Certain rather large Tom Thumbs belong to the group. In everyday life we see doll creatures, overgrown children, on every hand. Mental measurements of any large group of population reveal a remarkable percentage of it as below the mental age of 12. Juvenile traits and juvenile mind, separate or combined, should always suggest the possibility of the infantiloid constitution of one type of thymocentric also.

The eunuchoid or feminoid personality is also found often among artists. One must carefully distinguish the two because the ensemble of characteristics of the one may easily stimulate the other. Yet fundamentally they are as far apart as the poles. The infantiloid type never rises above the subnormal, which is its habitat, while the feminoid type (or masculinoid, in woman) often produces an abnormal personality which rises above the normal. The infantiloids become the slaves and the weaklings of society, the Mark Tapleys, and the Tom Pinches, while the eunuchoids have created splendid literature and immortal music.

The life reactions, and especially the sex reactions of the gonado-centric, are as complex and difficult as those of the thymo-centric. Straightforward homosexuality and the eunuchoid constitution have always been intimate. The homosexuality of the thymo-centric is more subtle and disguised, often buried under the stronger masculine component of the personality.

Homosexuality as a cult has appeared correlated with the production of the functional hermaphrodite by artificially creating the eunuchoid type of constitution. Among the Aztecs, homosexuals were produced in quantity for religious purposes by a deliberate fostering of the eunuchoid constitution. They called them the Mujerados. Their method consisted in making a healthy man ride horseback constantly, until an irritable weakness of the reproductive organs ensued, and a paralytic impotence followed. The exhausted testes would then atrophy, and the voice ring falsetto, muscular tone and energy diminish, inclinations and habits become feminine. The Mujerado lost his position in society as a man, assumed female clothing, manners and customs, and to all intents and purposes was treated as a woman. Their large breasts were said to be capable of lactation. Their only reward was the high honor paid them as religious consecrates.

Among the Phoenicians there was a similar sect, devoted to the worship of Astarte. Known as the Galli, they were men who had transformed themselves into the closest possible resemblance to women. At all times they were prepared to engage with members of either sex in sexual relations of the most depraved kind. They lived in idleness as prostitutes, cultivating and extending their skill in sex perversions as specialists. Their initiation into their professional careers was a part of a religious ritual. During the revels of great festivals, apprentices to the trade, wrought up by certain traditional songs and music, would be hypnotised into a frenzy, run amuck, throw off every garment, and, snatching up swords, deliberately placed in convenient spots, castrate themselves at one blow. In a wilder hysteria, screaming loudly, the self-made eunuchs would then run through the streets holding the severed organs high above their heads. At last, faint through loss of blood, they brought their madness to its climax by hurling the organs in their hands into the nearest houses, so forcing the owners to take them in, and provide them with female wearing apparel, and the other feminine accoutrements of war. Henceforth, this manner of dress was not to be changed. The physical changes followed. The hair of the face was lost, the breasts enlarged, the voice became high-pitched, and the other type-characters of the eunuchoid complex appeared.

These constitutions thus may be either congenital or acquired. Individuals apparently normal during childhood and adolescence may be transformed. Injuries to the reproductive glands, sometimes the slightest bruises, may lead to atrophy, and a change of personality follows in less than six weeks. Mumps may achieve the same results because of the inflammation of the gonads that may accompany or follow it.

Whole family and races may show some of the signs of the eunuchoid constitution for generations. According to Darwin (Descent of Man) "the development of the beard and the hairiness of the body differ remarkably in the men of distinct races, and even in different tribes, and families of the same race. On the European-Asiatic continent, beards prevail, until we pass beyond India, although with the natives of Ceylon they are often absent.... Eastward of India beards disappear, as with the Siamese, Kalmuks, Malays, Chinese, and Japanese. Throughout the great American continent the men may be said to be beardless: but in almost all tribes a few short hairs are apt to appear on the face, especially in old age...." Hair being an adrenal cortex trait, it is to be inferred that hairless families and races are more eunuchoid, and possess less of the adrenal cortex secretion than the more hairy.

Whatever the exceptions--and there have been eunuch generals in history--Marces, Chancellor of Justinian, who beat the Goths at Nocera, and Ali the Gallant who commanded the Turkish Army after the invasion of Hungary in 1856--the eunuchoid generally runs to type in his mentality and his sexuality. He is an introvert, his personality is shut in, he isolates himself from the world.

The lower eunuchoids exhibit a curiously child-like personality. Naively confiding, communicating to all comers all their joys and sorrows, they ask diffidently for confirmation of their statements, and they pass quickly from tears to laughter. About sexual matters they are extremely timid. A moral innocence pervades their speech and conduct. Usually they have no true conception of crimes of jealousy or passion. The occupations they go in for are those without responsibility away from crowds or observation, such as ship cooks, stewards, and so on. They marry to find a home, without the object of establishing sexual relations. When they are asked whether they think their wives will be pleased to look at the matter in the same light, and be contented to live with a man upon such conditions, they are puzzled or perplexed, as if they had never thought seriously about the matter before. Their simplicity has even extended to proposing to their wives to seek gratification from some other man. Naturally, such an arrangement often proves unsatisfactory, and desertion follows.

Concerning the children sometimes the offspring of these unions, scepticism as to the identity of the father is decidedly permissible. Still in some cases the best of evidence exists that fertility occurs. The vitality of the children then is subnormal and the mortality rate high. The eunuchoid tendency is transmitted. Variations and transitions of every kind are found among the undersexed eunuchoid personalities, depending upon the quality and degree of the secretions lacking.

When there is an excess of these sex secretions, a turbulent, tempestuous, sexually sensitive temperament, that may go on to satyriasis or nymphomania, is created. It has been shown that doves can be rendered overfeminine in their behaviour and characteristics by injections of ovarian material. Oversexed types of personality therefore may exist as well as undersexed.

COMBINATIONS AND PERMUTATIONS

The types of personality sketched--the thyrocentric, the pituitocentric, the adrenocentric, the thymocentric, the gonadocentric--are really prototypes, the great kingdoms of personality, to which individuals can be assigned, by hall marks which facilitate their classification. They may also be described as the pure endocrine types, which include a minority of a population. But the majority consist of dominant mixtures, hyphenates, groups which are the species and varieties of the greater classes. Combinations and variations of control among the adrenals and thyroid, pituitary or thymus, and so on, occur, with effects that are sometimes additive, reinforcing a particular trait of the person, and at others conflicting, and neutralizing. Quantitative variations of the same secretion may occur periodically in the same individual, which explains the multiplicity and complexity, the inconsistency and contradictions of conduct in a man or woman at the different episodes and crises of life, to a certain extent.

There should be a stable balance between the various endocrines, the stability expressing itself in what we are pleased to call the normal. There should also be a balance between the antagonistic elements in the same gland; for instance, the pituitary. The pituitary, built of two distinct portions, the anterior and the posterior, is in equilibrium when the two are nicely adjusted. But the accidents and vicissitudes of life (pregnancy for example) will upset the balance. And so there will result changes of physique, conduct and character. Like possibilities apply to all the other glands of internal secretion. In our ability to exercise a control over these disturbances of balance, to be developed in the future, lies one of the great hopes for a chemical perfectability of human life and nature.

NATURE'S EXPERIMENTS VS. MAN'S

The kinds of personality described, as prototypes and variants and the fundamental facts supporting the view that they are the reaction types of the human beings we meet in everyday life, represent simply a beginning of the work to be done. Putting into our hands a new powerful searchlight that penetrates the interiors of body and soul, a fresh attitude toward the complicated problems of Man in society grows imminent. The normal and the abnormal become illuminated with an effect as if our retinas were suddenly to get sensitive to the ultraviolet rays to which we are now blind. An apparatus is put in our hands which shows us not only a static condition at a given moment, but the whole life process of an individual, normal or abnormal, his past and his future.

Upon that fetich of the biologists, the struggle for existence, the struggle for survival, the struggle for possessions and satisfactions, for happiness, victory and virility, in short, for success, as success is measured by the biologists, a searching spectroscope can play, with a yield for our understanding and control of life, that will stand comparison with the astronomer's analysis of the stars. Toward the process of adjustment and adaptation, of the environment to the individual, as well as of the individual to the environment, attitudes will change from ***hopeless acquiescence in the inevitable to a complete self-determination of the self and its surroundings.*** The adventures of the personality, strung along as the episodes of his career, his friendships and sex reactions, his mishaps and diseases, and the final fate or fortune that overtakes him, be he normal, subnormal, supernormal, or abnormal, begin to become comprehensible, and hence controllable.

CHAPTER XI
SOME HISTORIC PERSONAGES

THE INTERNAL SECRETIONS IN HISTORY

According to the views, facts and guesses concerning human personality, as a body-mind complex dominated by the internal secretions, outlined in the preceding pages, biography, and human history as the interaction of biographies, become capable of interpretation from a new standpoint. If human life, in its essentials, is so much the product of the internal messenger system we speak of as the endocrines, then biography should present us with a number of illustrations of their power and influence. What is the evidence that, as Huxley anticipated, "the introduction into the economy of a molecular mechanism which, like a cunningly contrived torpedo, shall find its way to some particular group of living elements, and cause an explosion among them, leaving the rest untouched," and the multiplication of such cunningly contrived mechanisms, were responsible for those personalities, magnificent chemical compounds, with whose adventures historians are concerned?

THE CASE OF NAPOLEON

As a unique will and intelligence, Napoleon Bonaparte the First must be classed as one of the Betelegeuses of the race. H.G. Wells has called his career the "raid of an intolerable egotist across the disordered beginning of a new time." "The figure of an adventurer and wrecker." "This saturnine egotist." "Are men dazzled simply by the scale of his flounderings, by the mere vastness of his notoriety?" "This dark little archaic personage, hard, compact, capable, unscrupulous, imitative and neatly vulgar." There are other opinions. The Man of Destiny was worshipped by millions. Napoleona bring fortunes today. Interest in the man as a man has multiplied with every year. And certainly no one can deny him the quality of individuality in its most exaggerated form.

In the second place he belongs among the moderns. Modern science and methods of observation have had their chance at him, and have left a conscious record of their results. Napoleon was the central figure of his time, and was watched by trained medical eyes during his life, and after his death. Protocols of the examination of his body are accessible, and Napoleonic specimens, preserved by fixing agents, may still be viewed at the Museum of the Royal College of Surgeons, England. Dr. Leonard Guthrie has worked up the material at hand in a report which he presented to the historical section of the International Congress of Medicine, in London in 1913. I propose to relate his findings to some other facts and the general principles roughly sketched in this book.

There are a number of word portraits of Napoleon extant. But for our purposes certain of the notable features of his face and physique are to be considered. The first characteristic that struck everyone about him was the matter of his height. He was definitely sub-average, at death being about five feet six inches in height. As has been emphasized several times, deficiency or excess of growth will always direct attention to the pituitary. His sharply outlined features and a powerful lower jaw, combined with oddly small plump hands, long straight black hair, and dark complexion, all point to the pituitary, with a secondary adrenal effect. His pulse was slow, according to Corvisart, his personal physician, rarely above 50 to the minute. His sexual life, his libido, was abnormal. Curiously explosive in their appearance and manifestations were his sexual impulses. They "beset him on occasions which were sometimes inconvenient, and a peculiarity about them was that they subsided with equal suddenness if not immediately gratified, or if meanwhile something occurred to discourage his attention. All women were to him 'filles de joie.' Sexual rather than social attractions in women appealed to him." He was never in love, never possessed of permanent affection or tenderness for any woman. This explosive periodicity of the sexual life, "with a tendency to compression of it to the merely physical," is another mark of some pituitary-centered personalities.

Two other phenomena that persisted throughout his life throw light upon his endocrine constitution. One was trouble with his bladder which he told Antommarchi, another physician, bothered him as long as he could remember. Irritability of the bladder was so pronounced that he could not sleep for more than a few hours at a time. After battles, the trouble became worse so that it interfered with his riding. Constitutional difficulties in urination have been connected definitely with the function of the pituitary. The other pituitary disturbances which tinctured his life were certain "brain storms," attacks of vomiting followed by "stupor verging on unconsciousness" brought on by outbursts of temper, physical overexertion, mental strain, or sexual excitement. It has been shown that such epileptic tendencies are present in subjects of pituitary disease, particularly those with pituitary instability. In Napoleon's case the brain attacks may have been crises of pituitary insufficiency in a hyper-pituitary type. This supposition is borne out by the headache which followed them, the headache of an oversecreting pituitary compensating for a defect in its formation. During his prime, his intellect was mathematical, logical, and rational, and remarkable for a prodigious memory. Such an intellect is the product of an extraordinary ante-pituitary. That he never permitted feeling to interfere with the dictates of his judgment, a quality which rendered him the most unscrupulous careerist of history, must be put down to an insufficiency of the post-pituitary. What post-pituitary does to the brain cells and the organism as a whole to render them susceptible to sympathy and suggestion, the social sublimations of the maternal instinct, with its offsprings of religion and art, we have seen. Napoleon lacked a chemical trace of the religious instinct, his sympathy was nil, and his conquests were made possible only because he was blind to the suffering and misery his greed for glory and dominion generated. Post-pituitary insufficients of this type, patent or concealed, gradually become corpulent as they grow older. The increasing corpulency of Napoleon was commented upon by all observers.

A student of his make-up, and acquainted with present developments concerning the internal secretions, given an opportunity to observe him as we have when he was alive, and at the height of his success, would have had every reason for classing him a pituitary-centered, ante-pituitary superior, post-pituitary inferior, with an instability of both that would lead to his final degeneration. Besides, his insatiable energy indicated an excellent thyroid, his pugnacity, animality and genius for practical affairs a superb adrenal. Given the kind of pituitary he possessed, with its great intellectual potential energy and the relation between the two parts which would further the objects of an intellectual machine, plus a remarkable thyroid and adrenal, plus the military education Napoleon had, and the character of the Revolution into which he was plunged, and we have the conditions out of which his career emerged as inevitable.

That it was his pituitary which first failed him, rather than the thyroid or adrenal, which might have, is demonstrated by a number of considerations. Before he made himself Emperor, it was noticed that he was becoming fat, a pituitary symptom. A comparison of portraits at different stages of his rise and fall shows an increasing abdominal paunch, and a laying down of fat in the pituitary areas, around the hips, the legs and so on. The beginning of weakness in judgment that he was to exhibit soon in the invasion of Russia manifested itself at the same time. His keen calculating ability attained the peak of its curve at Austerlitz, Jena and Friedland. Thereafter, the descent begins. A rash, grandiose, speculative quality enters his projects, and divorces the elaborate coordination of means and end from his plans. That his thyroid energy capacity did not fail him is indicated by the fact that at St. Albans he would ride for three hours at the end of the day to tire himself sufficiently for sleep. That his adrenals were not affected is indicated by the brutality which remained characteristic to the end of his life.

The findings after death confirm the view of him as an unstable pituitocentric who succumbed to pituitary insufficiency toward the latter half of his life. We possess the account of the postmortem by Dr. Henry, who performed it. "The whole surface of the body was deeply covered with fat. Over the sternum, where generally the bone is very superficial, the fat was upwards of an inch deep, and an inch and a half or two inches on the abdomen. There was scarcely any hair on the body, and that of the head was thin, fine and silky. The whole genital system (very small) seemed to exhibit a physical cause for the absence of sexual desire, and the chastity which had been stated to have characterized the deceased (during his stay at St. Helena). The skin was noticed to be very white and delicate as were the hands and arms. Indeed the whole body was slender and effeminate. The pubis much resembled the Mons Veneris in women. The muscles of the chest were small, the shoulders were narrow and the hips wide." In other words, the typical feminization of the body which accompanies pituitary insufficiency was found. He died of a cancer of the stomach. But before his death there were noted the mental transformations that succeed deficiency of his central endocrine. Apathy, indolence, fatigability, and frilosity were what impressed his associates at St. Helena. The deterioration of his mentality was also exemplified in his literary diversions, the "Siege of Troy" and the "Essay on Suicide." The puerility of these productions, as well as of his conduct, a sulking before his captors, and the decline of his physical energy, once a bottomless well, all point to the same conclusion.

The rise and fall of Napoleon followed the rise and fall of his pituitary gland. No better illustration exists of the fundamental determination of a personality and its career by an endocrine, aside from other factors of education, environment, accident and opportunity. Without the sort of endocrine equipment he was born with, however, none of the other factors would have found the material to work upon. Born, say, with more of a posterior pituitary than he had, which would have rendered him more sensitive to the sufferings of his fellow-creatures, if nothing else, and the forces of the Revolution probably would have swamped him from the very first moment of his emergence at Toulon, when the whiff of grape-shot, symptom of an inexorable, merciless intellect and will, started him upon the road that led to the Napoleonic Era. Destiny is always ironic. For the deficiency of the internal secretions which made him eligible for glory was responsible as well as for his downfall.

EPILEPSY AND MIGRAINE IN GENIUS

In the annals of genius, there occur a number of instances of those who suffered from attacks that have been diagnosed epilepsy or migraine. Because their ailment was associated with their extraordinary ability, they attracted an attention that concerned itself not at all with the circumstance that genius has also been liable to measles, scarlet fever, and so on. Epilepsy and migraine certainly occur in people of no supernormal gifts, and often in degenerates and subnormals. Yet the fact remains that these affections of the nervous system, so terrible to feel and to behold, have afflicted the finest brains of the race.

About forty years ago the idea established itself that epilepsy, exhibiting itself in one form or another as "fits," and migraine, the severe periodic sick headache, were interconvertible manifestations of the same underlying morbid process in the brain. Nothing in the way of a concrete cause, attackable on the material side, was elicited by this generalization. Then the investigations of the pituitary in the last decade produced evidence of epilepsy-like and migraine-like symptoms in sufferers from tumors or other enlargements of it. Reasoning back, cases of epilepsy and migraine began to be examined for evidences of involvement of the pituitary in their troubles. These accumulated rapidly. The physiognomy and physique of the pituito-centric were discovered in them. The phenomena noted in Napoleon's case were often present: lowering of the pulse, chilliness, and an increased irritability of the bladder. In women the attack often coincides with the menstrual period, a typical time of endocrine unbalance. Finally X-ray examinations of the sella turcica, the bony lodging of the pituitary, clinched the matter: it often appeared small, or enlarged, with erosions of the bone, signifying a desperate attempt of the gland to grow, and meet the needs of the organism. The complex of appearances called migraine now becomes understandable. There are a number of factors, such as fatigue, intense cold, or high sugar food like chocolate, which will cause an engorgement of the gland with blood and swelling of it. But they do not concern us now. Intense mental occupation, concentration as the popular term has it, acts as a patent excitor of the attack.

Brain work drives more blood into the brain and the gland. Besides, mental activity is accompanied by increased function of the ante-pituitary, if intellectual, or of the post-pituitary if emotional. Brain work then causes a temporary enlargement of the gland. If, now, the bone container of the endocrine is too small to permit of much swelling, the bone will be pressed against or even worn into. This means headache, severe, easily going on to the kind known as sick-headache. The nerves which move the eyes in various directions lie next to the pituitary. If, in its expansion, it moves sufficiently outward, it may press upon, irritate them or paralyze, and so evolve various eye disturbances in association with the headache. No one can overrate this conception of migraine, for a number of men of genius have suffered from sick-headache and eye symptoms.

As for epilepsy, the problem is more complex. One has to rule out first those who have organic destructive disease of the brain. But they are out of our field: genius predicates at least an intact brain. Of the others a number may be interpreted upon an endocrine basis. At least they will, in their physiognomy, physique, mentality, conduct and character, document the glandular constellation under which they live, and a proper understanding of which is necessary for them to be helped. One frequently seen is the thymo-centric, with small enclosed sella turcica. The latter fact explains the occurrence of the epilepsy. Periodic variations in the secretory tides of the other endocrines, the ovaries, the thyroid, and so on, may determine the onset of the attack of "fits." The point is that when epilepsy plays a constant part in the life history of a man of genius, we are justified in assuming a disturbed balance among his hormones, and so a reasoned picture perhaps of the foundations for the erratic in his behaviour or his productions.

THE NEURASTHENIC GENIUS

The fin de siecle intelligentsia of the nineteenth century were quite stirred up by a publication of Max Nordau on "Degeneration," in which a number of revered artists and intelligents were held up to public scorn as degenerates and neurasthenics. So wrought up were they, in fact, that Bernard Shaw was moved to compose a defense entitled "The Sanity of Art." In spite of the Great Vegetarian's dialectics, it remains to be explained why a certain species of creative ability has been combined with the fatigability, variability and general wretched irritability of every organ and tissue in the body which taught them that they were sensitive souls imprisoned in the flesh. Going from doctor to doctor as from pillar to post, from this medical creed to that hygienic cult, lucky to escape the worst, often landing upon the bosom of New Thought for succor. We have noted in previous chapters the relation of neurasthenia to the glands of internal secretion in general, and to adrenal insufficiency in particular. A closer examination of neurasthenic genius will show it to consist essentially of a pituitocentric in whom for one reason or another, congenital (the persistence of the thymus) or acquired (shocks, accidents, diseases) there has been failure of the adrenals, thyroid or the interstitial cells, about in the order of their occurrence.

THE CASE OF NIETZSCHE

Friedrich Nietzsche is about as good a case as there is on record of a genius blasted by migraine. The originality and force of his mind, as well as the articulate music of an imaginative poet, places Nietzsche among the philosophic elect of the race. Showing that he was an unstable pituitary-centered of a certain type will throw light upon his malady, as well as upon his life and work.

In a set of volumes, entitled Biographic Clinics, Dr. George M. Gould of Philadelphia contended that the ill health of a number of men and women of genius of the nineteenth century was due to unconnected eye troubles. In attempting to bolster up his thesis he has collected biographic material useful to the student of personality. He never appears to have asked himself what was behind the eye trouble. The evidence relating to Nietzsche's endocrine personality is derived from some of the data he collected, as well as from the two volume life of the philosopher written by his sister, and the other biographies of him extant.

To reconstruct the endocrine formula or equation of Nietzsche inductively, one should analyze first the information available concerning his parents and relatives. His grandfather was a conservative bourgeois of a superior type, who was the author of treatises designed to narcotize the forces of rebellion of his time. What he was like physically, no epitaph declares. His father was a clergyman. A description of him reads ... "tall and slender, with a noble and poetic personality, and a peculiar talent for music ... short-sighted." That ranks him at once as a pituito-centric. The mother was dark and had a fiery temper and came of a family distinguished for the powerfully built anatomy of its members. In the heredity of Nietzsche, the father appears therefore to supply a pituitary predominating element, the mother an adrenal-pituitary predominating element.

Nietzsche himself worked strenuously at the intellectual life (after 20, when he probably stopped growing, and the brain tonic action of the ante-pituitary could manifest itself). Early distinction rewarded him with a professorship in philology at 24. One of Prussia's wars of conquest entangled him, and presented him with diphtheria. A friendship with Richard Wagner marked the turning point of his life, and the point of departure for his works on the most fundamental values of human life. Meanwhile, attacks of sick-headache of varying degrees of severity made him miserable periodically--they came about every two weeks and lasted two to three days--and left him wretched and exhausted. At last, at 44, a species of stroke terminated his sufferings, causing him to lose his speech and memory, and thenceforth there was progressive deterioration, physical and spiritual, with repeated attacks.

In the sister's biography there are several good photographs and reproductions of sculptures of Nietzsche at different ages. An examination of the frontispiece picture, which shows him in profile (profile views are the best for physiognomy), as well as of the bust of Nietzsche by Donndorf, exhibit the most striking traits of the head. To the student of internal secretions, the most prominent feature of the face, emphasized by both the camera and the artist, is the remarkable prominence of the supra-orbital arches, the bony protuberances from which the eyebrows spring. This is a definite pituitary character. The eyebrows themselves are luxurious and slope to meet, the bony development of the face as a whole is sharp and clean-cut, the skull tends to be long and narrow and the chin is square. All these point to a pituitary-centered personality. It is to be regretted that we have no picture or record of Nietzsche caught smiling, which would have preserved the state of his teeth for us. At any rate, considered as checks to my interpretation, his physiognomy and physique, the nature of his genius and the attacks which finally ruined his life, all fit into the conception of him as one whose life centered, like Napoleon's, around what was happening in his sella turcica.

The attacks of sick-headache, diagnosable symptomatically as migraine, were so devastating that in 1883, after the printing of his masterpiece, "Also Sprach Zarathustra," he wrote "My life has been a complete failure." Extracts from his letters, collected by Gould, provide some idea of his suffering. In 1888, just before his stroke, he said, "I have in my eyes a dynamometer of my entire condition."

The history of Nietzsche's eye trouble makes it probable that not simply a defect in his eyes themselves, but a deeper condition behind them was responsible. Up to the age of 15 he was a model scholar. Essential eye defects of refraction should make themselves felt during childhood. Then, with adolescence, he changed. Adolescence is one of the red-letter epochs for the pituitary, when its growth and enlargement precedes and stimulates the ripening of the sex cells in the reproductive organs. Until adolescence ended and physical development ceased, his intellectual interests were nil, and he was particularly backward in mathematics. Colds and coughs, and recurring pains in the head and eyes bothered him (colds and coughs are frequent in those whose pituitary expansion is limited by the bony sella turcica to any extent). After his puberty, migraine definitely became his demon companion. Following the diphtheria in the army (which must have damaged his adrenals), the attacks grew much worse, and complaints about them more bitter because the pituitary now, in addition to its own burden, had to compensate for the insufficient adrenals. So "his frequent illness made him more and more a subject of treatment and commiseration.... If only my eyes would hold out ... it seems to me at the age of 30 as if I had lived 60 years ... very frequent sufferings of stomach, head and eyes ... acidity oppresses me, and everything except the tenderest food becomes acid.... I cannot doubt that I am the victim of a serious cerebral disease, and that stomach and eyes suffer only from this central cause ... half-dead with pain and exhaustion." In December 1888, he fell, had to be helped home, lay silent for two days, then became loud, active and unbalanced. The attack was preceded by the drinking of much water.

The specific quality of the Nietzsche genius also directs attention to a pituitocentric, to a pituitocentric in whom both ante-pituitary and post-pituitary are extraordinarily well-functioning, but are in a state of unbalance in which the post-pituitary gets the upper hand. Now, as we have seen, the post-pituitary makes for that instability of association between the brain cells which must be at the bottom of originality and creative thought, as well as of phobias, obsessions, hysterias and hallucinations. Persons in whom the post-pituitary predominates have a lively fancy and are liable to suffer from the tricks of association. Nietzsche, as we have noted, was poor in mathematics and in the calm cool proportioned forward march of scientific thought in general. His most brilliant ideas came to him in flashes and gleams. That is why so much of his work has come down to us in the form of aphorisms and paragraphs. He was, essentially, a poet among the metaphysicians, which again favors the conception of him as a pituitary-centered with a dominant post-pituitary. Yet his incisive critical faculty, as well as his love of music, also document the supernormal ante-pituitary.

To sum up, the physique and physiognomy of Nietzsche, his migraine attacks and the later fate which overtook him, his likes and dislikes, his tastes, abilities and accomplishments followed from his composition as one pituitary-centered, with post-pituitary domination, a superior thyroid, and inferior adrenals.

DARWIN AS A NEURASTHENIC GENIUS

Charles Darwin, as the author of the "Origin of Species" and the greatest revolutionist of the nineteenth century, has naturally had a great deal of attention paid to his life and personality. Yet not until the publication of his Autobiography and his son's Reminiscences was it generally known that he suffered from chronic ill health for most of his adult life. Dr. W.A. Johnston, in an article in the ***American Anthropologist***, 1901, has marshalled a number of available facts, to sustain his thesis that Darwin was a victim of neurasthenia. Now neurasthenia, it is now accepted, is simply a waste-basket word, corresponding to the class miscellaneous in a classification of any group of real objects. And, as has been emphasized in preceding chapters, most neurasthenia rises upon a disturbed endocrine foundation, most often, an insufficiency of the adrenals. That is, a defect in the chain of co-operation, balance and compensation among the internal secretions is the basis for the weakness of the nervous system the term neurasthenia is supposed to explain, actually only names. Darwin's case was pretty certainly that.

There can be no doubt that Darwin had an abnormal fatigability, a lack of stamina and endurance in mental as well as physical application which plagued him from the late twenties to the sixties. As a child, he was strong and healthy, fond of outdoors, and though underrated by his teachers, noted to be possessed of intense curiosity, especially concerning natural objects. At school he was a fleet runner and cultivated a habit of long walks. Then he was surely no neurasthenic. Three years which, he himself afterwards said, were worse than wasted, at Cambridge, were filled with shooting, riding and hunting. His good health lasted until the time he probably stopped growing at 21 or 22. Thereafter his troubles began.

What was Darwin, so far as his endocrine composition was concerned? In the first place his father was a variety of pituitocentric, of the post-pituitary inferior type, six feet two inches tall, exceedingly corpulent, and, in the eyes of his son, the sharpest of observers and the most sympathetic of men. He wished to make a physician out of his son in order to carry on the medical tradition of the family: Erasmus Darwin was a physician before him. His son, however, showed no inclination for so learned and confining a profession and had to be reproached by his father in these immortal words: "You care for nothing but shooting dogs, and rat-catching, and you will be a disgrace to yourself and all your family."

Cambridge came after Edinburgh, as he was rushed from medicine into the clergy. But in vain. A friendship struck up with a naturalist, Henslow, settled his career for him. Henslow heard of a trip of general exploration the ship *Beagle* was to take and recommended Darwin as naturalist. The captain at first would not hear of the proposal because of Darwin's nose, a typical pituitary proboscis. But his prejudices were overcome, and Darwin sailed.

It was upon this voyage that Darwin made himself the greatest naturalist of all time, and at the same time infected himself with the virus of neurasthenia. At Plymouth, while waiting for the ship to sail, he complained of palpitation and pain about the heart, probably due to a transient hyperthyroidism, brought on by excitement. During the voyage, which lasted five years, he was afflicted often by sea-sickness. A ship-mate relates that after spending an hour with the microscope he would say

"Old Fellow, I must take the horizontal for it" and lie down. He would stretch out on one side of the table, then resume his labors for a while when he again had to lie down. Already fatigability had to be fed with rest. A serious illness that Darwin claimed affected every secretion of his body acted probably as the exhausting drain upon his adrenal potential.

The return to England was the date of onset for a record of continuous illness, aggravated by his marriage, apparently, for his misery increased progressively after it. So much so that he was forced to leave London altogether so as to avoid the strain of social life, even that of meeting his scientific friends or attending scientific society meetings fatiguing him to exhaustion. After such occasions there would be attacks of violent shivering, with vomiting and giddiness. It was necessary for him to impose upon himself an absolute regime of daily routine. Any interference with it upset him completely, and made it impossible for him to do any work. Early morning was the only time for physical as we; as mental exertion. Evening found him thoroughly used up, with every move an effort. Insomnia made him its prey. A curious sensitiveness to heat and cold distressed him. In 1859, when the "Origin of Species" appeared, he wrote to a friend that his health had quite failed, and that indigestion, headaches, with a looming hopeless breakdown of body and mind made his life a burden and a curse. The twenty years of research he devoted to the problems of evolution were one long torture. For sixteen more years, during which he worked upon and produced immortal classics of biology, he was the most wretched and unhappy sufferer from neurasthenia. His life was a continuous alternation of small doses of work and large doses of rest. So he was enabled to publish twenty-three volumes of original writing and fifty-one scientific papers. Living a sort of quasi-sanitarium life, with the rules and regulations of one undergoing a rest cure for thirty-six years, he thus accomplished infinitely more than the millions who have led the strenuous life. That he thus survived, as a genius, among the perils of an intellectual nature in an environment for which his adrenals sentenced him to destruction, must be put down in large measure to the ministrations and good sense of wife and children who supplied him with the endocrine energy he lacked. All these details I have given in the attempt to analyze the internal secretion constitution of this great man of genius, to establish that he really suffered from inadequate function of his adrenal glands, for the symptoms of chronic though benign adrenal insufficiency coincide in their mass effect with the story of his life. He was not a good animal, as Herbert Spencer declared was a first sine qua non of the successful life. He was a poor animal, the poorest of animals, because he possessed poor adrenals. What saved him was his congenitally superior pituitary (the nidus of genius) and the overacting thyroid, which combined to compensate to some extent for his fundamental lack. According to his son he rose early because he could not lie in bed, and he would have liked to get up earlier than he did.

What other hints have we that in spite of his fatigue disease he was a pituitocentric? The record of his physique and physiognomy, documentary and that left in portraits and photographs. He was tall and thin and his frame was naturally strong and large. Face was ruddy, and his grey eyes looked out from under deep overhanging brows and bushy eyebrows. The ears were large and prominent, the hair straight, the nose broad and well developed. All these are distinctive pituitary traits. The photograph of him taken by Maull and Fox in 1854 shows his chin to be the square firm kind that goes with the ante-pituitary type physique. (This photo is the frontispiece of the collection of essays entitled "Darwinism and Modern Science," edited by A.C. Seward and published in 1909). Charles Darwin, we may say, then, lived the life of one with a hyperfunctioning pituitary, the anterior portion dominating the posterior, a thyroid excess, and an adrenal much deficient, the combination settling the fate of a grand intellect in an invalid. It is interesting to note that an extant portrait of Erasmus Darwin, Darwin's distinguished grandfather, shows a pituitocentric, but with a rounder head and a fatter face, which point to a predominance of the post-pituitary over the ante-pituitary. Correspondingly, he was more speculative and poetic intellectually than his grandson, and more irascible and imperious in his moods.

After 1872, when Charles Darwin was sixty-three years old, a marked change for the better occurred in his health. For the last ten years of his life the condition of his health was a cause of satisfaction and hope to his family. "He was able to work more steadily with less fatigue and distress afterwards." This is probably to be explained as following the gonadopause hi him--the cessation of activity of the interstitial cells. After this event, the adrenals in the male nearly always function more efficiently, and well being is improved even though the blood pressure often rises coincidently. In the relative vigor of that decade we have another bit of evidence that the adrenals had much to say over Darwin's life.

EPILEPTIC GENIUS

He had a fever when he was in Spain
And, when the fit was on him, I did mark
How he did shake: 'tis true, this god did shake
His coward lips did from their color fly;
And that same eye whose bend doth awe the world,
Did lose his lustre: I did hear him groan.
                                        --Julius Caesar.

Epilepsy, the "falling sickness" or "fits," is generally associated with a deterioration or degeneration of mentality, and an inferior personality is frequently an ingredient. Progressively increasing data accumulate to incriminate more and more a disturbance of the endocrine balance, on the side of multiple deficiencies, as the basic mechanism at the bottom of a good many of them. Concurrent studies reveal that abnormalities of the thyroid, the parathyroids, the ovaries and testes, and even the thymus exist behind the attack. Investigation of the content of the consciousness of the different kinds of epilepsies from this point of view will doubtless bring to light some interesting information. There is much to be done for the epileptic with this new method of approach.

Epilepsy, just the same, may occur in men gifted with the sort of transcendent ability called genius. Mohammed, Lord Byron, Dostoyevsky, Flaubert, to name a few cases, are famous instances. The point to be settled is whether epileptic genius, that is epilepsy with superior ability, occurs most often in pituitocentrics, the epilepsy being symptomatic of a pituitary struggling against barriers, tugging against bonds. As mentioned, in such cases epilepsy appears as the twin brother of migraine in genius. Should that be established, we should have more evidence for the pituitary dominance of most specimens of intellectual power. As a case in point let us take the most famous of the epileptic geniuses--Julius Caesar, "When the fit was on I marked how he did shake; tis true, this god did shake."

According to Plutarch, Julius Caesar was of slender build, fair-complexioned, pale, emaciated, of a delicate constitution (reminding us of Darwin), subject to severe headache and violent attacks of epilepsy. In view of the work of Cushing, the concurrence of "severe headache and violent attacks of epilepsy" is sharply suggestive of a pituitary origin for both. In his seventeenth year he was already engaged to be married, which proves his precocity. An overactive, erratic pituitary could here also be held responsible. Soon after he was proscribed by the dictator Sulla, and the first of a series of epileptic convulsions is recorded. Shock tries the pituitary, as well as the adrenals.

His sexual libido was of the quality that stimulated his soldiers to sing celebrations of his exploits. The first woman he was engaged to be jilted. Cornelia, his first wife, he divorced on the ground that "Caesar's wife must be above suspicion." Matrimony committed twice thereafter landing him in the divorce court, he devoted himself to liaisons, one with Cleopatra. This sexual hyperactivity was probably another pituitary trait.

The compound of intellectual and practical ability he realized was of the rarest. It meant a most delicate balance between his ante-pituitary, post-pituitary, adrenals and thyroid. He was an orator, politician, historian, conqueror, and statesman. That his thyroid functioned well can be deduced from a career which involved more than three hundred personal triumphs as recognition from his native city. On horseback, riding without using his hands, he would often dictate to two or three secretaries at once. The masculine love of glory and ambition, expression of a well-working ante-pituitary, was combined with the effeminate echoes of an equally well-evolved post-pituitary. No prima donna was more concerned with the care of her skin, complexion and hair than he. The analogy extends even to superfluous hair which he had removed, not by the modern electrolysis, but by depilation with forceps and main force. The attendants at his bath would polish his epidermis, for his satisfaction, until it resembled alabaster or marble.

Caesar was not the kind of great man that Darwin was, and only a rather muddled careerist because he had too much adrenal and post-pituitary. But he was pituitocentric of a certain type. We possess no authentic portraits or busts of him to go by. But the bust in the Museum of Naples, for which he probably sat (some, H.G. Wells among them, will not accept this), presents the sort of face that is often seen in pituitary epileptics, and the features and skull of a pituitocentric: long, large, well-modeled head eyebrows prominent, with tendency to meet, aquiline nose and strong chin.

In these three, Napoleon, Nietzsche and Caesar, we have male pituitocentrics, exhibiting diversities of life and tastes because of differences in the co-working endocrine glands in their makeup. We shall consider now a female pituitocentric who presents the strangest contrasts in physique, physiognomy, conduct and character, dependent upon a variation in the balance between the two portions of the pituitary.

THE LEGEND OF FLORENCE NIGHTINGALE

All biographies consist of prevarications and all autobiographies of fiction. That summing up of a mass of literature over which industrious students have ruined their eyes, held good until after the War, when things changed. Then Mr. Lytton Strachey, at one fell blow, and with one magnificent masterpiece, hurdled the old idols and established a new standard of deliberate accuracy in print. In his "Eminent Victorians" he set the pace for the host of those who have been stimulated by his good example, like Lady Margot Asquith.

Of the four Victorian respectable worthies Strachey has dissected as ruthlessly as the anatomist a post-mortem, his portrait of Florence Nightingale, the founder of the modern science and art of nursing, is most interesting because it provides data of the utmost value to the student of the endocrine basis of human personality. In the conventional two-volume biography of this superwoman, she is pictured as an intellectual saint, stepped from a stained glass window upon her wonderful visit to a clay-smeared earth. The biographer, presenting all the ins and outs of her body and soul as he has, makes her live before us with a fresh vitality that is startling.

The species of life Florence Nightingale lived, involving as it did struggle with a masculine world, and conquest of it, implies the existence in her of certain masculine traits and marks, for the normal feminine psyche is submissive rather than aggressive toward its environment, human and otherwise. Belonging to a family in the highest circles, it was upon the table d'hote of her destiny that she should become a regulation debutante, careeristina, and successful wife and mother. Instead, she chose to question the whole routine of the life of her class, and in her diary she records her doubts and cravings, and her revolt against what is assumed by her family and friends to be the normal course of existence for her. The attitudes and

questionings in these passages, the religious feeling displayed, are distinctly masculine. Most easily could the following, for instance, pass as having been written by a
man: "I desire for a considerable time only to lead a life of obscurity and toil, for the
purpose of allowing whatever I may have received of God to ripen, and turning it
some day to the glory of His Name. Nowadays people are too much in a hurry both
to produce and consume themselves. It is only in retirement, in silence, in medita-
tion that are formed the *men* who are called to exercise an influence upon society."
In a note-book she puts May 7, 1852, as the date upon which she was conscious of a
call from God to be a saviour. Now the vast majority of women who have remained
spinsters at 32, in spite of considerable personal attractions and high natural ability,
are visited by waves of emotional fervor for a de-personalization of the self. But in
the case of the subject, as Strachey has so well shown, the call was pursued with a
self-willed, pitiless, unscrupulous determination, worthy of Satan himself upon the
most ferocious evil bent. In its pursuit indeed she became what her latest biographer has called a "woman possessed by a Demon." All necessary, not alone because
if she had been meek and mild she would have existed in futility, but because of the
high percentage of the masculine endocrines in her composition. It is most regret-
table that we have no statement of the findings of a gynecologic examination of her.
That she was almost consciously masculine may be inferred not only from the way
she bullied Lord Pannure and worked to death her dearest friend with the angelic
temper, Sidney Herbert, who was so amiable that he could be driven by one who
wrote: "I have done with being amiable. It is the mother of all mischief." She could
also write, "I attribute my success to this: I never gave or took an excuse. Yes, I do
see the difference now between me and *other men*. When a disaster happens, I act,
and they make excuses."

Lytton Strachey has painted superbly all this in his essay. But for us his most
significant passage is the following: "When old age actually came, something curious happened. Destiny, having waited patiently, played a queer trick upon Miss
Nightingale. The benevolence and public spirit of that long life had only been
equaled by its acerbity. Her virtue had dwelt in hardness, and she had poured forth
her unstinted usefulness with a bitter smile upon her lips. And now the sacredness
of years brought the proud woman her punishment. She was not to die as she had
lived. The sting was to be taken out of her: she was to be made soft; she was to be

reduced to compliance and complacency. The change came gradually, but at last it was unmistakable."

"*There appeared a corresponding alteration in her physical mould.* The *thin, angular* woman, with her haughty eye, and her acrid mouth, had vanished, and in her place was the *rounded, bulky form* of a *fat old lady*, smiling all day long. Then something else became visible. The brain which had been steeled at Scutari was, indeed, literally growing soft. Senility--an ever more and more amiable senility--descended."

We have here an absolutely typical pituitary history, with another case of pituitocentric natural ability. What happens when pituitary hyperfunction or superiority becomes underfunction or inferiority is precisely as Strachey has described so cleverly of the "ministering angel": the acrid, thin and keen degenerate every time into the amiable, fat and dull. Just as Napoleon was transformed by the mutations of his pituitary, so was the Saint with the Lamp. And in both instances the contrasting modifications, from one extreme of glandular function to the other, supply us with the clue to the secret hand of their inner being and becoming, which worked upon the twists and turns of circumstance about them as a sculptor upon clay.

The official biography by Sir Edward Cook contains three portraits, representing three different stages, which bear out the pituitocentric thesis of her personality and life history. One as she was at 25, and pictured by Mrs. Gaskell: "She is tall; very straight and willowy in figure; thick and shortish rich brown hair; very delicate complexion ... perfect teeth ... perfect grace and lovely appearance ... she is so like a saint." The face is long and oval, of the post-pituitary kind. Then gradually the ante-pituitary gained an ascendency in the concert of her internal secretions, so coloring her life with its masculine tints, and altering her face as well as her disposition. The photograph of her taken when she was 38 shows a quadrangular outline, and all the acridity that impressed Strachey. The last picture of her, a water color drawing made in 1907, shows a round visaged old dame, who might be the peasant grandmother of two dozen descendants. Little patches of red over the cheek bones remind one of myxedema and indicate that toward the very end of her life her thyroid failed her as well as her pituitary. So that our biographer relates: "Then by Royal Command, the Order of Merit was brought to South Street, and there was a little ceremony of presentation. Sir Douglas Dawson, after a short speech, stepped forward and handed the order of the insignia to Miss Nightingale. Propped up by pillows, she dimly recognized that some compliment was being paid her. 'Too kind--too kind!' she murmured; and she was not ironical." In the days of pituitary and thyroid hyperfunction we may be sure she would have been caustically and penetratingly ironical.

THE EXPLANATION OF OSCAR WILDE

The case of Oscar Wilde, as one of the high tragedies of English Literature and Life, attracted the attention of the whole world in its heyday, and even today evokes controversy. As a literary figure and artist, the poet of the Portrait of Dorian Gray, and "De Profundis," belongs without a doubt to the immortals. As a convicted criminal, who served for two years at hard labor in Reading jail, and afterwards, a prey to chronic alcoholism, died in obscurity in Paris, he still remains a subject of whispered conversation in private, and his crime a taboo to the public, mentionable only at the risk of arousing the terrible odium sexicum of the prurient majority. Oscar Wilde was a homosexual of a certain type. In view of the previously laid down considerations concerning the endocrine genesis of homosexuality, how are we to explain him, and his natural history?

As with the other exemplars of genius examined we need here, too, to gain some insight into his "internal secretion heredity." His father, Sir William Wilde, was a surgeon. Photographs of him show the long and broad face of a pituito-adrenal centered individual, with a corresponding duplex incarnation in the face, the upper half strikingly spiritual, the lower curiously animal.

He was active, practical and eminently successful. His wife recalls Florence Nightingale, in face, figure and conduct (people who are built alike as regards their internal secretions are those whom we recognize as similar physically and psychically). She, too, was a pituito-adrenal, and in so far resembled her husband. But as in a woman ante-pituitary and adrenal superiority make for masculinity, she must be classed as a masculinoid type of woman. She was socially aggressive, and took part in the revolutionary movement of her time in Ireland. Thus we find that Oscar Wilde was the result of a mating of internal secretions acting in the same direction. The process might be compared to parthenogenesis.

It is on record that when enceinte his mother often expressed the wish that her child be a girl. When a boy was born, she was immensely disappointed. To compensate for her disappointment, she brought him up a good deal like a little girl. She had him dressed in girls' clothes at an age when most boys are violent destroyers of clothing. She would hang massive jewelry upon him, for the delight of playing with the resultant stage picture as a satisfaction for her discontented desires. In the light of modern psychology, and our formulization of her endocrine status, we must put down her conduct to a suppressed homosexual craving. Had her son been built along the lines of strong emphatic masculinity, her influence, though vicious, would probably have found no congenial soil, and would have died out altogether after his contacts with the outer world, beginning with school. No matter how she would have conditioned his vegetative system temporarily, his internal secretions, released then from compression, would have asserted themselves and determined his fate differently. However, it is quite possible that if such had been the case Oscar Wilde, the aesthete, the paradoxer, the disciple of Walter Pater and Baudelaire, would have stayed in the land of the to be born. I mean that then we would not have had Oscar Wilde, but another person, genius or commonplace, who also might have borne the name of Oscar Wilde.

That was not to be. The singular assortment of endocrines that mingled their activities to make Oscar Wilde shaped a personality which we must classify as the thymocentric (thymus-centered). Why this should be so is an interesting question. Pituito-adrenal plus pituito-adrenal of his heredity should make two pituito-adrenals according to elementary arithmetic and the rule of three. A cancellation of the two factors of the equation rather than addition seems to have occurred. The result was a persistent thymus superiority, with an instability of the other two main glands involved.

How do we know that Oscar Wilde was a thymocentric? Because in his fullest development he exhibited all the earmarks of the thymus pattern. We possess a number of good pictures and descriptions of him, as he was really a contemporary, and would probably be alive today if he had been put in a hospital for proper treatment instead of in prison. An excellent description is that of Henri de Regnier's: "This foreigner (Wilde) was **tall**, and of **great corpulence**. A **high** complexion seemed to give still greater width to his clean shaven face. It was the **unbearded** (glabre) face that one sees on coins. The **hands** ... were rather **fleshy** and **plump**." The points of immediate interest are the height, the complexion and the beardlessness. One classic variety of the thymocentric is tall, has a baby's skin, and has little or no hair on the face. A passage from a narrative written by one of his warders confirms the last condition decidedly. "Before leaving his cell to see a visitor, he was alway careful to conceal, as far as possible, his unshaven chin by means of his red handkerchief." Bristles on the chin, with little or none on the cheeks, is the inference. It is important to stress the thymocentric significance of this glabrosity of the face. Another sign to be put in italics was the quality of his voice. It has been described as a beautiful tenor, when he had it under perfect control, and high pitched and strident when under the influence of passion or temper. Such a voice would be the product of a larynx remaining partly or completely in the infantile state, as in a woman's. That, and the large breasts he is said to have had, point again to the thymus-centered constitution. All in all, there can be no doubt that Oscar Wilde was a case of status lymphaticus, the technical name for the thymus-centered personality.

As happens in a number of thymocentrics, his pituitary must have attempted to compensate for the endocrine deficiencies always present in them. The exceptional size of his head was a pituitary trait. Finding, possibly making, plenty of room for itself to grow, for some unknown reason, in an extraordinary fashion, it reinforced the love of the beautiful that is part of the feminine post-pituitary nature, with an intellectual ability and maturity that was at first all-conquering. In the face of a society organized for pure masculine and pure feminine types, disgrace and disaster at last overtook him with almost the ruthlessness of natural selection wiping out an unadapted sport suddenly cropping up in an environment. In prison he suffered from severe splitting headaches, which were probably due to changes in his pituitary. Described as being directly over the eyes, they haunted him until his death, and may have had a good deal to do with the absinthe addiction he acquired.

THE TREATMENT OF GENIUS

The problem of Oscar Wilde raises an ethical question that still remains to be finally answered. Granting that all of society should one day see him and his kind as a peculiar and specific constitutional product of an odd intermixture of internal secretions, what should be done with him and them? It is easy to play with words like "degenerates." But still, we do not condemn imbeciles, idiots or defectives, or other substandard, subnormal creatures to the prisons. For the sake of the good opinion society would maintain of itself, it sends the latter nowadays to hospitals, sanitaria, or their equivalents, where protection for itself without punishment for them may be practised. But is confinement, or even treatment the solution? For we have to consider what society would lose by cutting such abnormals off from itself, and them from its stimulations. A number of artists have been built like Oscar Wilde, musicians in particular. Without them, would there not be a great gap, a yawning absence, in the world's culture?

Modern diagnosis and modern therapy might have done a great deal for Napoleon, Nietzsche, Julius Caesar, Florence Nightingale, Oscar Wilde. Were they alive today, and willing to submit themselves to scientific scrutiny, the X-ray would tell us of the state of the pituitary and thymus in them, chemical examinations of the blood the condition of the thyroid and adrenals, detailed investigation of the body and mind a flood of light upon their maladies as well as their personalities. Therapy might have relieved Napoleon of his attacks, and so, halting the creeping degeneration of his pituitary, made Waterloo impossible. But then, would we have had the Emperor at all? Would there have been enough of that instability that drives on the genius to his goal? Nietzsche might have been relieved of his headaches, and Caesar of his epilepsy--but then, would not--with correction of the underlying streams of activity on the part of the other glands of the internal secretion to compensate--their peculiar superiority and distinction, and the fruits of their lives as by-products, have been destroyed. Florence Nightingale, too, might have been a softer and more human person. But then would she have revolutionized the practice of nursing? Oscar Wilde possibly might have been made over into a heterosexual. But then would not the world be the poorer without "De Profundis," let us ask? To state the problem in the most general terms: how much abnormality are we to tolerate (I speak, of course, of malignant abnormality, and disregard benign abnormality altogether) for the sake of the valuable that is concomitant? How much are we to stand of that which degrades the germ-plasm while it raises the mind-plasm of the race? The Flowers of Evil. Destroy or modify the roots, change the seed, and the buds will bloom, if at all, not orchids, but dull brown commonplaces.

What means may be licensed for the attainment of a worthy end is perhaps the broadest aspect of the problem. The instruments of Man's ascent to divinity may arouse his instinctive repulsions, dislikes, and destructive passions. The study of the internal secretions is putting and will put the most powerful apparatus for the control of the abnormal into our hands. What are we going to do with them?

It does not follow that because we are beginning to understand the normal that we are to establish one fixed absolute standard of the normal. In view of all the possible mixtures, permutations and combinations of the endocrine glands, that may construct an individual, it is possible to conceive a million types of normals. For normality means harmony, the harmonious equilibrium between the hormones, which tends to continue itself, because it does no harm to itself. So there are all sorts and conditions of men and women who are classed as normals. We need create no inquiry into the value of raising the subnormal to the normal level. It is when we come to consider the possibility of lowering the supernormal (in certain respects) to the normal, that we pause and hesitate. Traditional morality assists not, but hinders us here.

Whatever the race may ultimately decide, it is safe to predict that it is now somewhat possible, and will become more and more possible, to regulate or even check the ills of genius, without interfering with its highest evolution and expression. For example, Bernard Shaw, to take a living man of genius, is pretty visibly a pituitocentric of the well-balanced variety. He has the height, the facial features, the hands, and the sort of mentality that run together in his endocrine make-up. He also has the headaches. It is quite probable that feeding him pituitary gland extract in the proper dosage would relieve him of his headaches. A process might be started in his pituitary, however, that would diminish its extraordinary output which has assisted to make his brain so brilliant. The possibility, nevertheless, is excessively remote as the pituitary predominance in him is so overwhelming, that nothing short of surgery, nature's or the medical graduate's, could really affect that overmastering eminence. The time will come, though it is not yet by a long, long road, when we shall be able to intervene, and perhaps meddle, in nature's most intimate plans. The right of the power to modify, like the power to kill, will be defined and limited by common agreement before that goal will be reached.

CHAPTER XII
APPLICATIONS AND POSSIBILITIES

The knowledge that the shape and action of a man's body as well as his mind depend on the internal secretions inspires the hope of the emergence of a hitherto inconceivable controlling power over human life in the future. For in the wake of chemical discovery there has always come chemical control. The nature of chemical research, the necessity for clear thinking, accurate measurement, and experience in the actual handling of materials, the fundamental tradition and technique of the science, have made and will make the practical applications about which we today may only speculate. What the study of the internal secretions suffers from, at the beginning of the third decade of the twentieth century, is insufficient appreciation of its meaning for mankind. It is true that there are thousands of workers scattered throughout the world contributing their mites to the general store. They increase yearly, almost daily, and their achievements, in spite of an uncritical enthusiasm in some quarters and a semi-charlatanism in others, have been and continue magnificent. But they are pecking at a mountain which requires organized, massive, engineering organization for its blasting.

The crying need is for an international institute, endowed and equipped for investigation upon the proper scale, with all the available appliances and methods already worked out and at hand. Such an institution would possess the right chemical laboratories for the making of blood analyses, metabolism examinations, and tests of endocrine functions. There would be X-ray machines and experts to radiograph the pituitary, pineal and thymus glands when possible. There would be psychologists to carry out intelligence tests, determine emotional reactions, and group mental aberrations, deficiencies and defectives. There would be statisticians, trained in biometrics, to criticize and compare data obtained. There would be anthropoligists to note and measure variations in angles and curves, ratios and quotients of the external conformation of the body. Internists would record the history and status of the organs and viscera. There would be librarians to collect, abstract and collate the vast, accumulating literature. In short, the mystery of personality, the most marvelous, complex, and variable process in the universe, would be attacked and at length penetrated systematically and persistently, with the ideal of absolute control of its composition as the goal in view.

The nature of the researches? They would be infinite in their variety and significance. Their practical by-products, dropped in the pursuit of knowledge by the scientist, as Atalanta's lover the golden apples in his race, to assuage the scent of the hard-headed business man, would be profitable enough for any country in peace or war, to pay for itself ten times over and at compound interest. A volume could be filled with suggestions for interesting and promising investigations. But we may glance at some of the immediately useful aspects that might exercise those concerned with the everyday life of men, women and children.

THE ENDOCRINE EPOCHS OF LIFE

There is no more famous classifications of the epochs of life that mark off the milestones of the individual's evolution than Shakespeare's Seven Ages. So different is he at those different stages of his development, so changed his body and mind that it has become a part of popular physiology that we are entirely made over every seven years, and that no cell in the organism lasts longer than that. The tradition certainly does not apply to the brain and nervous system, for the number of brain cells is fixed at birth, and cannot be increased, only decreased, because they are too highly specialized to reproduce themselves.

What transfigures the individual as the years go by is no simple wear and tear of the tissues, nor the replacement of old cells by new. It is the rearrangement of relationships among the ductless glands, the shifting of influences from the predominant to the subordinate, and vice versa, in the constellation of the internal secretions, that determines the unfolding of the personality. The transformations raise doubt sometimes as to the reality of personal identity. What actually happens in the changes from childhood to adolescence, from adolescence to maturity, and so on, is the sloughing of one internal glandular dominance for another.

Growth, as a general name for the mutations, the ensemble of somatic and psychic differentiation, from year to year, passes through five epochs that are standard for the normal. The normal is the being who harmonizes with his environment, and yet reacts with it because of recurring needs within him. His endocrine equation settles what is unique and different in him. But the gland which flourishes during the epoch as its time of triumph, when it has its day, determines what makes him like his fellows.

From this point of view it becomes permissible to speak of the five Endocrine Epochs. Similarities and resemblances of mind and body between people at a given period of life, childhood, youth, maturity must be put down to their common government by the salient endocrine of the epoch. So one may list:

Infancy as the epoch of the thymus
Childhood as the epoch of the pineal
Adolescence as the epoch of the gonads
Maturity as the epoch of whatever gland is left in control as the
result of the life struggle.
Senility as the epoch of general endocrine deficiency.

Infancy as the epoch of the thymus explains why, in any given geographic locality, the babies look alike and act alike. Specialists in the observation and treatment of infants have noted that not until after the second year is any tendency to differentiation discernible to any extent among them. It is only after the second year, or somewhere around that time, that the child begins to individuate, and distinct individual traits and a personality manifest their outlines. The thymus is the great inhibitor of all the glands of internal secretion. By its checking activity upon the other members of the endocrine system, the thyroid and pituitary in particular, it gives the baby time to grow in bulk, which is its chief business during the first two years of its existence. It quadruples its birth weight. The brain and nervous system complete their growth in mass by the end of the fourth year. Recall the experiments of Gudernatsch working with tadpoles, who showed that feeding with thymus produced giant tadpoles whose metamorphosis into frogs was inhibited, while feeding thyroid produced frogs the size of flies. Differentiation occurred without the preliminary increase in mass usual. As differentiation and bulk thus appear antagonistic, at least at the beginning of growth, the function of the thymus, at a maximum during infancy, seems then to be to restrain the differentiating endocrines, until sufficient material has been accumulated by the organism upon which the differentiating process may work.

After the second year, the thymus begins to shrink. That is to say, officially its involution begins. Careful dissection will demonstrate some thymus tissue even in a normal subject up to the fourteenth year. This refers to the average normal, for the large thymus may continue large and grow larger after the second year in the type of individual designated in a preceding chapter as the thymocentric.

If the thymus retrogresses after the second year, what takes its place as a brake upon the forward driving impulses of the other endocrines? We have every reason for assigning that role to the pineal. It performs its service mainly, in all probability, by inhibiting the sex stimulating effect of light playing upon the skin. Since it is especially a sex gland inhibitor, the thyroid and pituitary become freer to exert their influences than under the thymus regime. And so we find that it is after the second year that thyroid and pituitary tendencies manifest their effects. The Pineal Era, from the second to the tenth to fourteenth years, remains to be investigated from a number of viewpoints interesting to the parent, the educator, and the student of puericulture. Precocity is directly related to early involution of the pineal. For just as the thymus involutes at the second year, the pineal atrophies before the onset of adolescence.

Adolescence is the period of stress and strain throughout the somatic and psychic organism because of the volcanic upheavals in the sex glands. The history of the individual is dominated by them up to twenty-five or so, when maturity commences in the sense of a relative sex stability. They continue to exert a powerful pressure throughout maturity. But life episodes and crises, diseases, accidents, and struggles, experiences of pleasure and pain, as well as climatic factors, settle finally which endocrine or endocrines are left in control as a consequence of the series of reactions the period of maturity may be analyzed into.

THE INTERPRETATION OF SENILITY

Senility inevitably follows maturity, not as night follows day by a mathematical necessity, but because of the process of degeneration which ultimately overtakes all the glands of internal secretion, dominant as well as subordinate. Just why the degeneration must occur no one can say. Injury to the endocrine organs of one sort or another, ranging all the way from emotional exhaustion to bacterial infection, is the reason usually considered sufficient. Just why recuperation and regeneration do not preserve them in the elderly as they do in youth is a problem to be solved when we understand the laws of regeneration, at present almost totally beyond our control. Some say that it is a matter of the wear and tear of our blood vessels, those rubber-like tubes which transport food and drainage with nonchalant equanimity to all cells as long as they last. In the classic phrase: a man is as old as his arteries, ergo his ductless glands will be as old as their arteries. And the age of arteries is simply a matter of wear and tear, the resultant of the function which is universal among molecules. Arteriosclerosis, the hardening of arteries, might be the whole story.

But there are certain experiments and considerations which rather confute that easy explanation, or at least make clear that the mystery is not so simple. The work of Steinach, a Viennese investigator, has contributed most to the elucidation of the nonarterial factor in senility. No one has asserted more loudly the importance of the interstitial cells that fill in the spaces between the tubules of the testes in the male, and the follicles of the ovary in females. Rats have been his medium of study, for they are most easily procurable, live fastest, breed, and withstand experimental and operative procedures better than any other animal.

An old rat is like an old man in his dotage. His bald, shrivelled skin covers an emaciated body. His eyes are dimmed by cataracts and his breathing is labored and difficult because his heart muscle has lost its tone. Huddled in a corner, life to him has become concentrated into the desire for a little food, and immobility. If now, something is done to his sex apparatus, a marvelous transformation may be effected. That something no one could predict. It consists in slitting the genital duct, which leads from the germinal cells to the exterior. After the operation, the germinal cells, which grow into the spermatozoa, atrophy and disappear, since they can no longer function. As if released from some restraint, the interstitial cells, however, multiply enormously. With their multiplication, the miracle of rejuvenation is performed.

After some weeks the sluggish currents of being in the rat, which had slowed down as a preliminary to stopping altogether, flow fast and furious. Waves of new chemical substances inundate his cells. And they respond like the fields that border the Nile after the annual flood. All his tissues, skin, muscle, nerve, even bone, are restored. A vitality is created which makes him bound and dart like a youth of his species. In due time, though, senility returns. It is as if a storage battery, recharged, runs down and becomes dead again. Slitting the genital duct of the other testis, causing its interstitial cells to hypertrophy and multiply, repeats the effects of the first experiment. The organism responds again to the new waves of vitality that vibrate through it. That it is recharged is demonstrated again by a revival of sex appetite and sex activity. The female which had become an object of indifference is reinstated as a creature to be sought and pursued. The second period ends in its turn. And now entirely new interstitial glands, in the form of fresh testes removed from a young animal, are transplanted into the body of the old rat. Once more youth returns. But now it burns itself more quickly than even before. An acute exhaustion of the mind appears first. Then all the other phenomena of old age steal back upon the old rat, and senility, firmly established in the saddle, rides him to the end.

THE POSSIBILITIES OF REJUVENATION

Whatever other deductions may be extracted from these experiments, they prove beyond a doubt the existence of an endocrine factor in the process of aging, as well as an arterial. They also demonstrate that the internal secretion of the sex glands, well advertised as it has been as the Elixir of Youth that Ponce de Leon, and Brown-Sequard with so many others, pursued in vain, is not the whole story. For if it was, the duration of the new youth should be another span of life, whereas in actuality it is only a fraction of that time. This fact, together with a number of others, make clear that while the gonads may be the jeune premier of the drama, the vitality of the plot depends upon the other endocrines. Since old age is an exhaustion, permanent and irreparable of *all* the members of the ductless gland directorate, the reason becomes clear for the temporary quality of the rejuvenation effected by the procedures of Steinach.

Practically, then, the question at once arises: which of the glands in particular are involved? There is first that ubiquitous agent in the system, the thyroid. Chemical analysis of it has shown that the iodine content decreases with the age of the individual, and becomes specially low after forty. It is after the menopause in women that myxedema, the disease of complete degeneration of the thyroid, and of the physical and mental faculties, is most frequent. The thyroid of old people exhibits, in varying degrees, signs of a similar degeneration. Thyroid feeding, properly controlled, will clear up certain of the deteriorations of mind and body observable in the aged. The grossness of the features lessens, a number of the pains go, muscular endurance increases, memory and intelligence do not remind one so forcibly of the old dotard in his second childhood. Of course the improvement at present achievable is only relative. But in the prematurely aging, decay invading a half accomplished maturity, marvels have been achieved at times with feeding of the gland.

The pituitary, too, begins to retrogress after the period of maturity. And an early retrogression means a short maturity. In women, the onset of an obesity, and coincidently, of a lazy and dull morale, coincides with this declension of the pituitary powers. All the glands of internal secretion, in fact, shrink and shrivel as old age advances. Only, as in other relationships, the predominating endocrine stamps its signature more visibly upon the documents of decadence than the others. Pituitary types, as said, get fat and slow, thyroidal become bulky and stupid or thin and sour, the adrenal dark, shrunken and forever tired of life. So type emerges, even in all-around glandular deficiency.

The problem of rejuvenation is the problem of recharging, or replacing all of the glands of internal secretion, at least the most important, the thyroid, the pituitary and the adrenals, as well as the gonads. Longevity is perhaps largely a matter of preventing, or postponing their wane. Beside, there is the prophylaxis of bacterial infections, and their all embracing corrosions--which, too, have an endocrine aspect.

Persistence of youth or juvenility may be manufactured by nature in two ways. There may be a persistence of early glandular predominances. We have seen what happens to the thymocentric. That a pineal-centered juvenile or infantile type exists may be safely predicted. Nature's only other mode of securing perpetual youth seems to be by prolonging the time allotted to the sex gland crescendo.

As for the golden age of maturity itself, what humdrum people and poets have despised as middle age, the margin of reserve of the ruling hormone is a quantity almost malleable in our hands, but still to be regarded with respect as a hard cold proposition by the physiologist. In general, the continuance of any stage of development means the maintaining of the glandular administration peculiar to it. So the chubby debonair irresponsible whom nothing can touch is happy in the possession of a pineal uncorrupted by the years, while the genius who can turn out his best work at sixty-five must thank his pituitary for standing by him to the end.

THE SCIENCE OF PUERICULTURE

There is a specialty now growing in the womb of science which in its own good time will come to fruition as the study of the child's needs or puericulture. Even today there exists a scientific basis for the formulation of the principles upon which every child should be brought up. Though we have had marvelous results from the campaigns to lower infantile mortality, most of what has been done has been medical in its interest, and so largely negative in its accomplishments. The removal of the causes of evil no doubt gives the good its opportunity. But how to raise a child, endowed with satisfactory ancestral stuff, as a Grade A normal or supernormal, still remains to be erected into an exact science.

A number of attempts have been abortive in this field. Why they have failed to arouse the ardor of the parent has puzzled some of the pioneers. Child-culture as the foundation of all systems of education has continued more or less of a hope rather than an achievement because of a lack of appreciation of the different constitutional varieties of children. A certain amount of attention has been lavished upon children needing special attention, those mainly suffering from insufficient development of one sort or another. In the last decade or so, an endeavour to focus upon the exceptional child, exceptional in intelligence or some special creative endowment, has started an interesting movement. All of them have suffered from the fallacies and troubles of the pure psychologist who would handle mind as an entity in a vacuum.

A realization of the different physical and psychic educational needs of various children will arrive only when we see them as built differently. Just as shoddy and silk, cotton and wool, alone or in combination, all possess different qualities as wearing material, so different children have varying capacities for the wear and tear of education. The endocrine classification of the human race, applied to children, will here yield a harvest to the educator and to the country. Nothing is more evident than the diversified nature of the needs of the various internal secretion types, once they are realized as such.

The history of a thymocentric type, for instance, is predictable from the very first few months of his life. Difficulties in feeding, in habit formation and adaptation, in the reaction to infections, in social play and so on, one may expect for him. The course of events for the other endocrine types also follow laws of their own. It will be above all in the ***understanding*** of children, their make-up, reactions and powers, that the biologist will achieve some of his finest triumphs.

The educator will have to take account of the state of the pituitary in estimating the normal intelligence, or influencing the abnormal or subnormal intelligence. As well will he have to consider the thyroid in the child whose conduct is refractory, even though his proficiency in his studies is excellent. And the condition of the adrenal will be ascertained in the types that tire easily, and that seem unable to make the effort necessary or desirable. Periodic seasonal and critical fluctuations in the equilibrium among the hormones will have to be taken into account in the explanation of what have hitherto been put down to laziness, naughtiness, stupidity, or obstinacy.

A child's capacity for education, essentially its capacity for the highest and most productive kind of life, is limited by inherent factors. These factors are two: the quality of the nerve tissue, its ability to make a number of associations, and the quantity of the internal secretions, measured by the maximum obtainable in a given situation. These inherent factors explain, too, why children born and bred in virtually the same environment show the most extreme differences in educability. That the differences are inherited was made evident by Galton's finding that the chance of the son of an eminent man exhibiting eminent ability was 500 times as great as that of the son of a man taken at random.

Every baby, then, is born with a combination of nerve cells and ductless glands which determine its capacity for mental development, that might never be realized, but could never be exceeded. If, in any family, minor differences in educability are observed, they can be put down to disturbance of these two factors occurring after the fertilized germ cell had started to divide and reproduce itself. But any marked falling off in either the nervous or endocrine factors has to be considered pathologic, due to an impairment of them by adverse environment.

Recent studies have amply established that the proportion of certifiable mental defectives, and of a much larger class, the subnormal but not certifiable class, is progressing by leaps and bounds. It is perhaps the most absurd frailty of our present system of education that it takes almost no account of innate differences in educability. To spend money upon the teaching of these children along lines where they are unteachable is not only waste pure and simple, but crime, for it deprives the educables of their just due.

These, of course, are the crude and simple lines upon which the finer and more complex evolution of the endocrine problems of the school child will build. The fine art of education itself is crude and gross and simple compared with what it might be, even as a beginning. The science of education has yet to begin, as the off-spring of that science of the future, to which knowledge of the internal secretions will contribute no little, the science of puericulture.

VOCATIONAL EDUCATION

It is difficult, indeed, to avoid becoming merely enthusiastic upon the possibilities of the applications of the endocrines to the educational domain. Happiness for the average individual consists of a double success--success in his vocation (chosen or forced upon him) and success in his sex life. A certain hue and cry has been raised in the last few years concerning the vast and overwhelming importance of sex in the happiness and even in the successes of a man's everyday life. And no doubt there is a relation. Sublimation plays its part in the explanation of vocational idiosyncrasies. The fact, however, that perfect success in sex may occur with absolute failure in the career, however, splits the problem for good into its realities: a physiologic aspect as well as a psychologic.

So, as school education will have to take serious account of endocrine anomalies and possibilities, will the institution which selects and trains for a career. Vocational misfits have aroused the ardor of our efficiency experts. And again, the sweeping psychological attack has beaten its head against the stonewall of ignorance of constitutional predispositions and tendencies of material. The attempt to erect psychologic types for vocational selections could never make much headway because it could only flounder in a swamp of metaphors, product of the vices of its methods. Not that anyone would wish to discard at all the psychologic mode of approach. But no science, in the sense of accurate examination, was possible, in the matter of classification for vocation, without the insight into the physiology of the candidate that the analysis of his endocrine formula will provide.

One need not dilate upon the value of such an examination. Civilization has not yet learned how to pick its personnel. And so artists and scientists, philosophers and politicians, financiers and religious leaders, arise and survive by the operation of the laws of probabilities and chances, rather than by any intelligent selection and cultivation of material. The case, indeed, is simply a subdivision of the vast subject: haphazard muddle in the conduct of life. A cry has been raised for the superman, and a cry has been raised for a method of anthropometry. For the lack of these two, it has been said, all governments have been doomed to defeat. The study of the endocrines will by no means supply a panacea. But as it will furnish a means of approach to the determination of how men and women are built, and why they are built differently, no one can gainsay the tremendous advantages to the nation that will proceed to classify its population accordingly, and know its strength and weakness in terms of the actual generators of success and failure.

Suggestions have been offered in the preceding pages of concrete applications of endocrine knowledge to the understanding of behaviour, of the genius and commonplace, criminal and Puritan. And in the chapter on historic personages, we tracked some of the story in detail. This vein when explored will quarry untold riches. It has been observed that financiers of mark, like great musicians, are special pituitary types. Also that the financiers are voracious meat eaters and the musicians inordinately fond of sweets. Differences in anterior and posterior predominances might account for this. That we are playing here with no phantasy is proven by the fact that we can effect changes of tastes as well as of intellectual direction by appropriate feeding of various glandular extracts. Just as much, indeed, as we can influence sex susceptibility, and the reaction to sex stimulation, by the artificial introduction from without of the proper hormones.

FATIGUE AND INDUSTRY

In industry, business and profession, the biologist will come more and more to be called as consultant. Labor unions as well as the large employers of labor, and their employment managers have given much thought to the problem of fatigue. Just what fatigue is, why different individuals tire at different rates, why some are constructed for monotonous routine while others must have constant variety and change, the relation to accidents and to quantity output, are a few of the major lines of inquiry upon which the endocrines obviously have a large bearing. To the employment manager, labor turnover and the selection of personnel are adjacent fields of research.

Fatigue as an endocrine deficiency--a depressed state of one or more of the glands of internal secretion, abolished when its normal functioning is restored--is a general principle from which departures of exploration of sub-problems will proceed. An endocrine organ will secrete at a certain rate. When it is stimulated excessively, it will eject extra amounts of its secretion. How long the period of excessive stimulation may last must depend upon the secretion potential or margin of reserve of the cells, varying from organ to organ, and from individual to individual. After that, exhaustion and failure follows, with the onset of the symptoms of fatigue.

A pretty demonstration of this process has been worked out in the electrical stimulation of muscle. If a muscle, say the biceps, is irritated by an electric current, it will contract. As the strength of the current is increased, the degree of contraction becomes greater. A sort of stepladder effect of increasing contractions may be thus obtained. After a time, the electric shocks cannot cause a greater contraction, but only a lesser. And if continued, the muscle will cease to function because of fatigue. If now, when the muscle begins to lag in its response, and its contractions to decrease, one injects into a vein extracts of thyroid, parathyroid, or adrenal glands, they will immediately reinvigorate the failing contractions. The injections must be made before the fatigue is carried to the point of absolute exhaustion. It follows that these glands normally pour into the circulation substances which counteract the effect of fatigue substances, and in fact make possible muscular recuperation from fatigue throughout the day as well as in emergencies and crises.

Fatigue, conventionally recognized, is something acute and urgent. As such it means a violent draining of the endocrine wells. But there is also a chronic fatigue, which has been dignified with the name of Fatigue Disease. Bernard Shaw once asked for someone to tell him the name of the germ causing the symptoms of overwork. That being impossible, he will have to be satisfied with the answer that it is not a germ, but an internal secretion, or rather a defect of internal secretion that is the cause.

Whether or not the adrenals have been damaged by past experiences, and upon their capacity to respond to the necessities of an occasion, fatigue reactions primarily depend. A quotation from Sir James MacKenzie, most distinguished of modern English students of medicine, summarizes the matter neatly. "Abelous, and Langlois and Albanese have studied the relation of the adrenal bodies to fatigue.... They infer that the muscular weakness following removal of the adrenals is due to toxic substances. In view of our present knowledge of the physiological action of adrenaline in its various forms, it seems more probable that the weakness is to be explained by the absence of the normal tone producing internal secretions of the bodies in question." In other words, the adrenals regulate muscle tone. They produce nature's tonics for weary tissues. The chronic lassitude of thousands of our generation, suffering from "that tired feeling," may be put down to chronic adrenal insufficiency.

It requires no superlative imagination to see that an adrenal poor subject does not belong upon a job that involves muscle stress over a long period, or indeed fatiguing conditions of any sort. Nor that a thyroid poor individual is not the best choice for a position that demands a keen, alert body and mind. In the selection of executives, the nature and stamina of the pituitary will undoubtedly be taken very seriously in the near future.

A certain hocus-pocus concerning character reading, a perverted revival of the ancient phrenology and physiognomy, has invaded the employment territory in America as the newest charlatanism. The study of the internal secretions, including blood and X-ray examinations, will surely assist the demand for a truly scientific estimate of constitution and character that can be relied upon in the classification and distribution of personnel.

THE PROSPECTS FOR PUBLIC HEALTH

By their effects upon the endocrines, public health influences like food, clothing, sleep and overpressure and last but not least, *disease*, the so-called diseases of childhood, possess a tremendous importance in limiting the output of the educable. They act to subtract from and so to lower the rating, the capacity of the germ-plasm. Most material and vital of these influences are the common diseases of children, for they strike directly at the glands of internal secretion.

Measles, scarlet fever, diphtheria, mumps, and the others have long been accepted as providential visitations for sins known or unknown. That children had to have them and were better off when they had them has become part of the tradition of the laity, fostered by the lazy ignorance of previous medical generations. But today we are beginning to ask ourselves why children must have these endemic infections of their age. The pathologist goes farther and asks the reason for certain apparent immunities. He asks why the little boy who sleeps with his brother sick with scarlet fever does not contract the disease, even though not protected by a previous attack.

Determining why susceptibility to a special disease in a particular case exists will constitute the greatest line of advance for the understanding and prevention of disease, and so the perfection of public health. In the last influenza epidemic countless physicians were puzzled by the spectacle of men and women in the pink of condition carried off in twenty-four hours while puny associates were either passed over, or pooh-poohed their colds. Pathologists have spent their energies fruitfully upon the infectious causes of disease, the microbes and parasites especially. But now, having solved most of those problems, the vital question of why an organism permits itself to be attacked is pushing itself to the front. Why a peculiar ailment selects its victim, why the bacillus finds a fertile soil, is the neglected problem, which must be solved before the abolition of disease and its carriers will be remotely conceivable.

Long ago, Hippocrates, revered founder of the art of medicine, recognized that there was a specific affinity of disease for individuals with more or less the same characteristic somatic and psychic traits and trends. Tuberculosis, for instance, was noted for its frequency in long-skeletoned, thin persons, remarkably optimistic. And the plethoric, choleric nature of the sufferer from gout has become proverbial. Before the era of the great bacteriologic discoveries of the eighties and nineties, the concordance of esoteric racial and personal markings was a great help in diagnosis to the physician. For he realized, though he sometimes credited it to his clinical intuition, that it was a certain type of personality that was liable to the specific disease.

But personality and its reactions, normal and abnormal, are determined by the endocrines. So we should find that particular infections run with special internal glandular predominances. For the picture presented by an infection, temperature, rash, prostration, are the details of the general reaction of the organism in the face of a new situation, the presence of a powerful, destructive invader. Information has accumulated that the invader is powerful and destructive, as well as selective, because of endocrine deficiency of one sort or another in the body it has attacked. Work of a number of investigators has indicated that an individual's susceptibility or its reverse, resistance, is intimately subjected to the derangements or harmonies of the endocrine system.

Comparison of the endocrine type and the disease assaulting has yielded an even more interesting principle. Knowing the state of the internal secretion reservoirs enables us to predict the liability to certain of these infections of childhood. Diphtheria has been found to occur most virulently among adrenal poor individuals. Moreover, they are left poorer in adrenal afterwards. It follows that they would be assisted by the feeding of adrenal. Mumps is a sickness that sometimes permanently injures the gonads: the testes or ovaries. The thyroid dominant, whose system is rich in thyroid, will rarely suffer from any of the common diseases of children--if at all, from measles. Op the other hand, those who have every infection of the period, and who, as their mothers say, seem to get everything, are those whose system is thyroid poor. Thyroid poverty is a splendid enticement to the universal microbe. The thymocentric stands all diseases poorly. The pituitary type is more liable to epidemic meningitis and infantile paralysis, typhoid and scarlet fever.

The public health officer of the future will be armed with a new weapon in his fight against the spread of an epidemic. He will be able to classify the endocrine traits of the population exposed, and to advise a course of glandular feeding for the types specially liable. The Schick test for diphtheria susceptibility is an illustration of one method of approach to the problem of the epidemiologist in settling who needs protection. The endocrines will assist him in the great body of diseases for which no immunity test is at hand. Should another influenza epidemic come along, for instance, the proper handling, from the endocrine standpoint, of the thymocentrics and the related adrenocentrics would help considerably in lowering the mortality.

Endocrine types have other tendencies, which when studied and controlled, will decimate the great assassins of middle age: heart disease and kidney disease, with accompanying degenerations of the blood vessels and circulation. The adrenocentric tends to get up a hyperacidity of the stomach and a high blood pressure, besides certain forms of diseases of the lungs. The thyrocentric is predisposed to heart disease, as well as intestinal disturbances. The pituitocentric is liable to periodic and cyclic upsets in his health.

Narcotism, the craving for narcotic or stimulant drugs, and its subvariety, alcoholism, has been found most often among the thymocentrics. Any type of endocrine inferiority, interfering with success in life, may lead to the habit of drug addiction as one way out. But the blood and tissues of the thymocentric appear to become habituated to the narcotic stimulant more easily than the other types, and so to demand it with a physical imperative comparable to the food or sex urge. Among artists, philosophers and statesmen, on the other hand, actively productive and so contrasted with criminals and degenerates drug addiction has frequently been a mode of endocrine compensation. That is, the drug produced temporarily the effects of the internal secretion lacking or insufficient. Thus the effects of cocaine may be compared with the effects of thyroid. But while there is a normal mechanism for thyroid detoxication, the cocaine or heroin derivatives mark the tissues permanently with their scars and deform the personality.

THE HYGIENE OF THE INTERNAL SECRETIONS

All these protean expressions of endocrine determination may now begin to be looked upon with the hopeful and optimistic attitude of him who understands cause and effect and can control. The advances made in the last ten years in the practical manipulation of the ductless glands from without, the introduction of glandular extracts by feeding or injection, and the modification of their structure and function by surgery, the X-ray and radium, and other procedures, enable us to regard more confidently the problems hitherto accepted as the insoluble and intricate handiwork of Fate. Fate may have woven the patterns of our being. But as we commence to probe the machinery and to examine the looms more carefully, we begin to understand why the wheels creak, and why there are seconds and odd lots in the product as well as the rare and precious firsts. Moreover, we are learning how to handle the machinery ourselves. The abdication of Fate can therefore be confidently expected in due time.

However, we have yet to begin, and we can begin with prevention. The theory of Adler, that some organ inferiority is responsible for much unhappiness in life has received much advertisement in conjunction with the doctrines of the Freudians. It is a theory of little scope when applied to the eyes, ears, heart and so on because only a small minority of the cases are of that kind. But as we have seen, a deficiency of an internal secretion, an endocrine inferiority, reverberates throughout all the cells. Not only the mind, but all of the members of the organism must strain and co-operate to make up for the break in the balance.

Endocrine inferiority is indeed the most frequent organic inferiority. And we may explain a number of mental types upon that basis. Thus the inferior gonadocentric, who has something wrong with his reproductive organs, will evolve in one of two directions. If his adrenal and thyroid are of poor quality, he will become the secluded introvert, shut off from the interests of normal life. He will enter the borderland of insanity if pituitary difficulties supervenes. If, on the contrary, the adrenal, thyroid and pituitary are present in a certain proportion, he will become the active, aggressive, never-resting, keen, and relentless fanatic reformer. A woman who is gonad deficient with a superior adrenal will suffer from virilism and specialize in the extreme tactics and mythology of the feminist movement. A number of life reactions are classifiable as the strivings of endocrine inferior individuals to overcome their sense of inferiority. The unconscious vegetative system and the system of consciousness are both modified by the weakness of a link in the glandular chain.

What, therefore, is to be recommended in the prophylaxis of the natural deterioration of the wells of life, the ductless glands? For even if we may be able to replenish them when they dry up, would it not be better to delay their dessication? The hormones reply to every call of life and respond in every reaction. The normal constructive process of their cells remanufactures what has been lost, and the original capacity to respond is restored. If, though, the rate of destruction and loss outruns the rate of repair and construction, they will be permanently damaged. This is what occurs in shock, serious, severe accidents and injuries, prolonged infections and diseases, profound continued emotions, and the wear and tear of overwork. The prevention of these excessive fatigues of the endocrine system in one or all of its parts, and especially the prevention and enfeeblement of the diseases of children which injure them at a period when they are most sensitive to injury, is the task of the endocrine hygienist. Periodic examinations, to check up the balance sheets of the hormone factories and to measure the amount of their damage by means of blood analyses, will provide the most valuable method in the campaign to lengthen the productive and enjoying span of life.

THE TREATMENT OF CRIME

Endocrine hygiene will discover no wider or more fruitful area for exploration and control than that of crime. For more than a generation there have been attempts at a criminology, and a new understanding and control of crime. In the

United States a concomitant sentimentalism has concocted measures like the honor system which, naturally failing of their purpose, have undermined confidence in the idea of scientific diagnosis and treatment of crime. As someone has noted, to ask a criminal to promise not to misbehave, when discharged from prison, is like asking a typhoid fever patient to promise not to have a temperature above ninety-nine degrees the next morning. For a large proportion of criminals--the percentage has yet to be determined, although the most recent police commissioner of Chicago has estimated it at ninety per cent--punishment for a period of time and then letting him go free is like imprisoning a diphtheria carrier for a while and then permitting him to commingle with his fellows and spread the germ of diphtheria.

Of course, the doctrine of responsibility is all tangled up with our attitude towards and treatment of crime. Though clear thought makes mandatory the recognition of a universal cause and effect law, practical common sense has defined free will. Consent or the withholding of consent to a given course of action has been the criterion of responsibility.

In practice, the limitation of responsibility will depend upon the insertion of extraneous factors into the formula of consent. The pragmatic test has been and will be the probability that the correction of the somatic or psychic condition would have prevented or will prevent the consent to the crime. As long as no such condition will be demonstrable, society for its own protection will have to confine the unfortunate individual.

The character of the confinement, its duration, and the uses to which it will be put should be dominated by the idea of discovering the unknown criminal predisposition. If crime is an abnormality scientifically studiable and controllable like measles, court procedure and prison management will have to be transformed radically. There is scattered throughout the world now a group of people who are applying medical methods to the diagnosis and treatment of crime. They are the pioneers who will be remembered in history as the compeers of those who transformed the attitudes toward insanity and its therapy. The insane were once condemned and handled as criminals are in most civilized countries yet. The criminologic laboratory as an adjunct to the court of justice, like that associated with the court of Chief Justice Olson in Chicago, remains to be universalized. What contribution to a more rational treatment of the criminal will the study of the internal secretions make?

It has been shown that the greater number of convicts are mentally and morally subnormal. To explain the subnormality, the criminologist has conducted and will continue to conduct investigations into the heredity and early environment of the criminal, his education and occupation, the social and religious influences to which he was subjected, and the intelligence test quotient. The conditioning of the vegetative system and the endocrine status of the prisoner, however, will without a doubt come to occupy the leading positions in any interpretation of crime in the future.

Introspective observation of pre-criminal states of mind by so-called normal persons reveals that in many of them there is an impairment of reason and will power, in others an exaltation amounting almost to hysteria. What are these but endocrine states of the cells, experimentally reproducible by increasing or decreasing the influence of the thyroid, the adrenals, the pituitary? Crimes of passion may be traced in no small part to disturbances of the thyroid. A psychologic examiner of a Pittsburgh court, interested in the subject, has found an enlarged thyroid in over ninety per cent of delinquent girls. Similarly, crimes of violence may be ascribed to a profound break in the adrenal equilibrium. Criminal tendencies in women during menstruation and pregnancy, periods of deep-seated mutation in the internal glandular system, have long been noted. A kleptomania, uncontrollable desire to steal, confined to the duration of pregnancy alone, has been described. We have seen how the thymocentric, especially if he possesses a small bony case for his pituitary, is predisposed to crime. A recent study of twenty murderers in the State of West Virginia showed them all to have a persistent thymus and the thymocentric constitution. A study of the recidivists, those who return for second and third offences, in one institution, disclosed that a large majority had a subnormal temperature and an increased heart and breathing rate. These are endocrine-controlled functions. Conduct, normal or abnormal, being the resultant of the conflict of conscious and subconscious impulses and inhibitions, the internal secretions as controllers of the susceptibility of the brain cells to impulses and inhibitions, must be held accountable for a portion at least of the chemical reactions behind crime.

It is possible, by X-ray treatment of the thymus, to cause it to shrink to more normal proportions. It is possible, by feeding various glandular extracts, to correct deficiencies or excesses of their function, and so to remedy the underlying basis for a criminal career. Here and there work of this kind has been successfully carried out in selected instances. What a suitable drive upon the whole matter would yield in happiness to the individual and dollars and cents to society, time alone will show.

CHAPTER XIII
THE EFFECT UPON HUMAN EVOLUTION

The ubiquitous and deep-seated influence of the internal secretions upon life and personality comprises but a fraction of what is known, and only a hint of what is to become known. There is an endocrine aspect to every human being and every human activity, normal and abnormal, internal process and its external expression, regulated by laws of which we are beginning to catch a glimpse. Their control promises us now a dominion over the most intimate and inaccessible recesses of our lives in a way comparable only to the control we now exercise over the forces and energies once revered as the instruments of the gods--light, heat, magnetism, electricity. We have learned how to control and change our environment. We are now learning, endocrine research is now discovering, how to control and change ourselves.

The story of the evolution of the two types of control has many analogies. When man ceased looking upon his surroundings as inhabited by spirits of good and evil, as he conceived himself, and discovered that they were composed of things malleable and analysable in his hands, he became their master. When now he drops the old superstitions about himself as a spirit, an emulsion of a spirit of good and spirit of evil, and sees himself more and more clearly as the most complex of chemical reactions, regulated and determined as are the simple and complex chemical reactions around him, he will begin to rule and modify himself as he rules and modifies them. Whether or not he will ultimately come to this final lucidity of thought and action, it behooves us to consider some of the uses to which our present knowledge might be put.

Since every step of the daily routine or adventure, from waking to sleeping, eating, drinking, marrying and giving in marriage, working, idling, fighting, playing, feeling, enjoying, sorrowing, every shade of emotion and nuance of mood, in short every phase of happiness and unhappiness, are endocrine episodes in the life history of the individual, the sphere of applications is as long and broad and deep as life itself. Not only do the internal secretions open up before us the great hope-- that Life at last will cease to stumble and grope and blunder, manacled by the iron chains of inexorable cause and effect. They provide tools, concrete and measurable, that can be handled and moved, weighed and seen, for the management of the problems of human nature and evolution.

Every department of human life, the questions of labor and industry, science and art, education, puericulture, international problems, crime and disease, may be illuminated. War and Sex, those two master interests of mankind, may be understood and handled sympathetically as they have never before. The reactions of man alone, and man in the crowd, will be clarified. The red thread of individuality which runs through the woof and warp of all human affairs will be unraveled.

Inevitably, customs, morals, codes of procedure and practice, institutions, all those expressions of opinion which make conduct, all the currents which contrive the infinite variety of life, will be transmitted into another set of values.

A remoulding, a remodeling will take place all along the line. Manifestly an unstable thymocentric should not be treated as a criminal, but treated in a sanitarium. A masculinoid woman needs satisfactions not vouchsafed in the old "love, honor and obey" home. How absurd it is to found codes of morality upon sermons or even the latest psychologies. During the nineteenth century progress in physics and mechanics overturned traditions thousands of years had painfully toiled to erect. What is to happen when man comes at last to experiment upon himself like a god, dealing not only with the materials without, but also with the very constituents of his innermost being? Will he not then indeed become a god? If he does not destroy himself before, that is surely his destiny. For better or for worse, we possess now in the endocrines new instruments for swaying the individual as individual, and as related to other individuals, as a member of a type, family, nation, species and genus.

THE BASIS OF VARIATION

The sense of likeness and the sense of unlikeness plays a decisive role in the diurnal schedule of the individual. His sense of resemblance to his father and mother, his kin and clan, mark him and them off against the cosmos as an alliance of defense and offense. Yet no matter how closely he is like them and they like him, he differs and varies, they differ and vary, with a sort of mutual forgiveness, because the amount of resemblance overtops the degree of variation. In a paper on the "Rediscovery of the Unique," H.G. Wells emphasized the unique quality of the individual, and how, in spite of the cleverest devices of classification, living things ultimately escaped the classifying net by virtue of their tendency forever to vary.

The individual is unique. Yet when all is said and done, the fact remains that between individuals there is resemblance, and among them variation. What is the reason for their resemblances and what is the cause of their variation?

The conception of a particular chemical make-up of the individual, stable and relatively controllable in terms of the internal secretions, supplies a more rational and satisfactory method of approach to the problem than any so far suggested as far as vertebrates are concerned at any rate. In effect, the differences between individuals may fundamentally thus be grouped among the differences which distinguish other chemical substances. The difference between water, technically known as hydrogen monoxide, and the antiseptic fluid labeled hydrogen dioxide lies wholly in the possession by the latter of an extra atom of oxygen in its molecules. All the peculiarities and qualities by which hydrogen peroxide is separated from water are referred to that additional quantum of oxygen. So the diversity of constitution and appearance of two brothers, alike in that they have inherited the same internal secretion trends, may be traced to the superiority of the pituitary of the one over the other.

Variation and resemblance are large issues, crucial material of the science of biology upon which much has been thought and written. That the proportion of the endocrines determines variation and resemblance, heredity and evolution is a hypothesis advanced, supported by a large amount of facts, and capable of the most interesting experimental verification and observation. If a child resembles particularly either of its parents, grandparents or relatives, there is good reason for believing that it is because their endocrine formulas are very much alike. When people apparently not blood-related at all resemble one other, the same law must hold. Resemblances may be partial or complete, and the degree will depend upon the amount and ratio of the internal secretions involved.

The same endocrine constitutions will produce corresponding physiques, physiognomies, abilities and characters. Deviations in endocrine type from that of the original stock, more of one endocrine and less of another, is at the bottom of the phenomenon of variation, basic for the origin of new species as well as the extinction of the old. In short, viewing the internal secretions as determinants, by their quantitative variations, of a host of biologic phenomena furnishes a concrete and detailed foundation for Darwin's theory of pangenesis.

INHERITANCE OF ACQUIRED CHARACTERS

Darwin's theory of pangenesis was an attempt to harmonize everything known in his time about heredity. It supposed that the various organs of the body gave off into the blood substances, themselves in miniature, which were taken up by the sex cells, and so became responsible for the development of their mother-organ in the newly forming individual. Modern knowledge cannot accept all this as a whole. But in a modified version, it has become the germ of a theory of heredity of which J.T. Cunningham, of Oxford, is the chief backer.

Beginning with the traits and qualities which distinguish the sexes, grouped as the secondary sex characters, he showed that they are correlated with the special sexual function of the species in which they occur. These traits appear only when the hormones occur which are present in one sex and that only when the gonads of that sex are mature. In some cases they appear only at the period of the year when reproduction takes place, disappearing again after the breeding season. Their presence makes certain cells develop in excessive numbers at a particular spot in the organism (as in the growth of breasts from a few sweat glands) or causes them to specialize (to make hair on the face in man, or to grow antlers on the head of a stag). After castration, the hormones being absent, all these points of contrast between the sexes fail to appear. So by analogy we may explain all somatic and psychic differentiation as functions of the glands of internal secretion. Contemplated from the angle of the effect of environment upon the endocrines, and a reflected action upon the germ cells, we may outline a mechanism of the inheritance of acquired characters at certain times and consequent adaptation. The cycle of events would be as follows:

1. A state of lability of cells at a point because of increased or decreased use.

2. An increased or decreased appropriation by them of the hormone control-

ling their function.

3. A corresponding increase or decrease in function of the gland of internal secretion and so,

4. An increased or decreased representation of it in the reproductive sex cells in the gonads.

To take a classic illustration, the long neck of the giraffe. The neck of certain animals living in a district populated by trees with high branches would be in state of instability. If at the same time the pituitary, for some reason, was unstable and reacted with an extra supply of its secretion, it would stimulate the neck cells to reproduce themselves. In turn the pituitary would become stabilized in the direction of increased secretion, and hand on the component of increased secretion to the sex cells. That component, in conjunction with other factors, would therefore determine the emergence of a definite species character. In other words, the glands of internal secretion, as intermediaries between the environment and body, and between the body and the reproductive sex cells or germplasm, tender the clue to a phase of the puzzle of heredity, adaptation and evolution. It is only a dotted outline of an explanation to be sure, but one certainly capable of being filled in.

THE BEARING ON BREEDING

Since the endocrine glands are so subtly sensitive and responsive to environment, and are at the same time so intimately concerned in the process of inheritance--a law which sums up their influence upon resemblance and variation in animals--there is no need to stress their importance for the practical science and art of good breeding, eugenics. Another mode of approach to its problems is opened up, and fresh enthusiasm instilled into its hopes and aspirations. A method of analysis of the factors involved, together with rules for the prediction of the outcome of certain matings, when finally worked out, will elevate its procedure to the level of the more exact sciences.

A man's chief gift to his children is his internal secretion composition. The endocrines are truly the matter of breeding as they are of growth. They are the material carriers of the inherited physical and psychic dispositions, powers, abilities and disabilities from the soma to the germplasm and back from the germplasm to the soma. All kinds of questions arise as soon as one attempts to consider the bearing of this underlying principle upon concrete situations. What happens, say, when a pituitocentric mates with a thyrocentric? Or when a pituitocentric marries a pituitocentric? Is there a reinforcement or a cancellation of the dominant endocrine? Is there a quantitative addition of internal glandular tendencies in the germplasm, or a more complex rearrangement dependent upon reactions between all the internal secretions?

The term endocrine dominants brings up the inquiries of Mendelism, and the relation of Mendelian conceptions of dominant and recessive to the internal secretions. The Mendelians have emphasized the role of the unit factor in heredity, and the conservation of the unit factor as an entity through all the adventures of matings. Also, that when unit factors, say of the color of the eyes, come into conflict, brown or black being mixed with blue or grey, one, the recessive, is submerged and overlaid but not destroyed by the other, the dominant. So brown or black eyes, dark hair, curly hair, dark skin, and so on, are dominant, while blue or grey eyes, light or straight hair, light skin are recessives. A nervous temperament is dominant to the phlegmatic. A number of psychic qualities have been declared to be Mendelian unit factors: memory, mechanical instinct, mathematical ability, literary ability, musical ability, and even handwriting.

As architects of human qualities the endocrines must be involved in the Mendelian unit factors. Moreover, they seem to act upon a particular locale in different degrees, which is the strongest argument against the resolution of a number of structural traits into Mendelian unit characters. Most characters, somatic or psychic, are the products not of the action of one internal secretion alone, but of the interlinked activities of all of them. The amount of fat deposited under the skin, for instance, is influenced by the pituitary, the thyroid, the pancreas, the liver, the adrenals and the sex glands. Other qualities, likewise, are resultants of a compromise between all the endocrine factors comprising the equation of the individual. If we are to look for unit factors at all in endocrine heredity, we must look more deeply into constitution, and measure the hormone potentials and their mobilization or suppression.

It will, in all probability, be found that the stability or instability of an endocrine will have a good deal to do with the part played by it in inheritance as well as in the life of the individual An unstable pituitocentric marrying another unstable pituitocentric will have children either exceptionally small or tall, or abnormally bright or stupid. The instability tends to right itself in the next generation, or that following. Genius as a sport, as well as sudden degeneration of family stock, the whole problem of mutation, may be closely connected with this tendency.

It has been noted that the extinction of species has been preceded by a great increase in their size, for example, the case of the great reptilia of prehistoric time. That possibly represented pituitary stabilization, and so an abeyance of the ability to vary, necessary for fresh adaptation to a changing environment. Indeed, endocrine instability appears the fundamental condition of the tendency to vary, endocrine stability the opposite.

Certain endocrine facts in relation to heredity should be mentioned. The daughters of mothers who menstruated early, themselves menstruate early. Animals fed upon thyroid during pregnancy, comparable to the thyrocentric, give birth to offspring with a very large thymus, comparable to the thymocentric. Women with partial thyroid deficiency, or myxedema, bear cretins. These are suggestive of what the internal secretions may do to an individual in inheritance and development. Inherited endocrine potential is the maximum reaction of which a gland is capable. This matter of potential is comparable to the factor of reserve power or margin of safety demonstrated up to the hilt for such organs as the heart and kidney as varying from individual to individual. A low potential, like instability of an internal secretion gland, may be latent, and not made manifest until the proper stimulus, the maximum amount of stress and strain, like accident, disease, shock or war, arrives.

When the individual is tested the effects may be purely local because there is always in the organism a point of least resistance. Physical changes alone may be prominent. Or because somatic changes are minor, the psychic will dominate the picture. An attack of the "blues," unaccompanied by any demonstrable transformation of the bodily processes, may be the sole symptom of an endocrine failure somewhere in the chain due to hereditary weakness or low potential.

So we may account for family trends and streaks, for varieties and strains among individuals, upon more precise lines based upon endocrine analysis. Family disturbances of the internal secretions of the extreme sort denominated disease are well known. Indeed, a number of family diseases or predispositions to diseases, have been traced to them. Predisposition in any direction will probably be shown to be caused by them, within limits. Research here has its opportunity.

THE IMPROVEMENT OF RACIAL STOCK

A vast new territory of inquiry and achievement, as yet totally unexplored, is opened by the endocrines to the eugenists, and those idealists whose most earnest aspiration is the improvement of racial stock as a necessary preliminary to improvement of racial life. Beginning with Galton, they have brought to light a great collection of data to prove that human traits and faculties, good and bad, are inherited. Ability has been shown to run in certain families and degeneracy in others. Yet all of the practical net result has been summed up in the term "negative eugenics," the eugenics of prohibition and warning.

Now the concept of personality, as woven around a system of chemical reflexes, handed on from generation to generation, is bound to change all that, and to create a structure of positive eugenics. It has been said that what radium is to chemistry, the internal secretions are to physiology. Just as radium enlightens the chemist about the history of matter, and the integrations and disintegrations constituting the life of an element--the internal secretions illuminate the history of the individual as part of the life of the race, and of its integrations and disintegrations. Seeing the individual as a system of chemical substances interacting will assist enormously to predict the nature, character and constitution of his descendants, which is essentially what the eugenist is after.

The study of matings, the heart of the matter, will concern itself with the investigation and comparison of the kind of endocrine personalities that mate, the internal secretion predominances that cross, and the consequent endocrine personality of the offspring. Data bearing upon physique and physiognomy, details of anatomy and function, mind and behaviour will so be co-ordinated as no eugenist has hitherto succeeded in doing. Laws of endocrine inheritance will emerge that will bring the control of heredity within measurable distance. Standards and norms of a new kind would be obtained.

A beginning of this study of endocrine inheritance, on the pathologic side, has been made. Some of these have been along Mendelian lines. Following up abnormal growth (making giants and dwarfs) and abnormal metabolism (goitre, diabetes, and so on), it has been stated that it would seem that abnormal growth is dominant in the male, and recessive in the female, while abnormal metabolism is dominant in the female and recessive in the male. If an endocrine abnormality like a goitre, or cretinism, or a dwarf or giant appear in a family as a sign of endocrine instability, other members of that family will very likely show internal secretion abnormalities.

If one gland of internal secretion acts as the centre of the system and the others as satellites, we should be able to trace what happens to it in the different generations. Does it maintain its supremacy? Or will it be ousted by another member of the group? The time will come when we shall thus be able to advise prospective parents of the consequences of procreation and to forecast the meaning for the race of a particular marriage. Internal glandular analysis may become legally compulsory for those about to mate before the end of the present century.

What are desirable and undesirable matings? The general law followed by nature in her helterskelter way seems to be the production of the greatest number of hybrids and variations possible, whether for good or evil does not matter. Certain endocrine types appear to be specially attracted to others belonging to the same group. Thus thymus-centered types frequently marry. The ante-pituitary type of male, the strongly masculine, mates often with the post-pituitary type of female, the markedly feminine. The children exhibit the lineaments of the pituitary-centered type. The general trend seems to be the establishment of a better balanced, equilibrated type. Yet the children often are apt to segregate into pituitary dominants or pituitary deficients. Happiness and unhappiness in marriage should be examined from the standpoint of endocrine compatibility or incompatibility. Likewise those divorced or about to be divorced.

The correction of endocrine defects, disturbances, imbalances and instabilities, before mating, presents another field. It remains to be seen whether we shall thereby, in one generation, be able to affect at all the germplasm, hitherto revered by all pious biologists as an environment-proof holy of holies. No one can deny, in the face of the multitude of evidence available, that internal secretion disturbances occur in the mother, which, when grave, offer in the infant gross proof of their significance, and therefore when slight must more subtly work upon it. Endocrine disturbances in infancy have been traced to endocrine disturbances in the mother during pregnancy. Pregnant animals fed on thyroid give birth to young with large thymus glands. The diet of the mother has been proved conclusively to influence the development and constitution of the child. As the internal secretions influence the history of the food in the body, they affect development in the womb indirectly as well as directly. Certainly, whether or no we learn how to change the nature of germplasm within a short time, we have in the endocrines the means at hand for affecting *the whole individual that is born and sees the light of day*.

THE CONTROL OF MUTATIONS

The true physical and intellectual evolution of man depends upon the production of mutations of a desirable kind that can survive. The information furnished by the study of the endocrines concerning the genesis of personality provides the foundations for a positive eugenics, a eugenics of the encouragement of desirable matings, with the proper legal and social procedures. Selective breeding for the production of the best endocrine types should become practicable.

But the biologist should be able to go farther. If the eugenist is to limit himself to the method of the animal breeder he will have to rest satisfied with the characters or hereditary factors given, that turn up spontaneously in an individual. But with the internal secretions as the controllable controllers of mutations, the outlook changes. It should become possible to produce new mutations, good and bad, to speed up their production at any rate. The feeding of thyroid to a gifted father before procreation might enhance immeasurably the chances of transmission of his gift as well as of its intensification in his offspring. A field of investigation is opened that would embrace in due time the deliberate control of human evolution.

All the physical traits, stature, color, muscle function, and so on, offer themselves for improvement, as well as brain size, and the intellectual and emotional factors which have dominated man's social evolution. The general prevalence of nervous disorders in civilized countries, visible even in the nervous infants the specialist in children's diseases is called upon to treat, shows that the nervous system of the better part of mankind is in a state of unstable equilibrium. It may be another example of the curious coincidences that have been called the Fitness of the Environment that the investigation of the endocrines promises to put into our hands the instruments of the control of the future of the nervous system. In general, meanwhile, the eugenist should strive for raising the level of the endocrine potential, and discourage its lowering. That means the encouragement of matings in which all the internal secretion activities are reinforced. On the other hand, those internal secretion combinations, generally leading to a deficiency of all of them which produce types of mental defectives, delinquency and crime should not be allowed to occur.

THE INFLUENCE OF ENVIRONMENT

What suggestions now are there for the euthenist who would control the influence of environment upon child culture. There are certain pertinent facts and leads that are worth considering.

In analyzing environment, one must distinguish sharply in the jungle, the nonliving factors from the living. For while the nonliving act upon the endocrines directly, the living act upon the vegetative system, as a whole. The non-living factors are those with the intimate scrutiny of which physics and chemistry have busied themselves: food, water, air, light, heat, electricity, magnetism. The living are the animals that prowl all over the planet, the predatories spreading the gospel of fear.

The dietetic habits of a person, for instance, are known to have an influence upon the glands of internal secretion. Meat-eating produces a greater call upon the thyroid than any other form of food. In time this ought to produce a degree of hyperthyroidism in the carniverous populations. Pre-war statistics concerning meat-eating in different countries show the greatest meat-eating among the English-speaking groups, who all in all must be admitted the most energetic.

Countries	*Meat per Day per Capita in Grams*
Australia	306
U.S. of America	149
Great Britain	130
France	92
Belgium and Holland	86
Austria-Hungary	79
Russia	59
Spain	61
Italy	29
Japan	25

Sea-water contains iodine. People living in contact with sea-water would be apt to get more iodine in their systems, and so a greater degree of thyroid activity. On the other hand, certain bodies and sources of inland water hold something deleterious to the thyroid, so that whole populations in Europe, Asia and America drinking such water have become goitrous and cretinous, and a large percentage straight imbeciles. Endemic cretinism is the name given to the condition. In parts of Switzerland, Savoy, Tyrol and the Pyrenees, in America around some of the Great Lakes, there are still such foci. Marco Polo described similar areas he encountered in his travels through Asia.

Certain foods with aphrodisiac qualities may act by stimulating the internal secretion of the sex glands. A type of pituitocentric has an almost uncontrollable craving for sweets. Alcohol and the endocrines remain to be studied.

Light, heat and humidity stand in some special relation to the adrenals. Pigment deposit in the skin as protection against light is controlled by the adrenal cortex. The reaction of the skin blood vessels to heat and humidity is regulated by the adrenal medulla. A change in the adrenal as a response to changes of temperature and humidity in an environment would result in a number of concomitant transformations throughout the body. So variation and adaptation are probably connected. Most Europeans living for a sufficiently long time in the tropics suffer from a combination of symptoms spoken of as "Punjab head" or "Bengal head." The condition is probably the result of excessive adrenal stimulation by the excessive heat and light of the tropical sun, followed by a reaction of exhaustion and failure, with the consequent phenomena of a form of neurasthenia. In the section on the pineal gland there was mentioned the relation between light and the pineal gland in growing animals, and how it serves to keep in check the sex-stimulating action of light. The earlier puberty and menstruation of the warmer climates may be explained as due to an earlier regression of the pineal under the pressure of a great amount of light playing upon the skin.

All these, and many more could be cited, are instances of the direct influence of environmental factors upon one or more of the endocrines, and so upon the organism as a whole. Indeed, stimuli may be considered to modify an organism only in so far as they modify the glands of internal secretion. Consequently, climatic factors will tend to make a population possess certain points of resemblance in common.

Varieties of the human race exist as do varieties of dogs. The pekingese and the fox terrier are as different as the Slav and Latin are different: because of differences in internal secretion make-up. The Slav peasant is definitely subthyroid in his general effect: round head, coarse features, stubby hands, and his stolid, brooding intellectual and emotional reaction. The Latin shows a pronounced adrenal streak in his coloration, his emotivity, his susceptibility to neurosis and psychosis. H. Laing Gordon, a Scot physician, reported that of 700 cases he studied, more than twice as many of duplex eyed individuals (brown or black, i.e., adrenal-centered most often), were susceptible to the mental disturbances of war as the simplex (blue or gray-eyed, i.e., thyroid-centered most often). He also pointed out that such individuals tend to have a narrow and abnormally arched palate. The Anglo-Saxon tends to be more sharply pituitarized, his features are more clean-cut, his mentality more stable. The Frenchman is rather a cross between the Anglo-Saxon pituitary-centered and the Italian or Spanish adrenal-centered.

So national resemblances, traceable to climatic influences being repeated from generation to generation upon the endocrines, may be explained physiologically. The physiologic interpretation of history will indeed be found the broadest, including as complementary Buckle's climatic theory, Hegel's ideas on the influence of ideas, and Marx's on the superiority of the economic motives and forces.

THE RACES OF MANKIND

Arthur Keith, conservator of the Museum of the Royal College of Surgeons of England, was the first to apply the principle of endocrine differentiation to the problem of the color-lines--the lines which have divided mankind crudely into the yellow, the red, the white and the brown, the Negro, the Mongol, the Caucasian, the copper tinted American. It has long been recognized by anthropologists that the differences of color march with differences in every comparable trait. Thus the ideal Negro is built upon a pattern in which all the elements are specific and singular. When the looms revolve that make him, there is produced a gleaming black skin, kinky black hair, squat wide-nostriled nose, thick protruding lips, large striking teeth, prominent jaws, and staring eyes. As his upright carriage and bone-muscle-fat proportions are distinctive, so are his musical voice and his easily wrought upon nerves. In contrast the Caucasian has a good deal of hair on his body, his skin is a pale tan-pink, his lips are thin, and his nose especially has the definite bridge which narrows it. The Mongol, like the Negro, has the hairless body and the beardless face, but unlike him has lank straight hair on his head, while his features are flattened and fore-shortened.

Upon the basis of these structural, functional and mental differences, the qualitative and quantitative evolution of which in the race as in the individual is guided by the glands of internal secretion, Keith presents a very good case for the view that the white man is an example of relative excess of the pituitary, thyroid, adrenal and gonad endocrines. "The sharp and pronounced nasalization of the face, the tendency to strong eyebrow ridges, the prominent chin, the tendency to bulk of body, and height of stature in the majority of Europeans" are the signs of pituitary dominance. Keith is also of the opinion that "the sexual differentiation, the robust manifestations of the male characters, is more emphatic in the Caucasian than in either the Mongol or Negro racial types ... in certain negro types, especially in Nilotic tribes, with their long stork-like legs, we seem to have a manifestation of abeyance in the action of the interstitial glands." As for the adrenal superiority of the white man, "it is 150 years since John Hunter came to the conclusion ... that the original color of man's skin was black, and all the knowledge that we have gathered since his supports the inference he drew. From the fact that pigment begins to collect and thus darken the skin when the adrenal bodies become the seat of a destructive disease we infer that they have to do with the clearing away of pigment, and that we Europeans owe the fairness of our skins to some particular virtue resident in the adrenal bodies." Finally, as regards the thyroid, a comparison of the face of a cretin with that of the Negro or Mongol tells the story. A certain variety of idiocy, Mongolian idiocy, in which the face simulates cretinism so closely as to deceive practised clinical observers, is characterized by a Chinese cast of the features and eyes, hence the name. And in the Bushman of South Africa, the cretin's face is even more startlingly recalled.

There is every reason then for believing that the white man possesses more of pituitary, adrenal, gonad, and thyroid internal secretions as compared with the yellow man or black man. And since these endocrines control not only physique and physiognomy, anatomic and functional minutiae, but also mind and behaviour, we are justified in putting down the white man's predominance on the planet to a greater all-around concentration in his blood of the omnipotent hormones. While the Negro is relatively subadrenal, the Mongol is relatively subthyroid. Their relative deficiency in internal secretions constitutes the essence of the White Man's Burden.

MAN'S ATTITUDE TOWARD HIMSELF

A last, but by no means least, application we may consider of the developing knowledge of the internal secretions in relation to human evolution is its effect upon Man's attitude toward himself and so toward his fellow men. Whatever else he is, man is a land animal with ideas. That makes him a thought-adventurer among materials. In a word, he is the last word of mind working upon matter. But persistently he has refused to recognize himself as matter and as subject to the laws, to the physics and chemistry of matter.

History consists of the protocols that record the high lights of the interactions of materials and ideas which is the adventure of man in time and space. Materials and ideas have reacted, the record shows; materials come upon have begotten strange fantasies. Ideas that flashed from nowhere into a consciousness have transformed utterly the face of the earth. The herd-brute, agglutinated with his fellows by a magnetism beyond his ken, could be infected with thought, and so cast in the heroic mould. The possibility of communion,--that possibility of possibilities, for without it none other could be possible--has rendered man the heir of a divine destiny. For the progressive education of the race, a single discoverer here, an inventor there, and thinkers everywhere have been inspired. In due time their inspiration becomes the possession of even the lowest brain but capable of grasping it.

Man's attitude toward himself, his self-consciousness, and his attitude toward his fellow creatures has grown and varied and evolved with his education about himself. According to the theory he formulated concerning his being, his why and wherefore, he directed and governed, punished and mutilated himself and them. But the pressure of his curiosity, and the inexorable quality of the truth would not let him stand still. The poetic genius within him, as Blake called it, struggled on from one dogma concerning his nature to another. Behaviour malignant or beneficent, horrible in its tragedy and pitiable in its comedy, flowed inevitably on. Witchcraft trials and the tortures of the Spanish Inquisition belong among the more mentionable consequences of some of man's theories about his own nature and its requirements.

Heretofore the imaginative spirit has had its day in the matter. And, curiously enough, an obsession to subjugate the natural has made it exalt the supernatural. Visions, dreams, portents, revelations, all symptomatic of an order of things above nature, are the stuff of what more than ninety-nine per cent of the millions of the race believe about themselves and their fate. Man's cruelty to man, through the ages, is a comment upon how vast and ramifying may be the consequences of a delusion.

But now for a couple of centuries the critical spirit, which is the spirit of science, has been invading the affairs of men. Humble but persistent corrosive of delusion, it has infiltrated the furthest bounds of ignorance and superstition. It has not dared to assert the supremacy of its fundamental views upon the everyday problems of human life because it was without concrete means of vindicating its claims. That lack is now supplied by the growing understanding of the chemical factors as the controllers and dictators of all the legion aspects of life.

The profoundest achievement of the physiologist will be the change his teachings and discoveries will bring about in man's attitude toward himself. When he comes to realize himself as a chemical machine that can, within limits, be remodeled, overhauled and repaired, as an automobile can be, within limits, when he becomes saturated with the significance of his endocrine-vegetative system at every turn and move of his life, and when sympathy and pity informed by knowledge and understanding will come to regulate his relationships with the lowest and most despised of the men, women and children about him, the era of the first real civilization will properly be said to be born.

Morality, as society's code of conduct for its members, will have to change in the direction of a greater flexibility with the establishment of organic differences in human types. There is nothing that is more emphasized to the pathologist than that one man's meat is another man's poison. In the family, as nature's laboratory for the manufacture of fresh combinations of the internal secretions, allowances will be made for divergences in capacity and deportment from a new angle altogether. Schools will function as the developers, stimulators and inhibitors of the endocrines, as well as investigators of the individuals who have not enough or too much of one or some of them. Prisons will have the same function, only they will be named detention hospitals. The raising of the general level of intelligence by the judicious use of endocrine extracts will mean a good deal to the sincere statesman.

The average duration of life will be prolonged for an enormous mass of the population. If the prevention of war depends upon the burning into the imagination of the electorates what the consequences of war are, a high intelligence quotient and revaluation of life will count for a good deal.

Man is the animal that wants Utopia. So long as human nature was looked upon as fixed constant in the ebb and flow of life, a Utopia of fine minds could be conceived only by the dreamer and poet. The desire for such a Utopia could only be regarded as a tragic aspiration for an impossibility. The physiology of the internal secretions teaches that human nature does change and can be changed. A relative control of its properties is already in view. The absolute control will come.

Nor need anyone fear that the science of the internal secretions in its maturity will signify the abolition of the marvelous differences between human beings that create the unique personalities of history. A derangement of the endocrines has been responsible for masterpieces of the human species in the past and will be responsible for them in the future. The equality of Utopia can be the equality of the highest and fullest development possible for each of its inhabitants. The applications of endocrine control will not necessarily interfere with the life of the individual. There will be breeding of the best mixtures of glands of internal secretion possible. And there will be treatment for those born with a handicap, or who have become handicapped in the life struggle. There will be a stimulation of capacity to the limit. But beyond that, compulsory equalization is a theorist's bogey.

The internal secretions are the most hopeful and promising of the reagents for control yet come upon by the human mind. They open up limitless prospects for the improvement of the race. A few hundreds of investigators are engaged upon their study throughout the world. That is one of the ironies of our contemporary civilization. A concerted effort at the task of understanding them, backed by the labors of tens of thousands of workers, would, without a doubt, accomplish as much for humanity as the vast armies and navies that consume the substance of mankind. If we could not obtain Utopia then, we might, at least by abolishing the subnormals and abnormals who constitute the slaves and careerists of society, render the human race less contemptible and more divine.

INDEX

www.**bookjungle**.com *email: sales@bookjungle.com fax: 630-214-0564 mail: Book Jungle PO Box 2226 Champaign, IL 61825*

QTY

The Rosicrucian Cosmo-Conception Mystic Christianity by *Max Heindel*   ISBN: *1-59462-188-8*   **$38.95**
The Rosicrucian Cosmo-conception is not dogmatic, neither does it appeal to any other authority than the reason of the student. It is: not controversial, but is: sent forth in the, hope that it may help to clear...   New Age/Religion Pages 646

Abandonment To Divine Providence by *Jean-Pierre de Caussade*   ISBN: *1-59462-228-0*   **$25.95**
"The Rev. Jean Pierre de Caussade was one of the most remarkable spiritual writers of the Society of Jesus in France in the 18th Century. His death took place at Toulouse in 1751. His works have gone through many editions and have been republished...   Inspirational/Religion Pages 400

Mental Chemistry by *Charles Haanel*   ISBN: *1-59462-192-6*   **$23.95**
Mental Chemistry allows the change of material conditions by combining and appropriately utilizing the power of the mind. Much like applied chemistry creates something new and unique out of careful combinations of chemicals the mastery of mental chemistry...   New Age Pages 354

The Letters of Robert Browning and Elizabeth Barret Barrett 1845-1846 vol II   ISBN: *1-59462-193-4*   **$35.95**
by *Robert Browning* and *Elizabeth Barrett*   Biographies Pages 596

Gleanings In Genesis (volume I) by *Arthur W. Pink*   ISBN: *1-59462-130-6*   **$27.45**
Appropriately has Genesis been termed "the seed plot of the Bible" for in it we have, in germ form, almost all of the great doctrines which are afterwards fully developed in the books of Scripture which follow...   Religion/Inspirational Pages 420

The Master Key by *L. W. de Laurence*   ISBN: *1-59462-001-6*   **$30.95**
In no branch of human knowledge has there been a more lively increase of the spirit of research during the past few years than in the study of Psychology, Concentration and Mental Discipline. The requests for authentic lessons in Thought Control, Mental Discipline and...   New Age/Business Pages 422

The Lesser Key Of Solomon Goetia by *L. W. de Laurence*   ISBN: *1-59462-092-X*   **$9.95**
This translation of the first book of the "Lernegton" which is now for the first time made accessible to students of Talismanic Magic was done, after careful collation and edition, from numerous Ancient Manuscripts in Hebrew, Latin, and French...   New Age/Occult Pages 92

Rubaiyat Of Omar Khayyam by *Edward Fitzgerald*   ISBN: *1-59462-332-5*   **$13.95**
Edward Fitzgerald, whom the world has already learned, in spite of his own efforts to remain within the shadow of anonymity, to look upon as one of the rarest poets of the century, was born at Bredfield, in Suffolk, on the 31st of March, 1809. He was the third son of John Purcell...   Music Pages 172

Ancient Law by *Henry Maine*   ISBN: *1-59462-128-4*   **$29.95**
The chief object of the following pages is to indicate some of the earliest ideas of mankind, as they are reflected in Ancient Law, and to point out the relation of those ideas to modern thought.   Religion/History Pages 452

Far-Away Stories by *William J. Locke*   ISBN: *1-59462-129-2*   **$19.45**
"Good wine needs no bush, but a collection of mixed vintages does. And this book is just such a collection. Some of the stories I do not want to remain buried for ever in the museum files of dead magazine-numbers an author's not unpardonable vanity..."   Fiction Pages 272

Life of David Crockett by *David Crockett*   ISBN: *1-59462-250-7*   **$27.45**
"Colonel David Crockett was one of the most remarkable men of the times in which he lived. Born in humble life, but gifted with a strong will, an indomitable courage, and unremitting perseverance...   Biographies/New Age Pages 424

Lip-Reading by *Edward Nitchie*   ISBN: *1-59462-206-X*   **$25.95**
Edward B. Nitchie, founder of the New York School for the Hard of Hearing, now the Nitchie School of Lip-Reading, Inc, wrote "LIP-READING Principles and Practice". The development and perfecting of this meritorious work on lip-reading was an undertaking...   How-to Pages 400

A Handbook of Suggestive Therapeutics, Applied Hypnotism, Psychic Science   ISBN: *1-59462-214-0*   **$24.95**
by *Henry Munro*   Health/New Age/Health/Self-help Pages 376

A Doll's House: and Two Other Plays by *Henrik Ibsen*   ISBN: *1-59462-112-8*   **$19.95**
Henrik Ibsen created this classic when in revolutionary 1848 Rome. Introducing some striking concepts in playwriting for the realist genre, this play has been studied the world over.   Fiction/Classics/Plays 308

The Light of Asia by *sir Edwin Arnold*   ISBN: *1-59462-204-3*   **$13.95**
In this poetic masterpiece, Edwin Arnold describes the life and teachings of Buddha. The man who was to become known as Buddha to the world was born as Prince Gautama of India but he rejected the worldly riches and abandoned the reigns of power when...   Religion/History/Biographies Pages 170

The Complete Works of Guy de Maupassant by *Guy de Maupassant*   ISBN: *1-59462-157-8*   **$16.95**
"For days and days, nights and nights, I had dreamed of that first kiss which was to consecrate our engagement, and I knew not on what spot I should put my lips..."   Fiction/Classics Pages 240

The Art of Cross-Examination by *Francis L. Wellman*   ISBN: *1-59462-309-0*   **$26.95**
Written by a renowned trial lawyer, Wellman imparts his experience and uses case studies to explain how to use psychology to extract desired information through questioning.   How-to/Science/Reference Pages 408

Answered or Unanswered? by *Louisa Vaughan*   ISBN: *1-59462-248-5*   **$10.95**
Miracles of Faith in China   Religion Pages 112

The Edinburgh Lectures on Mental Science (1909) by *Thomas*   ISBN: *1-59462-008-3*   **$11.95**
This book contains the substance of a course of lectures recently given by the writer in the Queen Street Hall, Edinburgh. Its purpose is to indicate the Natural Principles governing the relation between Mental Action and Material Conditions...   New Age/Psychology Pages 148

Ayesha by *H. Rider Haggard*   ISBN: *1-59462-301-5*   **$24.95**
Verily and indeed it is the unexpected that happens! Probably if there was one person upon the earth from whom the Editor of this, and of a certain previous history, did not expect to hear again...   Classics Pages 380

Ayala's Angel by *Anthony Trollope*   ISBN: *1-59462-352-X*   **$29.95**
The two girls were both pretty, but Lucy who was twenty-one who supposed to be simple and comparatively unattractive, whereas Ayala was credited, as her Bombwhat romantic name might show, with poetic charm and a taste for romance. Ayala when her father died was nineteen...   Fiction Pages 484

The American Commonwealth by *James Bryce*   ISBN: *1-59462-286-8*   **$34.45**
An interpretation of American democratic political theory. It examines political mechanics and society from the perspective of Scotsman James Bryce   Politics Pages 572

Stories of the Pilgrims by *Margaret P. Pumphrey*   ISBN: *1-59462-116-0*   **$17.95**
This book explores pilgrims religious oppression in England as well as their escape to Holland and eventual crossing to America on the Mayflower, and their early days in New England...   History Pages 268

QTY

The Fasting Cure *by Sinclair Upton*   ISBN: *1-59462-222-1*   **$13.95**

In the Cosmopolitan Magazine for May, 1910, and in the Contemporary Review (London) for April, 1910, I published an article dealing with my experiences in fasting. I have written a great many magazine articles, but never one which attracted so much attention... New Age/Self Help/Health Pages 164

Hebrew Astrology *by Sepharial*   ISBN: *1-59462-308-2*   **$13.45**

In these days of advanced thinking it is a matter of common observation that we have left many of the old landmarks behind and that we are now pressing forward to greater heights and to a wider horizon than that which represented the mind-content of our progenitors... Astrology Pages 144

Thought Vibration or The Law of Attraction in the Thought World   ISBN: *1-59462-127-6*   **$12.95**

by William Walker Atkinson   Psychology/Religion Pages 144

Optimism *by Helen Keller*   ISBN: *1-59462-108-X*   **$15.95**

Helen Keller was blind, deaf, and mute since 19 months old, yet famously learned how to overcome these handicaps, communicate with the world, and spread her lectures promoting optimism. An inspiring read for everyone... Biographies/Inspirational Pages 84

Sara Crewe *by Frances Burnett*   ISBN: *1-59462-360-0*   **$9.45**

In the first place, Miss Minchin lived in London. Her home was a large, dull, tall one, in a large, dull square, where all the houses were alike, and all the sparrows were alike, and where all the door-knockers made the same heavy sound... Childrens/Classic Pages 88

The Autobiography of Benjamin Franklin *by Benjamin Franklin*   ISBN: *1-59462-135-7*   **$24.95**

The Autobiography of Benjamin Franklin has probably been more extensively read than any other American historical work, and no other book of its kind has had such ups and downs of fortune. Franklin lived for many years in England, where he was agent... Biographies/History Pages 332

Name	
Email	
Telephone	
Address	
City, State ZIP	

☐ **Credit Card**   ☐ **Check / Money Order**

Credit Card Number	
Expiration Date	
Signature	

Please Mail to: Book Jungle
                  PO Box 2226
                  Champaign, IL 61825
or Fax to: 630-214-0564

ORDERING INFORMATION

web: *www.bookjungle.com*
email: *sales@bookjungle.com*
fax: *630-214-0564*
mail: *Book Jungle PO Box 2226 Champaign, IL 61825*
or PayPal *to sales@bookjungle.com*

Please contact us for bulk discounts

DIRECT-ORDER TERMS

**20% Discount if You Order
Two or More Books**
Free Domestic Shipping!
Accepted: Master Card, Visa,
Discover, American Express